Schrag   Enz / Messinger / Wolf   Taxacher · Healthy Calves – Healthy Cattle

# Healthy Calves-
# Healthy Cattle

## The most important diseases in rearing and fattening

**Recognition, Prevention, Treatment**

by
**Dr. med. vet. Ludwig Schrag**

Dr. med. vet. Hermann Enz
Dipl.-Ing. agr. Hartmut Messinger
Dr. med. vet. Franz Wolf
in collaboration with
Dr. phil. Dr. med. vet. Johannes Taxacher

Translation by W. Mehlig

**With 534 illustrations, including 476 colour photographs**

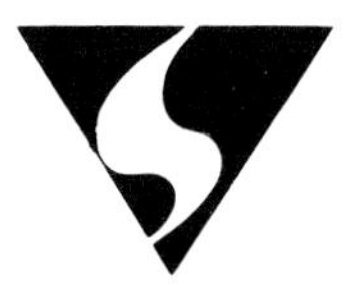

Verlag L. Schober, D-8355 Hengersberg · A-5400 Hallein · CH-5105 Auenstein AG

**Origin of Illustrations**

All illustrations have been provided by the authors, except for:
Figs. 140, 147, 239, 240, 242 and 243
by Denkavit International B.V., Voorthuizen,
Figs. 406, 421, 422, 423, 424, 425 and 426
by Dr. R. Lawrenz, Untersuchungslabor Scheyern,
Figs. 62, 64, 65, 66, 70, 71, 308, 309, 312, 313, 333, 334, 335, 358 and 361
by Prof. Dr. K. Zettl, Head of the Staatliches Veterinäruntersuchungsamt, Kassel.

CIP-Kurztitelaufnahme der Deutschen Bibliothek

**Healthy calves – healthy cattle** : the most
important diseases in rearing and
fattening ; recognition, prevention, treat-
ment / by Ludwig Schrag ... In collab. with
Johannes Taxacher. – Hengersberg ; Hallein ;
Auenstein : Schober, 1981.
Dt. Ausg. u. d. T.: Gesunde Kälber – gesunde
Rinder
ISBN 3-88620-104-X (Buch);
ISBN 3-88620-105-8 (Buch mit Diaserie)

NE: Schrag, Ludwig [Mitverf.]





Graphic Design: Leo Gehra, Munich
Offset reproduction: Repro Studio, E. Kieslich, Gersthofen
Setting, print and binding: Sellier Druck GmbH, Freising

Printed in West Germany
1982

ISBN 3-88620-**104**-x (Book)
ISBN 3-88620-**105**-8 (Book with set of slides)

# Introduction

The title 'Healthy Calves – Healthy Cattle' is the guideline of this book which aims at preserving and restoring the health and performance of calves and cattle in rearing and fattening.
The major diseases of calves and cattle, their prevention and treatment are presented succinctly with the aid of illustrations. The carefully planned graphic presentation together with the extensive pictorial material will help the reader to learn how to recognise diseases. In order to keep the material clear and free from unnecessary detail, less common diseases have purposely been omitted.
The drugs mentioned under methods of treatment are those with which the authors Enz, Schrag, Taxacher and Wolf have gained extensive experience in their own veterinary practice. It goes without saying that other active products or combinations of such products of the same or similar composition may likewise be used with success.
In keeping with the aim of this book, special emphasis has been placed on practical, effective prevention which calls for an accurate assessment of the possibilities of disease in calves and cattle at the time of particular stress.
Our special thanks are due to the publishers, L. Schober, for the excellent presentation of this book and for their kind understanding and readiness to meet all our requirements.

The Authors.

# Preface for the English edition

The legal provisions mentioned in the book are those valid in the Fed. Rep. of Germany. As the present edition is intended for an international readership, such passages could not be adapted to the legal provisions of other countries. However, the publishers are planning several other editions in English for certain countries in which the relevant passages will cover the legal provisions applicable locally.
For the latter editions, moreover, additional health problems peculiar to certain areas, and different housing conditions should be considered, and the drugs mentioned in the treatment tables should be checked for availability and, if necessary, replaced by equivalent ones.
We also wish to express our special thanks for the co-operation of Mr. W. Mehlig and for his accurate translations.

The Authors

# Contents

## Part 1

### The most important diseases 1st to 4th week of life

# Part 2

## The most important diseases 5th to 12th week of life





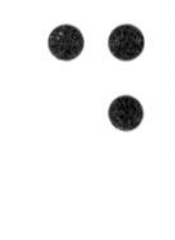

# Part 3

## The most important diseases from the 13th week of life Rearing and fattening.

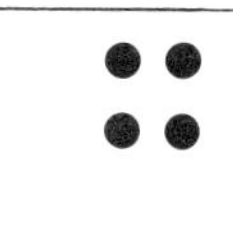

# Part 4

## Guidelines for treatment

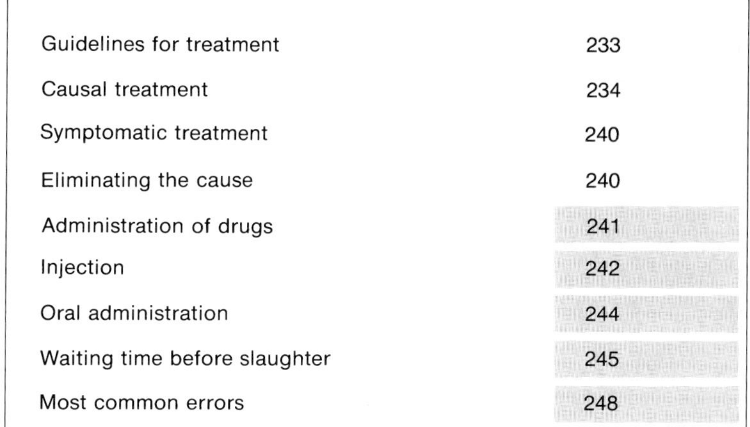



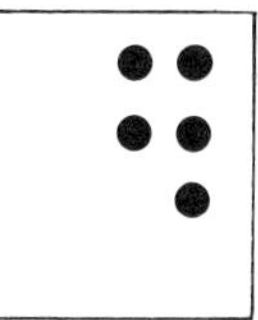

# Part 5

## Prevention and preventive treatment

# Using this book

The arrangement and presentation of this book aim to help the reader to find information quickly. For this reason particular attention has been paid to classification of the subject matter.
The book consists of 5 parts each of which is marked with an appropriate number of dots. Each part of the book is subdivided into several chapters. Each chapter has been given a colour code of its own. Within the coloured area which is repeated on every page of the chapter, the number of dots indicates the relevant part of the book.
Parts 1, 2 and 3 are each preceded by a summary which is presented in the form of an examination for important signs in healthy and sick animals.
The illustrations are described in the first column and provide information on typical, outwardly visible symptoms.
In the second column, reference is made to further observations and examinations leading to a diagnosis. The third column shows the diseases concerned and gives the relevant page number in the book.
The chapters are subdivided by means of sub-titles which are colour-coded in the margin to facilitate reference.

**Term** Brief explanation of the nature of the disease.

**Incidence** Distribution and duration of the disease according to animal species and age.

**Pathogen / Cause** Explanation of precipitating factors and causative organisms of the disease. Description of the life cycle of the pathogen.

**Importation / Route of Infection** Possibilities of infection and transmission, incubation period, precipitating factors.

**Symptoms and Course of the Disease** Visible signs of the disease, duration of disease stages.

**Diagnosis** Diagnosis of the disease or its cause from outward signs, demonstration of the pathogen and possible examinations.

Differentiation from similar diseases.

**Similar symptoms**

Dosage, therapeutic time schedule, combating pathogens and their intermediate hosts; elimination of causes of the disease.

**Treatment**

Possibilities of preventing disease. Protection of animals not yet affected. Disinfection and hygienic measures in the animal and in the environment.

**Prevention**

Possibility and assessment of active or passive immunisation against the disease.

**Vaccination**

Possibility of transmission to other animal species and to man.

**Danger to animals and livestock farmers**

Legally required measures*: Treatment, slaughter of diseased animals, quarantine measures, compensation.

**Legal provisions***

To enable the reader to gain a general conception of therapeutic and preventive measures against the various diseases, these measures are presented in summarised form. For this purpose symbols are used which have been given their own colour code for ease of reference.

In parts 4 and 5 of this book, the different sections of the chapters are introduced in the margin in the form of key-words. For quick reference, these key-words are always shown against the colour code of the chapter.

In part 4, the medicinal products mentioned in the book are listed on pages 246 and 247. This tabulation includes the active ingredients and waiting times, thus dispensing with the need to give this information in the body of the text.

Part 5 includes a preventive plan in summary form arranged in accordance with the three life periods being considered.

---

* Valid in W. Germany

## Important characteristics of healthy calves

### 1st to 4th week of life

#### General behaviour

Size and development corresponding to age; lively, alert and inquisitive behaviour; upright posture, lively facial expression, alert eye and ear movements; shining short coat.
Calves readily approach visitors and are alert to what is happening around them.

#### Body temperature

38.5 to 39.5° C

#### Pulse

Rate 72 to 92, strong and regular.

#### Breathing

Calm, regular, even. Respiratory rate: 20 to 40 per minute

#### Elasticity of the skin

Raised skin folds immediately level out again (within 1 or 2 seconds)

#### Urine

Thin clear amber fluid.
Daily volume: $^{1}/_{2}$ to 1 litre
pH value: 5.8 to 8.3
Specific gravity: 1,010 to 1,040

#### Faeces

Yellow to light brown, ranging from pappy to greasy and viscous, without solid components.
Daily quantitiy: 250 to 500 g.
First faeces: Greenish-black, viscous, without solid components

#### Blood volume

Approx. 80 ml blood per kg body-weight.

#### Digestive system

Single-compartment stomach (abomasum), coagulation by chymosin; beginning of change-over to multi-compartment stomach system in approximately the 3rd week of life.

Fig. 1

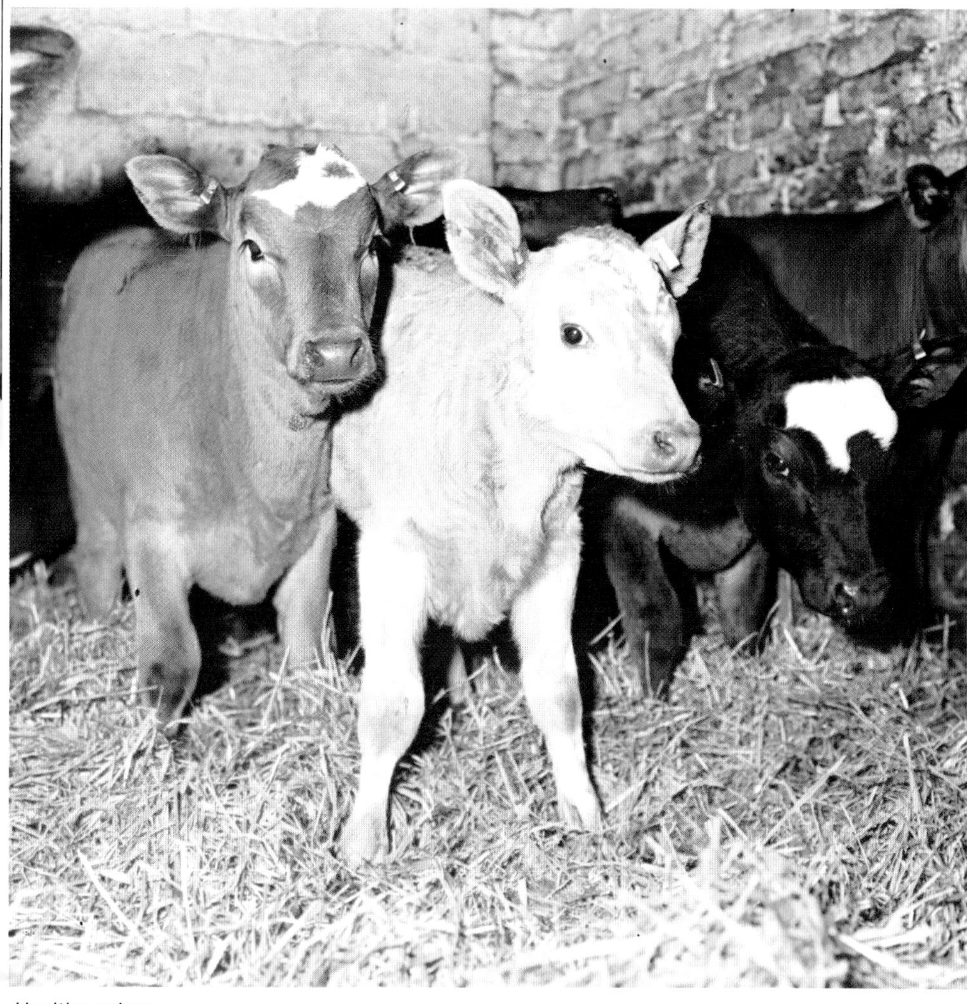

*Healthy calves*

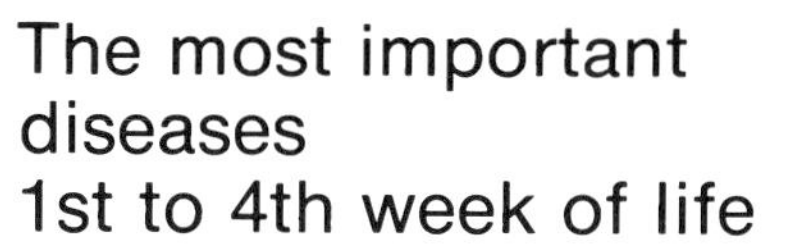

# Part 1

The most important diseases
1st to 4th week of life

## Summary of important signs in sick calves

### 1st to 4th week of life

| | Fig. 2 | Fig. 3 |
|---|---|---|
| | 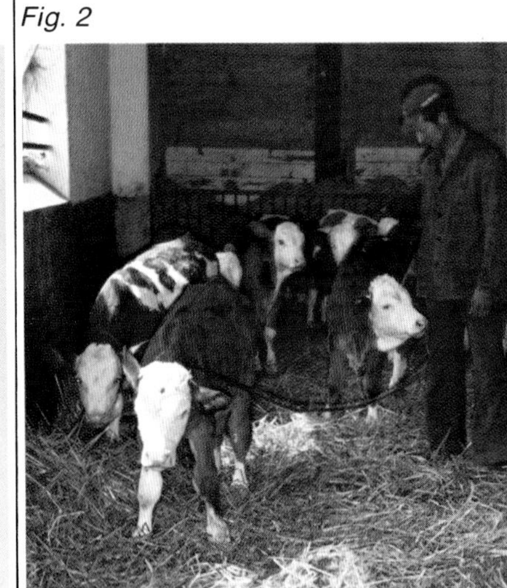 | 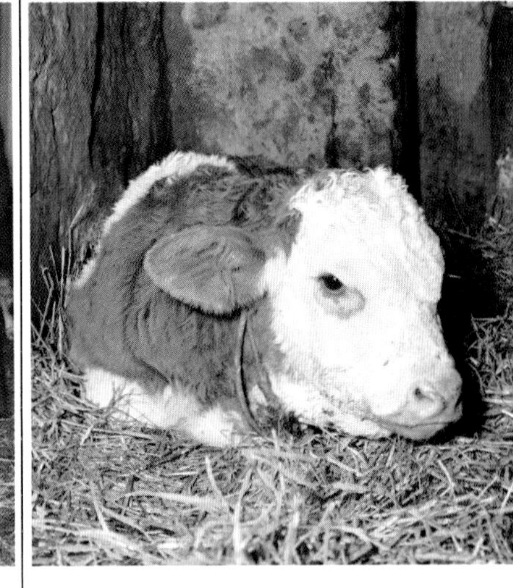 |
| Outwardly visible symptoms | Listlessness, limp posture, head bowed, inattentive look, drooping ears, standing apart from group of animals. | Dyspnoea, head bowed, nostrils opened wide, tongue stuck out, stretched head and neck posture; forelegs spread wide. |
| Diagnosis by examination | Temperature above 39.5° C. Respiratory rate increased. Drinking normally at first, later reduced fluid intake; finally drinking refused. | Temperature raised in infections; inspiration greatly prolonged with audible sounds and additional forward movement of the body; anal breathing. |
| Read up diseases that may be involved | Incipient general disease. Infectious bronchopneumonia in calves, page 82. | Pneumococcosis, page 34. |

*Fig. 4*

**Symptoms:** Abdomen drawn in because of great pain in the abdominal region; diarrhoea.

**Examination:** High temperature possible, perhaps above 40° C. Skin tension poor. Raised skin folds level out slowly (more than 2 seconds).

**Read up:**
Rota/corona/coli infection, page 26
Salmonellosis, page 36
Navel-ill, page 52
Nutrition-induced diarrhoea, page 48.

*Fig. 5*

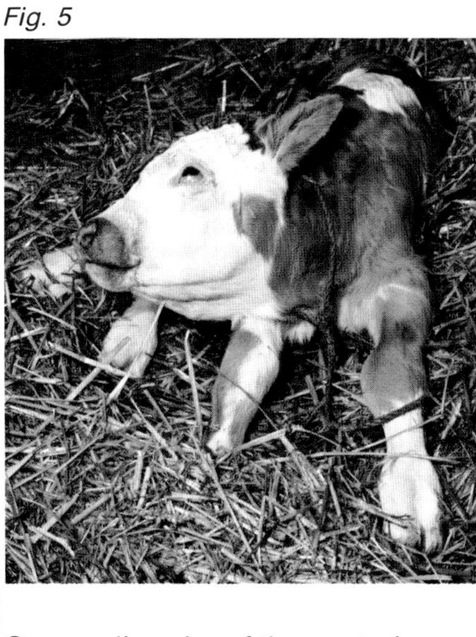

**Symptoms:** Severe disorder of the central nervous system; cramped posture; paralysis, typical retroversion of the neck.

**Examination:** Temperature normal or increased. Reflexes reduced or raised. Refusal of drink. Salivation.

**Read up:**
Coli infection, page 26
Salmonellosis, page 36
Listeriosis, page 104
Vitamin $B_1$ deficiency, page 102.

*Fig. 6*

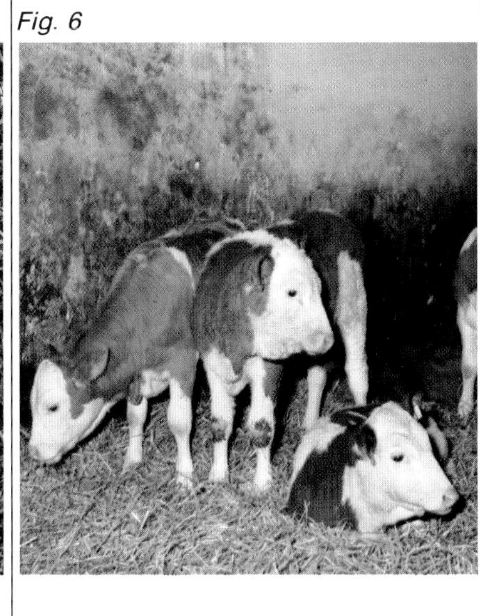

**Symptoms:** Stunted sucking calf; size and development not corresponding to age. Unduly large, "old-looking" head; rough coat.

**Examination:** Check: Feed intake, faeces (bacteriological and parasitological tests), navel; check coat for parasites.

**Read up:**
Condition following pneumonia, prolonged diarrhoea,
pages 26 and 34, 48,
Not completely cured diseases,
Worm infestation, page 62.

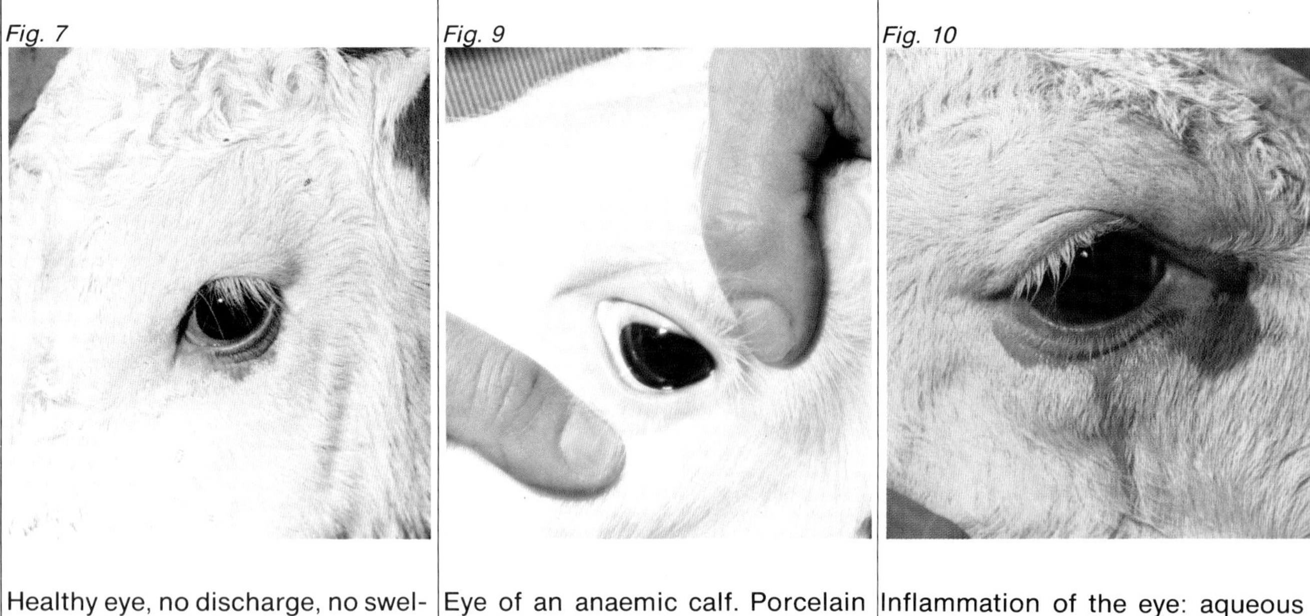

*Fig. 7*

**Symptoms**: Healthy eye, no discharge, no swelling of the eyelid, no changes around the eye.

**Examination**: Opening eyelid: Pale pink, well moistened palpebral conjunctiva without erythema.

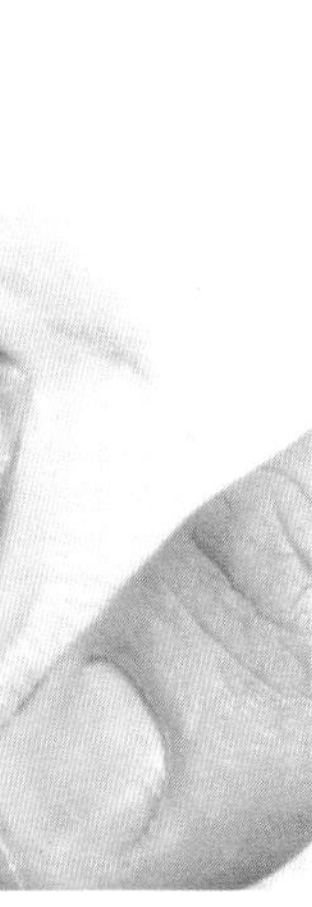

*Fig. 8*

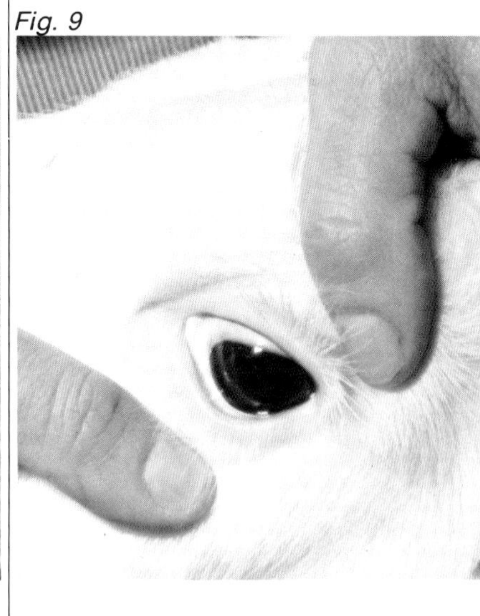

*Fig. 9*

**Symptoms**: Eye of an anaemic calf. Porcelain colour of palpebral conjunctiva; no discharge.

**Examination**: Buccal mucosa also pale. On exertion (rounding up animals) respiratory rate increases immediately.

**Read up**: Coccidiosis, page 108
Worm infestation; pages 62, 183, 192.

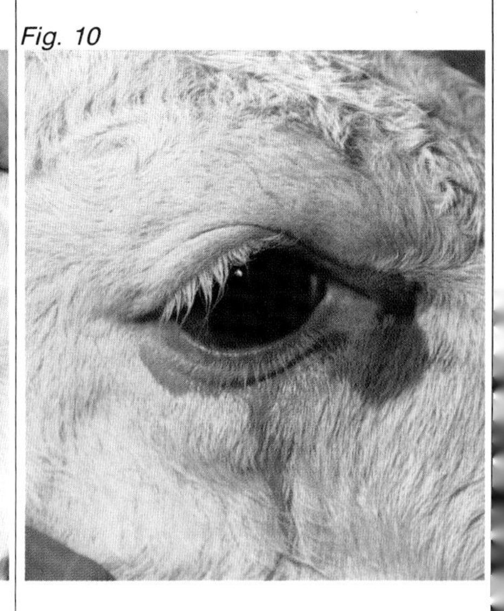

*Fig. 10*

**Symptoms**: Inflammation of the eye: aqueous discharge, lacrimation, swelling of eyelid, later adhesion of eye lashes; shunning light and squeezing eyelids together.

**Examination**: Reddening and inflammation of the palpebral conjunctiva; protruding blood vessels on the sclera. Take temperature!

**Read up**: Infectious diseases.
Pneumonia, page 34
Inflammation of the eyes due to chill (draughty cattle house, transport), page 82

| | *Fig. 11* | *Fig. 12* | *Fig. 13* |
|---|---|---|---|
| | 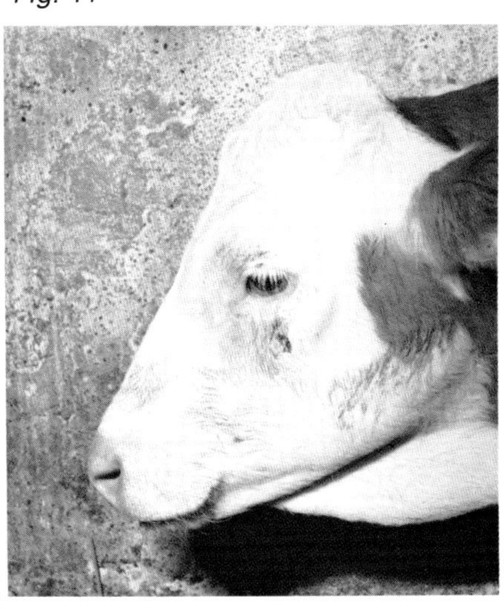 | 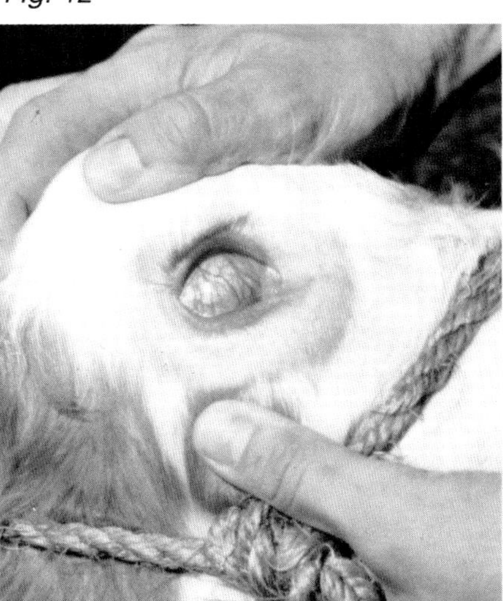 | 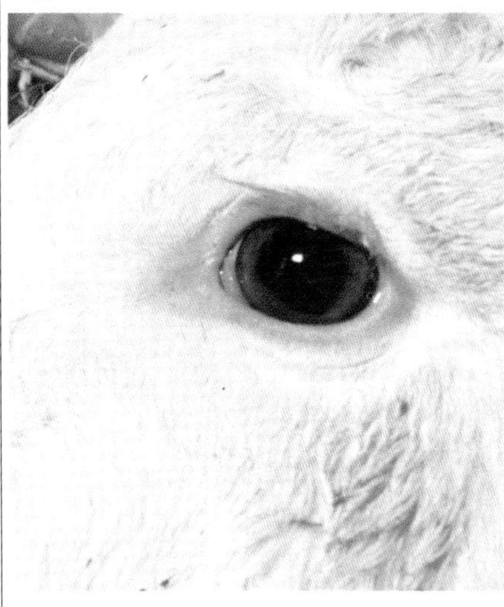 |
| **Symptoms** | Inflammation of the eye with purulent discharge, loss of hair along line of secretion, adhesion of eye lashes. | Vessels of sclera greatly congested with blood; swelling of eyelid. | Eye lying deep in its socket, making the orbit stand out and giving the impression that the eye is getting smaller. |
| **Examination** | Reddening and inflammation of palpebral conjunctiva. Protrusion of the blood vessels on the sclera. Take temperature! | Temperature frequently raised. Check other visible mucosae and faeces. | Desiccation of the connective tissue due to loss of fluid. Skin tension reduced (cf. illustration No. 42). Take temperature! Diarrhoea? |
| **Read up** | Infectious bronchopneumonia, page 82. | Cerebrocortical necrosis, page 102<br>ISTME, page 172<br>Mucosal disease, pages 138 and 162. | Diarrhoea, particularly Rota/corona/coli infection, page 26. Salmonellosis, page 36. High temperature in infectious bronchopneumonia, page 22. |

| | Fig. 14 | Fig. 15 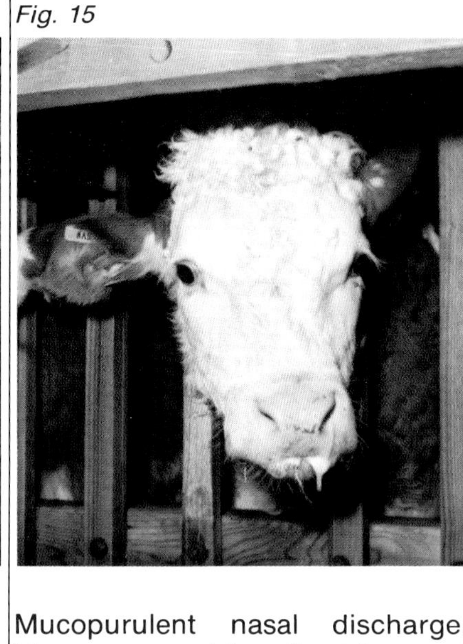 | Fig. 16 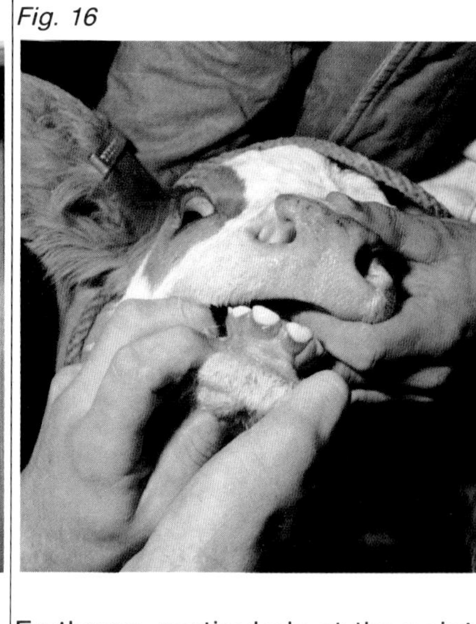 |
|---|---|---|---|
| **Symptoms** | Aqueous nasal discharge; outflow of clear, somewhat mucoid fluid. | Mucopurulent nasal discharge. Viscous mucoid yellowish nasal secretion. | Erythema, particularly at the point of transition from the haired skin to the muzzle. Cheek pouch and gum margin inflamed. |
| **Examination** | Temperature above 39.5° C. Husk, possibly accelerated breathing; listlessness. | Difficulty in breathing. Temperature above 39.5° C. Strained facial expression, poor feed intake. | Raised temperature (above 41° C) with aqueous intractable diarrhoea. Subnormal temperature. |
| **Read up** | Infectious bronchopneumonia, page 82. | Advanced stage of infectious bronchopneumonia, page 82.<br>Secondary bacterial infection, page 89. | Mucosal disease, page 162. |

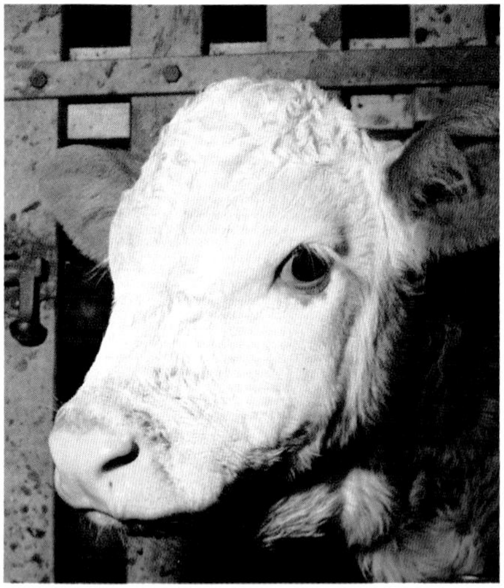

*Fig. 17*

**Symptoms:** Healthy navel, well dried out. On palpation the healthy umbilical cord is approximately as thick as a pencil.

**Examination:** Navel not painful to the touch.

*Fig. 18*

**Symptoms:** Inflamed, thickened navel.

**Examination:** Navel painful to the touch. Increased temperature possible (above 39.5° C).
Check joints for swelling!

**Read up:** Inflammation of the navel, page 52.

*Fig. 19*

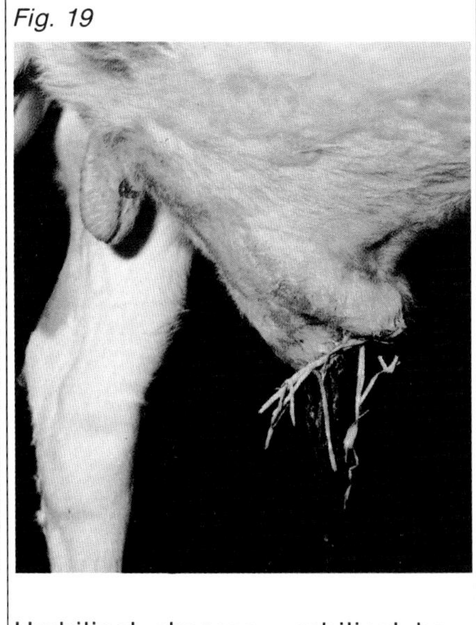

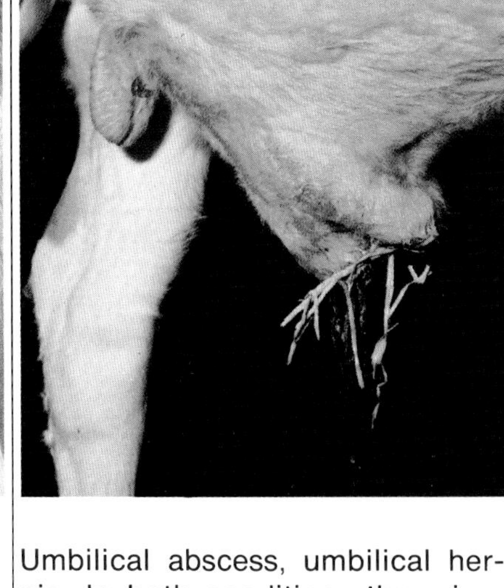

**Symptoms:** Umbilical abscess, umbilical hernia: In both conditions there is a sac-like extension of the skin above the navel.

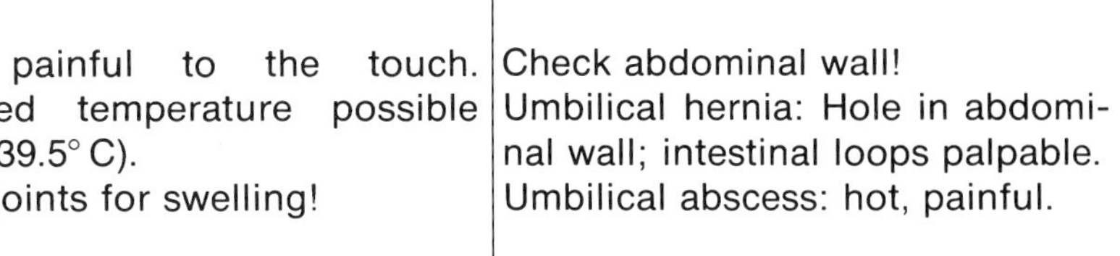

**Examination:** Check abdominal wall!
Umbilical hernia: Hole in abdominal wall; intestinal loops palpable.
Umbilical abscess: hot, painful.

**Read up:** Umbilical abscess, page 54.

| | *Fig. 20* | *Fig. 21* | *Fig. 22* |
|---|---|---|---|
| **Symptoms** | Trichophytosis (ringworm) in the sucking calf: Round bald patches, initially reddened, later asbestos-like crusts. | Infestation with lice: Bald areas; sucking sites and lice visible. | Incipient mange on the head: Irregular bald, raised areas with scab and crust formation. |
| **Examination** | No itching.<br>Demonstration of pathogen possible in the laboratory. | Itching.<br>Collect hairs for microscopic examination for nits. | Itching.<br>Skin scrapings for demonstration of mites in the laboratory. |
| **Read up** | Trichophytosis, page 112. | Infestation with lice, page 208. | Mange, page 200. |

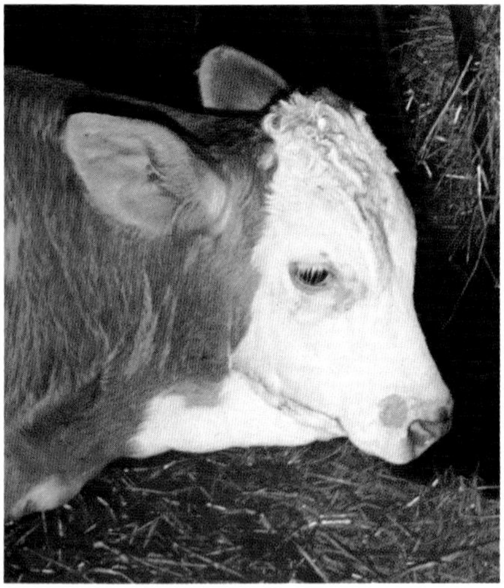

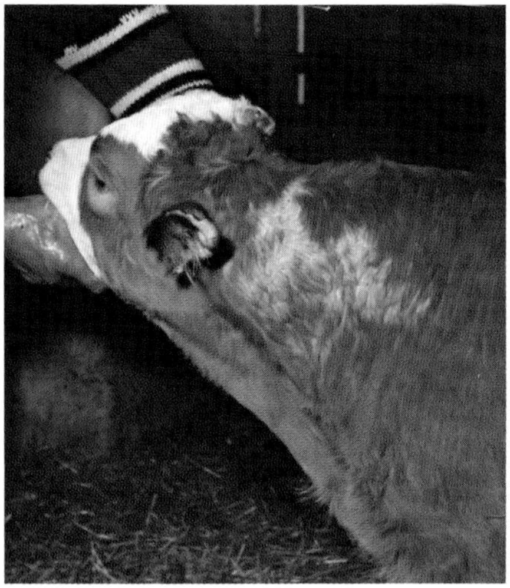

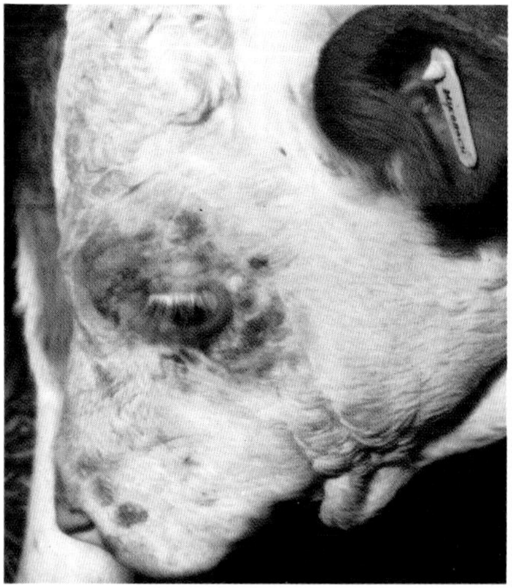

*Fig. 23*

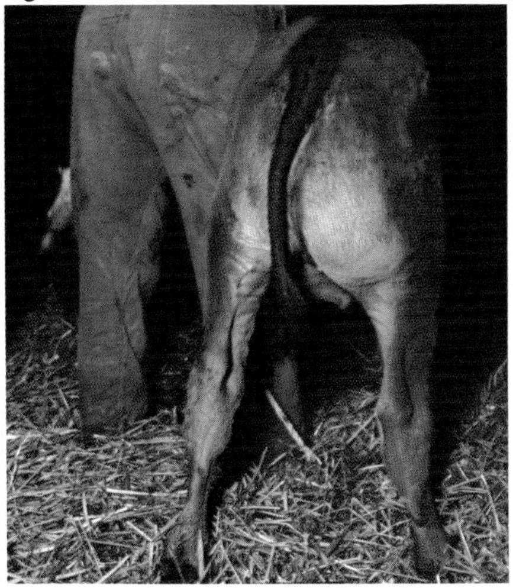

**Symptoms:** Subdermal abscess: Circumscribed boil-like distension; site of puncture or other injury sometimes visible.

**Examination:** Palpation: initially painful, increasingly hot; "wobbling" accumulation of fluid under the skin, usually not displaceable.

**Read up:** Abscess, page 222
Haemorrhage.

*Fig. 24*

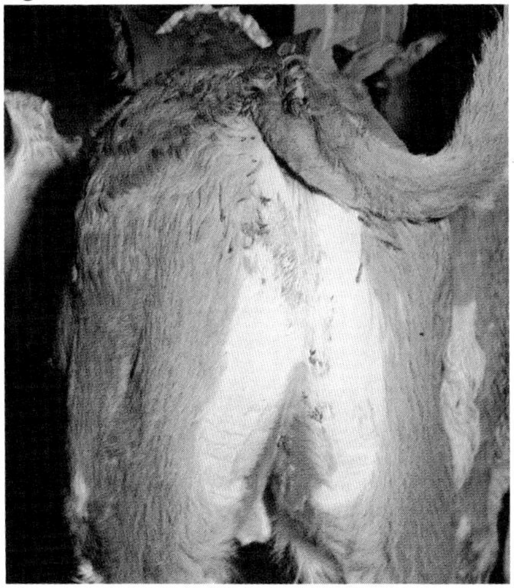

**Symptoms:** Bald patches on the thighs as a result of protracted diarrhoea.

**Examination:** Check faeces! Bacteriological and parasitological examination of faeces for the demonstration of salmonellosis and parasites.

**Read up:** Rota/corona/coli infection, page 26.
Late sequelae of salmonellosis, page 61.
Nutrition-induced diarrhoea, page 48.
Worm infestation, page 62.

*Fig. 25*

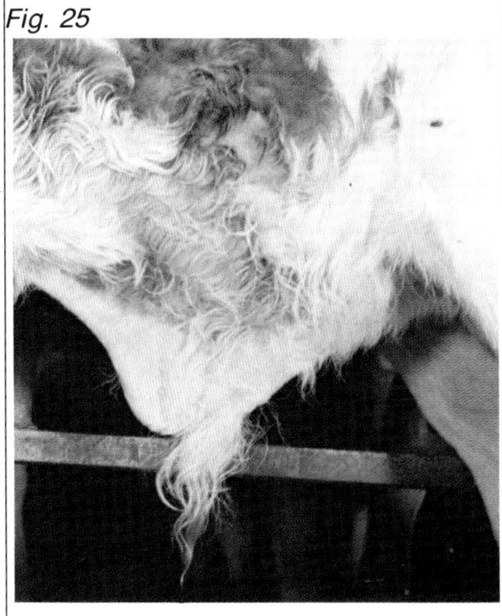

**Symptoms:** Sucking of navel: Bald skin patches around the umbilicus; sac-like extension due to sucking.

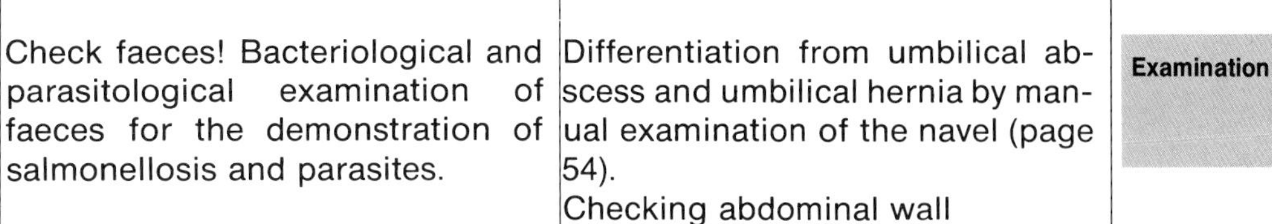

**Examination:** Differentiation from umbilical abscess and umbilical hernia by manual examination of the navel (page 54).
Checking abdominal wall (page 54)

**Read up:** Read page 54.

Fig. 26

**Symptoms**

Normal faeces. 1st week of life: yellow to light brown colour, consistency pappy to greasy/fatty and viscous, without solid components.

**Examination**

First faeces after birth: greenish-black, viscous; formed by the calf before birth and usually excreted on the first day.

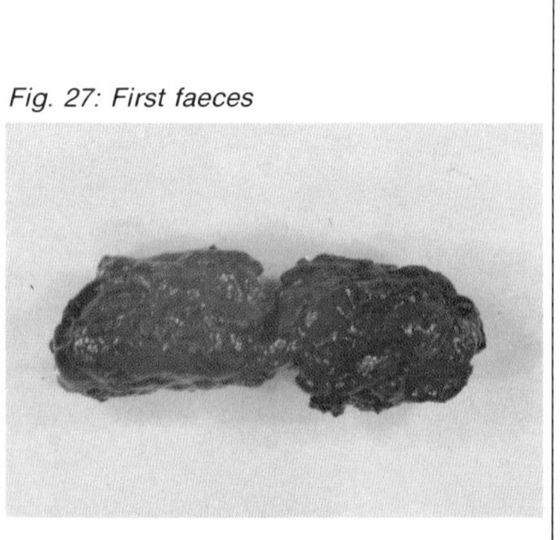

Fig. 27: First faeces

Fig. 28

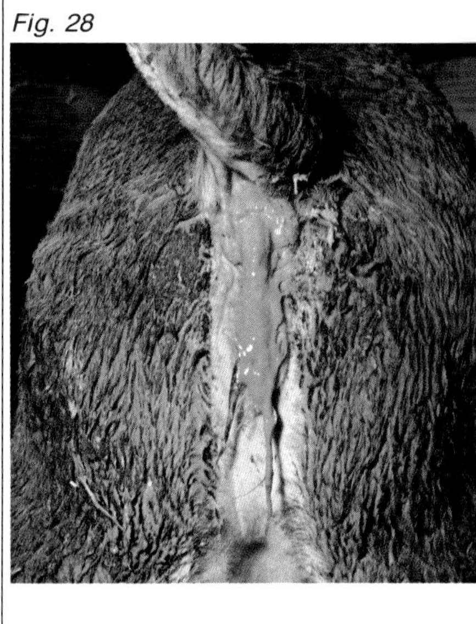

**Symptoms**

Soft faeces on change-over to milk substitutes, colour yellow to grey. Take-up of hay or straw; greasy/fatty, paste-like consistency, with solid components.

**Read up**

Read page 42.

Fig. 29

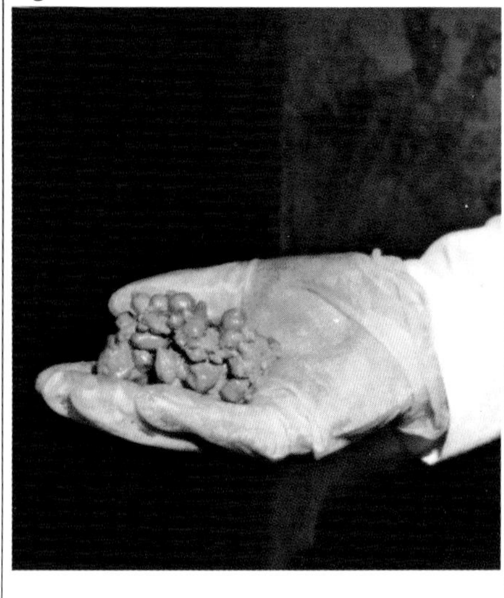

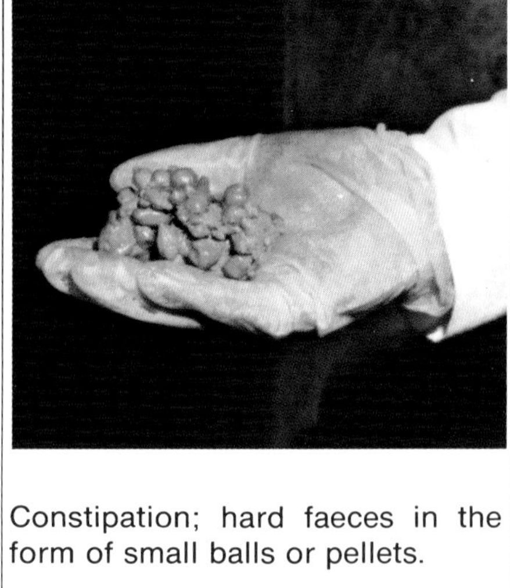

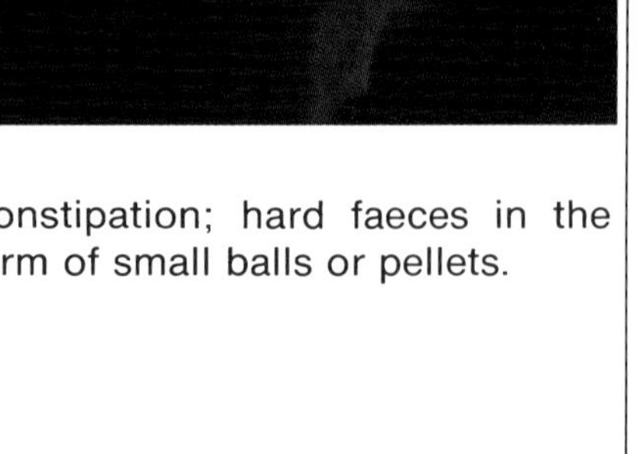

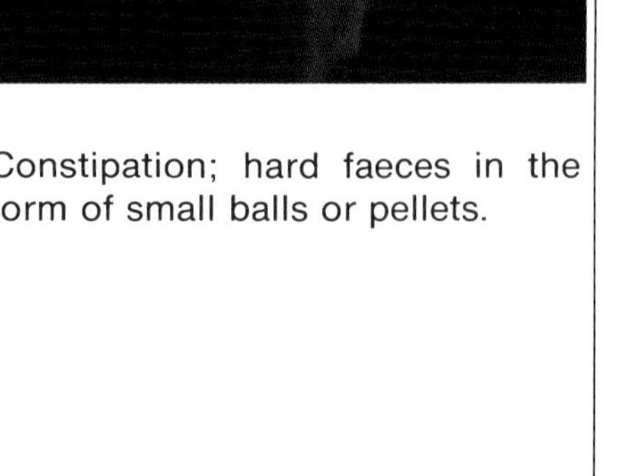

**Symptoms**

Constipation; hard faeces in the form of small balls or pellets.

**Examination**

Increased body temperature, inadequate fluid intake.

**Read up**

Febrile conditions,
pages 34 and 82.

*Fig. 30*

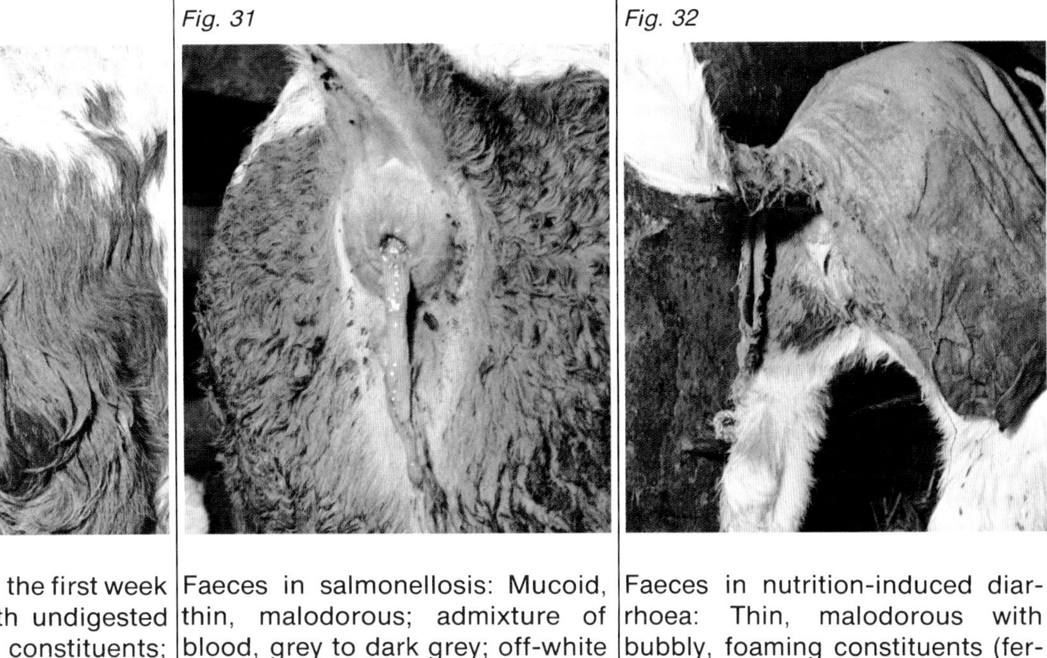

Incipient diarrhoea in the first week of life: Aqueous, with undigested coagulated milk constituents; admixture of blood.

Increased temperature possible. Examination of faeces.

Rota/corona/coli infection, page 26.

*Fig. 31*

Faeces in salmonellosis: Mucoid, thin, malodorous; admixture of blood, grey to dark grey; off-white mucoid flakes (Fibrin).

Increased temperature (41° C). Bacteriological examination of faeces.
Test for resistance.

Salmonellosis, page 36.

*Fig. 32*

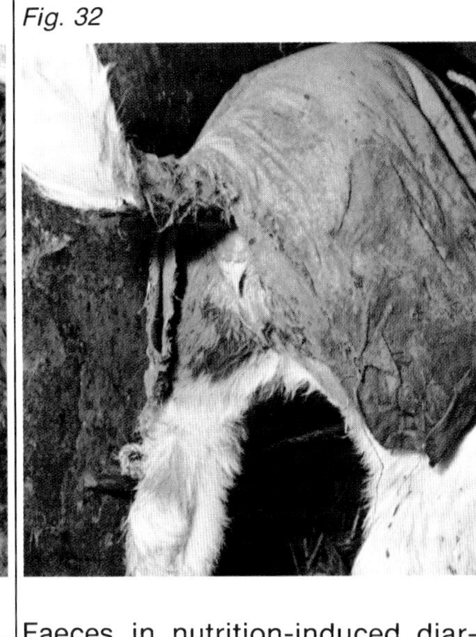

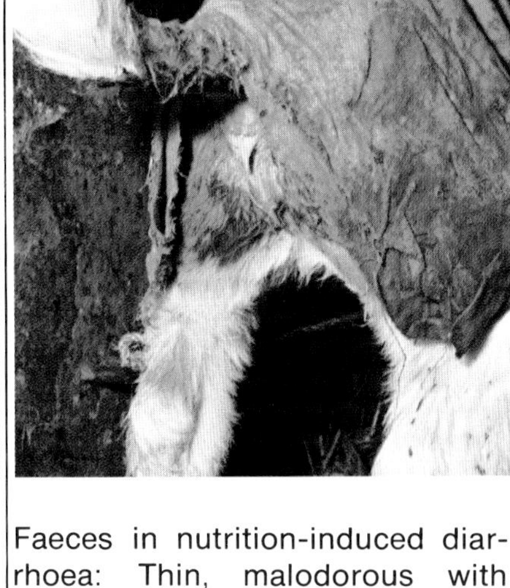

Faeces in nutrition-induced diarrhoea: Thin, malodorous with bubbly, foaming constituents (fermentation diarrhoea).

Initially temperature not increased. Check feed and feeding.

Nutrition-induced diarrhoea, putrescent and fermentation diarrhoea, page 48.

**Symptoms**

**Examination**

**Read up**

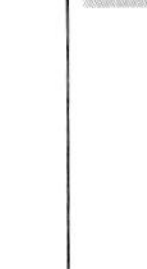

*Fig. 33*

**Symptoms**
Normal joints: Dry, well contured, strong; straight posture.

**Examination**
Palpation of the joints; walking the animals to detect any lameness.

*Fig. 34*

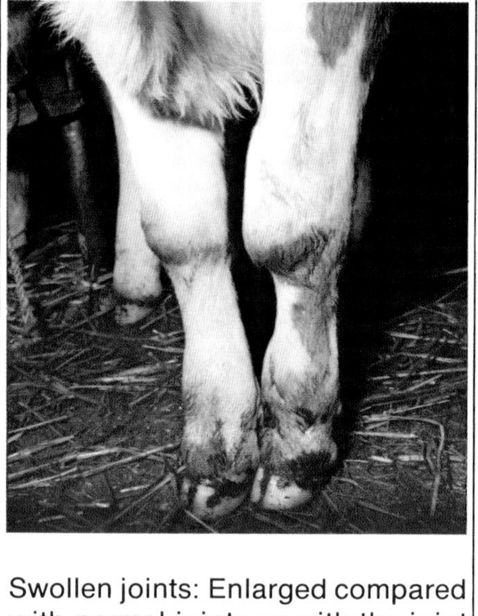

**Symptoms**
Swollen joints: Enlarged compared with normal joints or with the joint on the other side. Lameness, the calf does not rise when the animals are roused.

**Examination**
Palpation for increased heat and painfulness. Examination of the navel. Checking for signs of diarrhoea.

**Read up**
Salmonellosis, page 36
Septicaemia of newborn calves, page 60
Umbilical infection, page 52.

*Fig. 35*

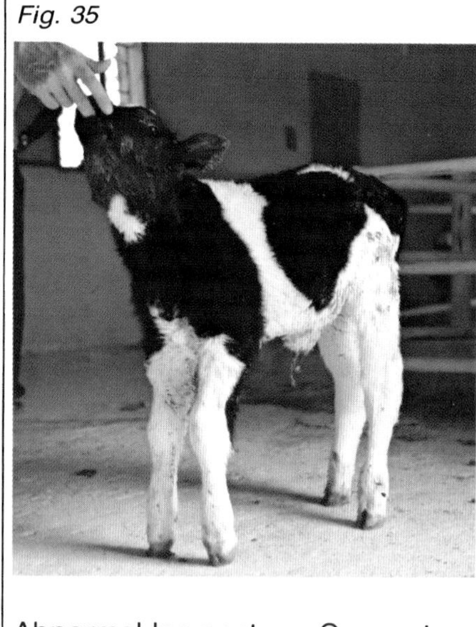

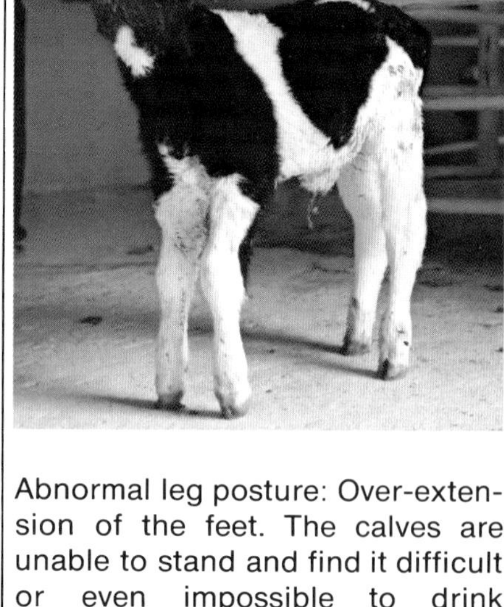

**Symptoms**
Abnormal leg posture: Over-extension of the feet. The calves are unable to stand and find it difficult or even impossible to drink unaided.

**Read up**
Congenital postural anomalies, page 66

*Fig. 36*

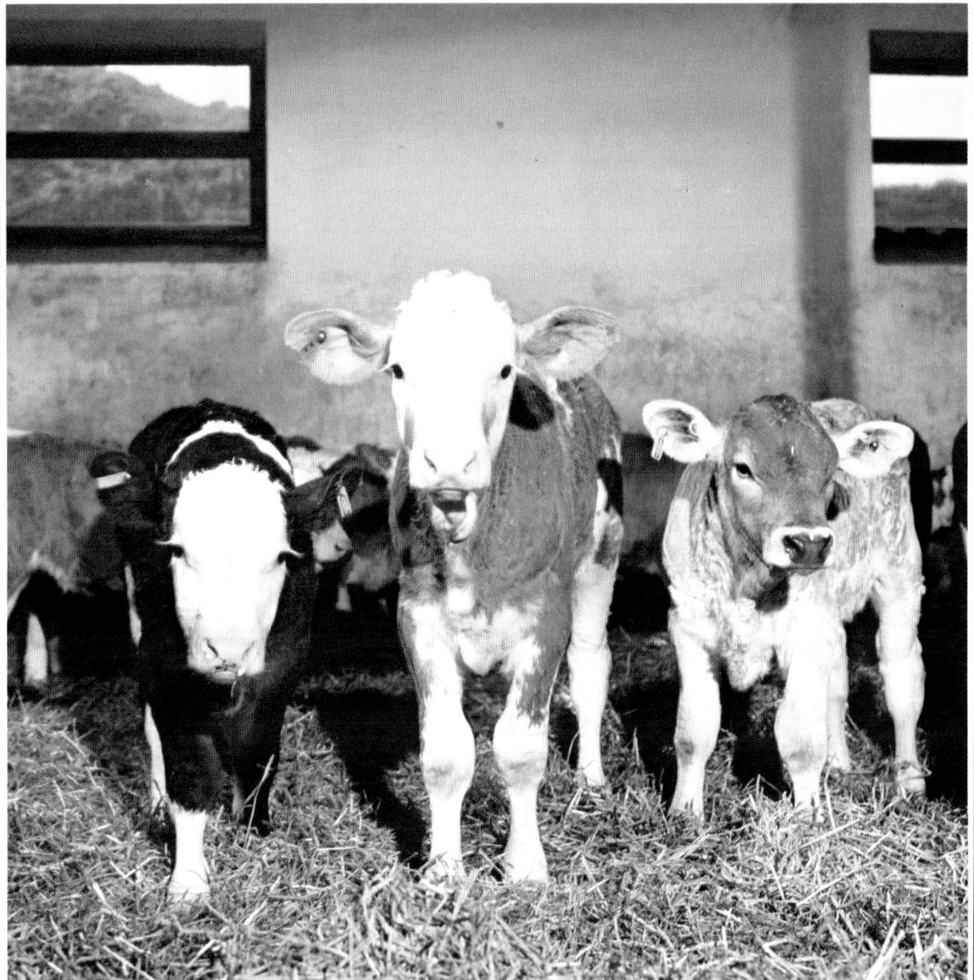

*Alert, curious calves. Regular observation is necessary to detect any impairment of their general condition at an early stage.*

# The most important diseases 1st to 4th week of life

# Scours in sucking calves

## Rota/corona/coli infection

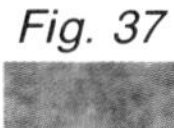

Fig. 37

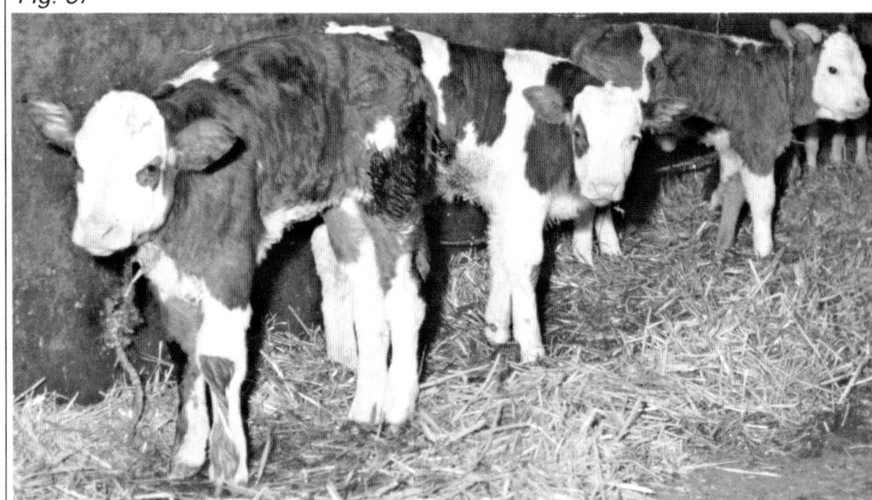

**Term**

A few years ago it was shown in the USA that diarrhoea in sucking calves is caused by certain viruses and that this condition is not, as had previously been assumed, exclusively due to bacterial infection (particularly E. coli). This severe infectious diarrhoea is precipitated by rota and corona viruses.

**Incidence**

The disease occurs frequently among calves in dairy herds where the causative organisms are nearly always present. An increased incidence of the disease is observed in cattle houses where several calves are born within a short period. With each additional calf the clinical picture deteriorates and death ensues in an increasing number of cases.
This type of diarrhoea is also seen on farms purchasing their calves at under 3 weeks of age.

Fig. 38

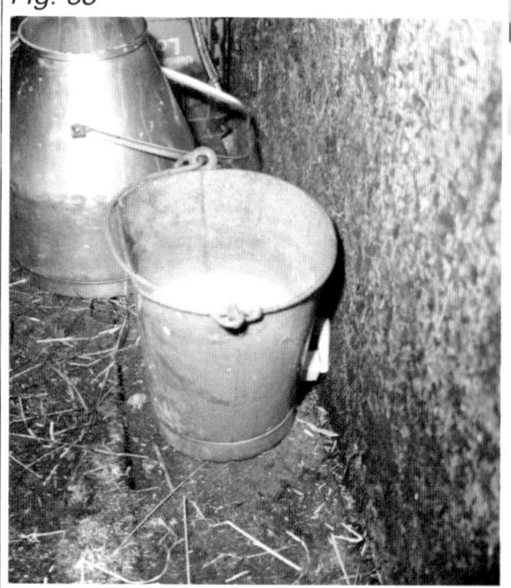

**Pathogen / Cause**

The actual cause of the diarrhoea are viruses belonging to the rota and corona group. Rota and corona viruses also occur in pigs, horses and sheep. The causative organism of transmissible gastro-enteritis of pigs (TGE) is also included in this group of viruses. In addition to the viruses precipitating the disease, bacteria occur (particularly E. coli) which aggravate the condition.

*Fig. 37: Inappropriate, but frequently seen location of calves. Calves tied up behind the cows along the dung passage are constantly in contact with the virus-containing faeces of the cows and neighbouring calves. The chain of infection is thus maintained.*

*Fig. 38: Drinking bucket with kinked suction drain standing at the faeces-soiled wall. This stops the milk from running out, but increases the danger of infection.*

*Figs. 39 and 40: Running faeces at the start of the disease.*

*Figs. 39/40*

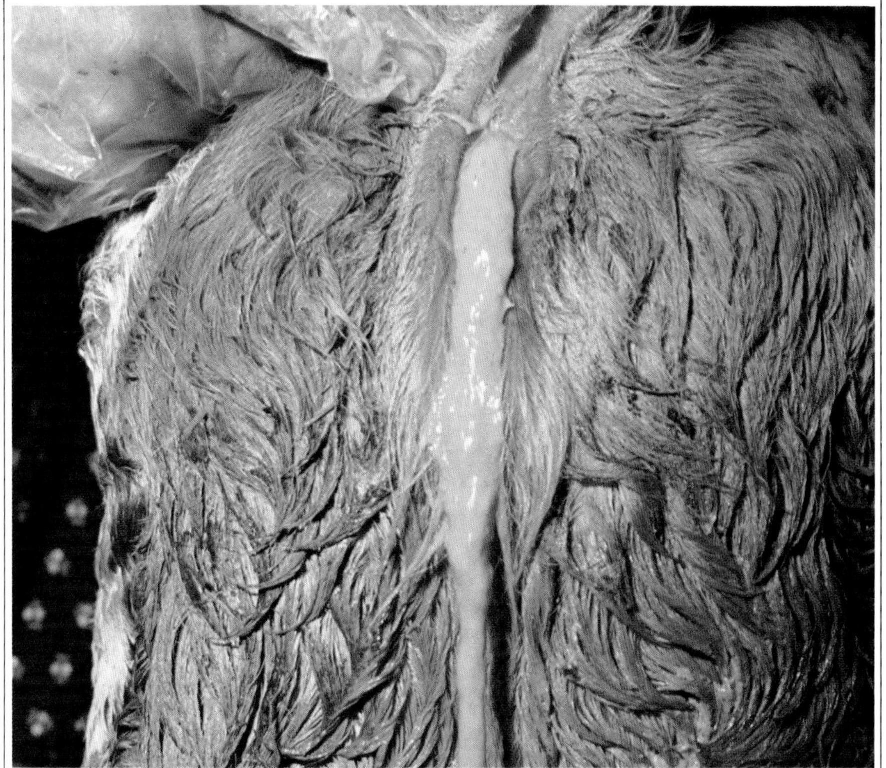

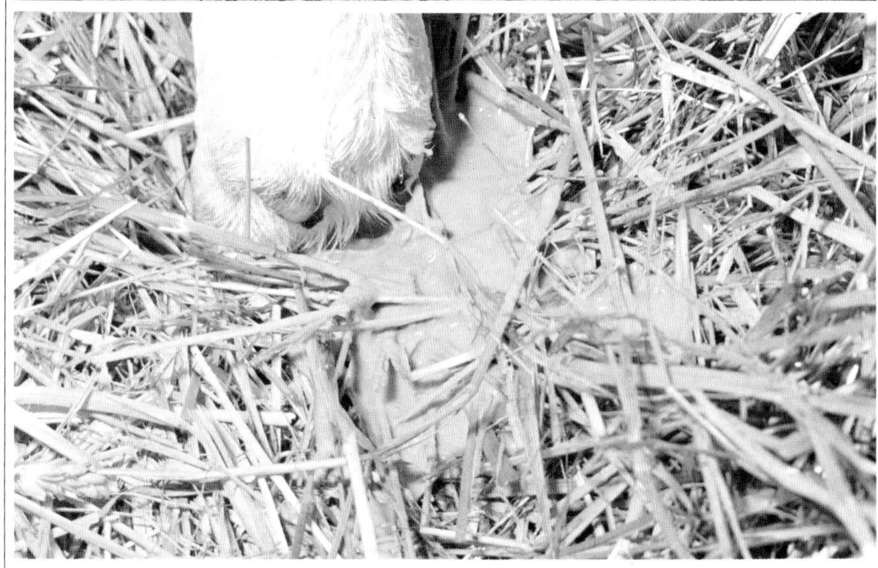

Since the pathogens are present in virtually all cattle stocks, any calf may contract the disease. The following factors increase the exposure to infection and thus the susceptibility of calves:

**Importation / Route of infection**

- Insufficient and incorrect care after birth.
- Incorrect removal of mucus from the mouth with dirty fingers.
- Late and inadequate feeding with colostral milk.
- Unhygienic milking of colostral milk.
- Incorrect temperature of drink.
- Inappropriate location of the newborn calf, such as: Tying calves to cold, moist external walls of the cattle house. Standing in or near the dung passage (close contact with virus-contaminated faeces).
- Inappropriate calf housing: Incorrect temperature, excessively high humidity of the air, draughtiness, calves placed too close together (infection through contact with neighbouring calves).

*Fig. 41*

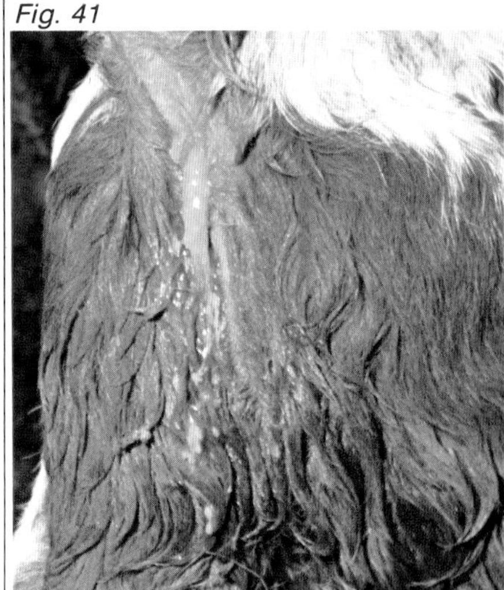

**Symptoms**

The period from the first appearance of the pathogens in the intestine to the visible signs of the disease is 12 to 14 hours (incubation period).

The disease initially manifests itself in dullness and loss of appetite. By this time the virus has attacked the villi of the intestinal mucosa and has partly destroyed them.

Diarrhoea occurs with the aqueous and foaming faeces being forcefully ejected. As a result of the intestinal irritation, the calves are constantly straining to pass faeces. The pain may be seen from the drawn-in abdomen.

Following the partial loss of the intestinal mucosa, utilisation of food is reduced or no longer possible. In addition to nutritive substances, vital salts (electrolytes) and trace elements are lost. This results in desiccation of the body and electrolyte deficiency. This desiccation is characterised by deep-set eyes and reduced elasticity of the skin.

*Fig. 42*

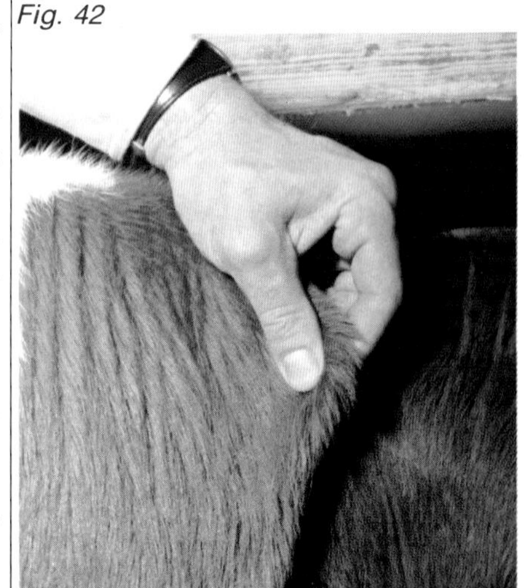

Fig. 43

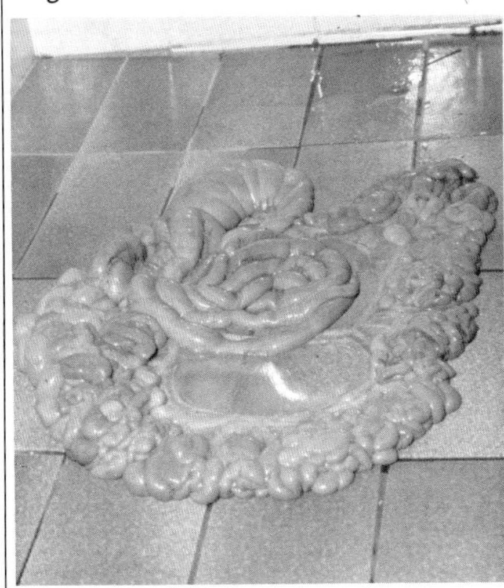

Fig. 44

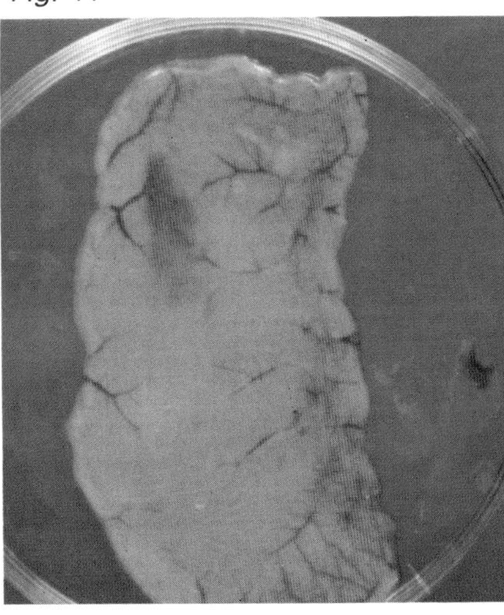

Fig. 45

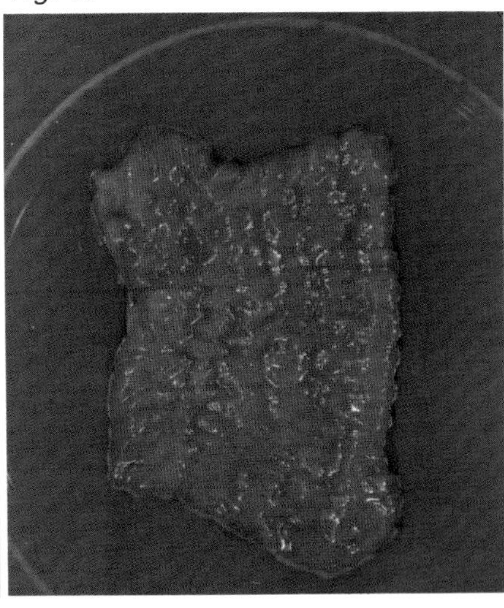

Symptoms

The undigested food with its high content of milk protein is an ideal growth medium for bacteria (particularly E. coli). The bacteria and their toxins can easily penetrate the intestinal mucosa damaged by viruses, pass into the blood stream and thus spread throughout the animal organism. This results in bacteraemia and septicaemia. Joints of the limbs are preferred sites of attack. This condition is generally described as septicaemia of newborn calves (cf. page 60).
The diarrhoea persists and the faeces now become malodorous because of decomposition in the intestine. In some cases admixture of blood and mucosal fragments are visible.
Treatment is rarely successful in this stage of the disease and the mortality rate is high.

*Fig. 41: Advanced stage: Aqueous faeces with flocculent, undigested milk components.*

*Fig. 42: Checking skin elasticity by raising a skin fold: With protracted diarrhoea the skin fold levels out slowly.*

*Fig. 43: Pronounced enlargement of the intestinal lymph nodes (arrows); gas-filled paper-thin small intestine.*

*Fig. 44: Viruses almost completely destroy the intestinal mucosa, hence the transparent appearance of the intestine.*

*Fig. 45: For comparison: Unchanged intestine of a normal calf.*

Diagnosis

The characteristic course of the diarrhoea in the stock, particularly its very early appearance in sucking calves during the first few days of life, is typical of this infection.

Demonstration of the virus is very difficult. In the live animal it is successful only if a faecal sample is taken as early as 2 to 4 hours after the first appearance of diarrhoea symptoms. The sample must be deep-frozen immediately and must not be thawed until the time of the examination which can only be carried out in specially equipped laboratories.

In dead calves, the gas-filled, paper-thin intestine is typical. Microscopic examination shows the shrinkage of the intestinal villi. The virus cannot be demonstrated in dead animals. This is possible only at the start of diarrhoea in freshly killed calves.

**Similar symptoms**

Similar symptoms are caused by salmonellosis, but this disease does not occur in any number until the second week of life. Inappropriate feeding (Fig. 85) also produces similar symptoms. The main distinguishing features are summarised on page 42.

*Fig. 46*

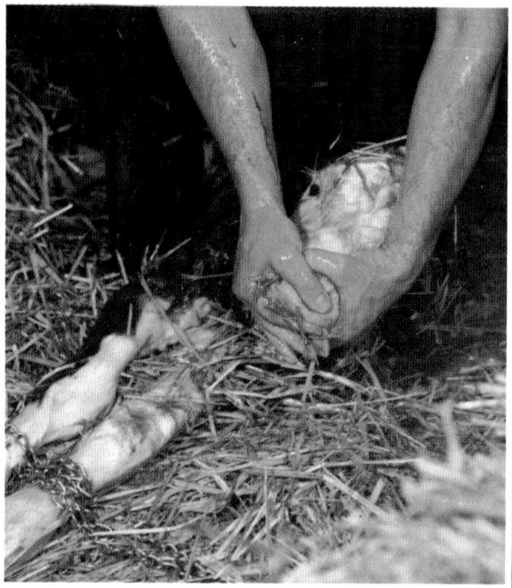

**Treatment**

Three important aspects need to be considered for treatment:

- **Normalisation of the water and electrolyte balance**
  In severe diarrhoea the loss of water leads to a deficiency of body salts, especially potassium and sodium. Without these electrolytes the body functions cannot be maintained. The administration of water and electrolytes therefore constitutes the most important measure in the treatment of diarrhoea. This is done by adding suitable electrolyte solutions to the drinking fluid. In the advanced stage the electrolytes need to be injected, since take-up via the damaged intestine is no longer sufficient and the electrolytes are absorbed more quickly in this way. The water volume of 2 litres twice daily taken up with the electrolyte solution, does not meet the water requirements of the calves at the start of treatment. Supplementary administration of tea and glucose is necessary. Do not give ordinary household sugar!

- **Withdrawal of high protein feed**
  The protein substances contained in milk and milk substitutes are no longer utilised. They form an ideal growth medium for pathogenic bacteria, particularly E. coli, in the intestine. As a result of the withdrawal of milk or milk substitute, the bacteria are deprived of this growth medium.

Fig. 47

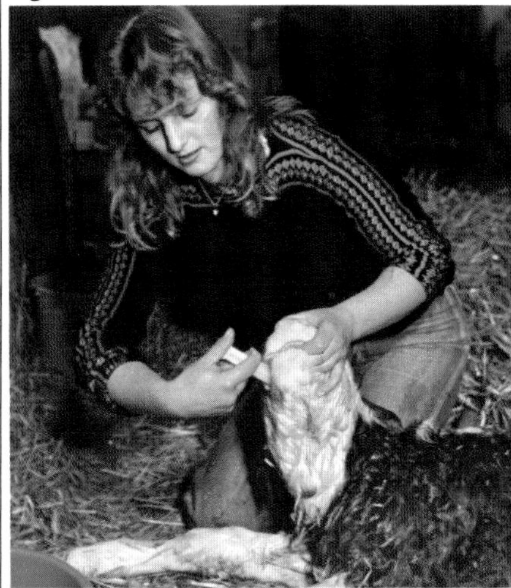



## Administration of antibiotics and sulphonamides

Any secondary bacterial infection present or likely to occur is contained with substances having an antibiotic effect. In selecting the drugs to be used, it should be considered that sucking calves, like human babies, are very sensitive and require medicinal products that are well tolerated and cause only mild side-effects.

Fig. 48

| | | |
|---|---|---|
| 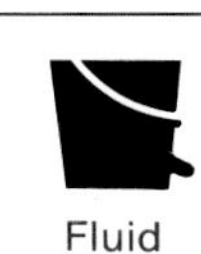 Fluid | **Replacement of milk substitute or milk** by electrolyte solution (90 g ELRISAL + 15 g BUSAL in 2 litres of water) twice daily; between feeds: 1 litre of tea twice daily. | 1st and 2nd day |
| 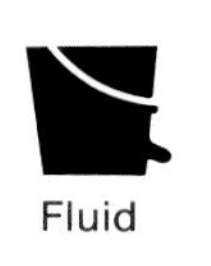 Fluid | **Change-over to milk:** 1 litre of milk or milk substitute and 1 litre of electrolyte solution (45 g ELRISAL + 15 g BUSAL in 1 litre of water) twice daily. | 3rd and 4th day |
| 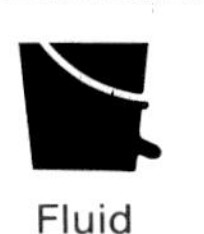 Fluid | **Change-over to milk:** $1^1/_2$ litres of milk or milk substitute and $^1/_2$ litre of electrolyte solution (25 g ELRISAL + 10 g BUSAL in $^1/_2$ litre of water) twice daily. | 5th and 6th day |
| 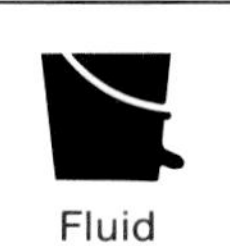 Fluid | **Follow-up treatment:** 10 g CHEVICALF per day and per calf in the drinking fluid, for 14 days. | From the 7th day, for 14 days |
| 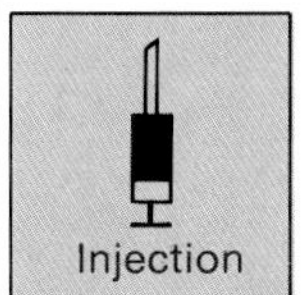 Injection | **Severely ill calves:** In addition to drinking fluid, 250 ml GLYKOFUSAL s.c. (divided over several sites) and 1.5 ml PENBROCK or KELFIZIN/10 kg body-weight i.m. | Twice at an interval of 24 hours |

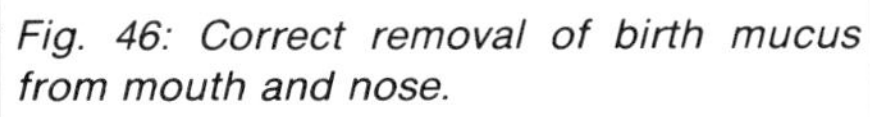

*Fig. 46: Correct removal of birth mucus from mouth and nose.*

*Fig. 47: Administration of gammaglobulin and vitamins before giving the first colostral milk.*

*Fig. 48: Treatment schedule for rota/corona/coli infection.*

*Fig. 49*

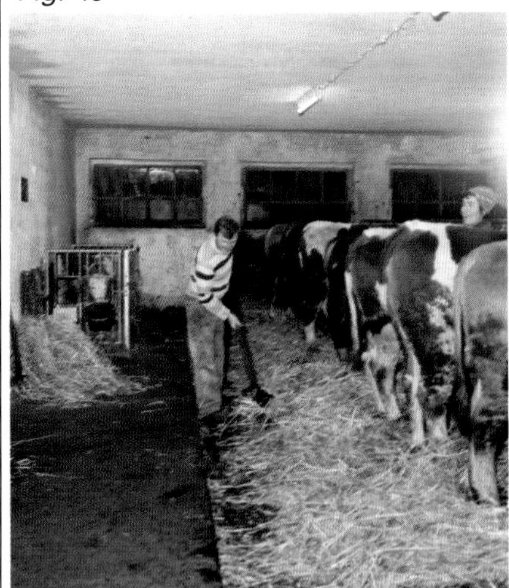

*Fig. 50*

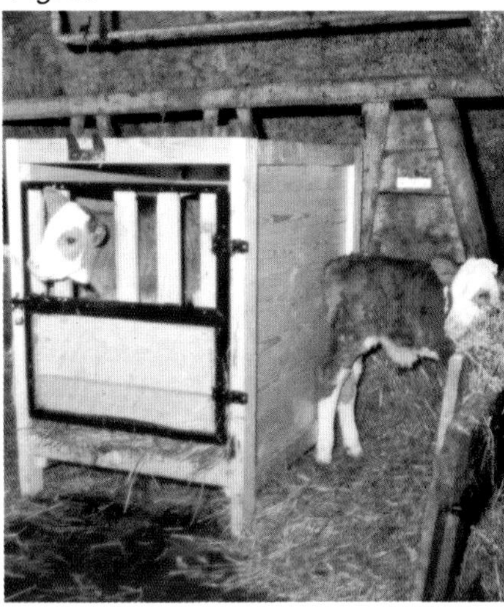

*Fig. 51*

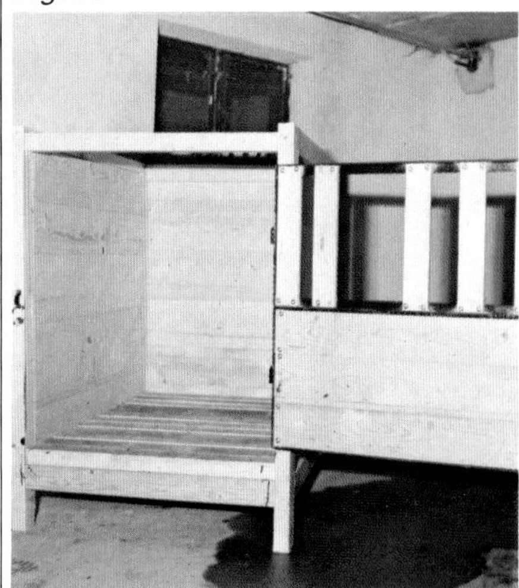

**Prevention and disinfection**

We have found the following 4-stage programme to be very successful in problem stocks:

- **Immediate removal** of the calves from the calving shed and placing in a carefully cleaned, disinfected, isolated and heated calf house (air humidity: 70%, temperature: 16 to 20° C for straw litter, 22 to 24 °C for slatted floors). Special care should be taken to ensure that in the calving shed the newborn calf has as little contact as possible with the faeces of the calves and cows kept there.

- **Before** the first colostral milk is given, the calves receive 20 ml bovine gammaglobulin and 20 ml of an aqueous vitamin A-$D_3$-E mixture (500,000 to 1 million I. U. of vitamin A) both orally and – in the same dosage – injected subcutaneously.
  Gammaglobulin contains the natural protective substances from the blood and the colostral milk of adult cattle in particularly high concentration. Vitamin A strengthens the skin and mucosae and plays an important rôle in the calf's defence mechanism against infections. Bovine gammaglobulin and vitamin A are given before the first colostral milk, because it is only at this time that the gastric and intestinal cells are ready to absorb them.

- Administration of a well tolerated antibiotic product (10 g CHEVICALF/day) from the 1st day of life to the 3rd week. The water-soluble drug is added to the drinking fluid.

Fig. 52

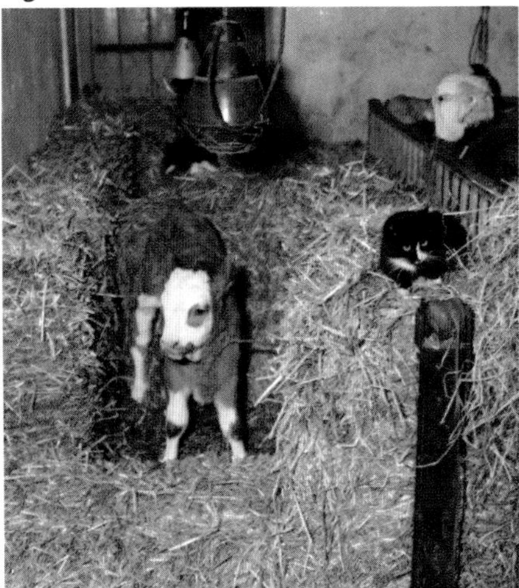

■ **Additional measures:**
When milking the colostrum, special attention should be paid to cleanliness. Within the first 4 hours of life the calf should drink at least 2 litres of colostral milk. Contact of the calf with the milk cattle house and attendants should be avoided. The best method is for one particularly attentive person to look only after the calves. Special clothing, particularly shoes, should be worn only in the calf house.

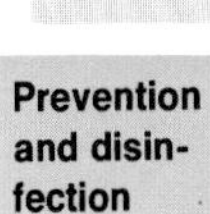



Fig. 53

| | | |
|---|---|---|
| 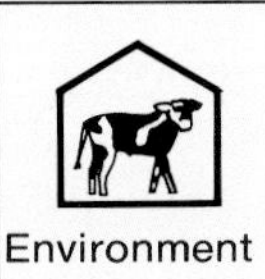 Environment | Avoid contact with faeces of other cows and calves. Immediate removal from the calving shed. Use at least a calf pen. | |
| 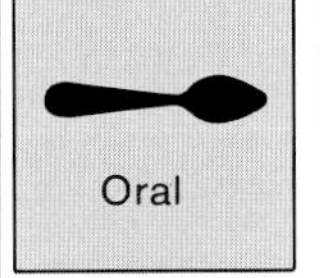 Oral | **Before administration of colostral milk:** 20 ml GAMBUL and 10 ml VITAMIN-$AD_3$EC-100 per calf. | immediately, by 2nd hour if possible |
| 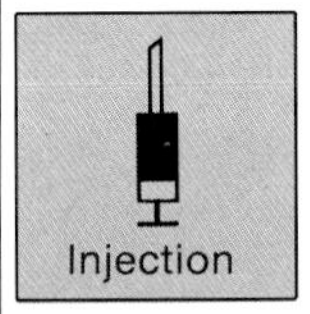 Injection | **Before administration of colostral milk:** Give 20 ml GAMBUL and 10 ml VITAMIN-$AD_3$EC-100 per calf subcutaneously. | immediately, by 2nd hour if possible |
| 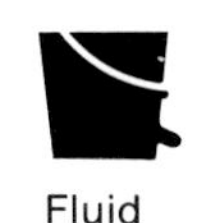 Fluid | **Colostral milk:** At least 2 litres within the first 4 hours of life. | by 4th hour if possible |
| 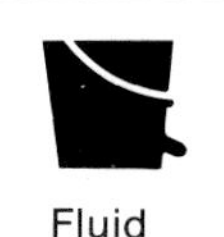 Fluid | Preventive treatment: 10 g CHEVICALF/calf/day, for 14 days, via the drinking fluid. | 1st to 14th day |

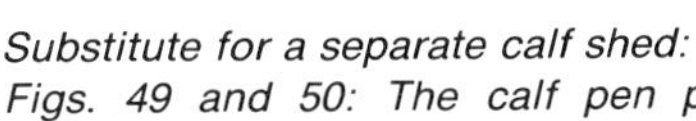

*Substitute for a separate calf shed:*
*Figs. 49 and 50: The calf pen provides appropriate conditions for the calf. This separation from the other animals is sufficient in small stocks to prevent infection during the first few hours and days of life.*

*Fig. 51: Home-made calf pen (For dimensions, see part 5).*

*Fig. 52: Emergency solution for immediate separation of calves.*

*Fig. 53: Preventive schedule for rota/corona/coli infection.*

# Pneumonia of sucking calves

## Pneumococcal infection

Fig. 54

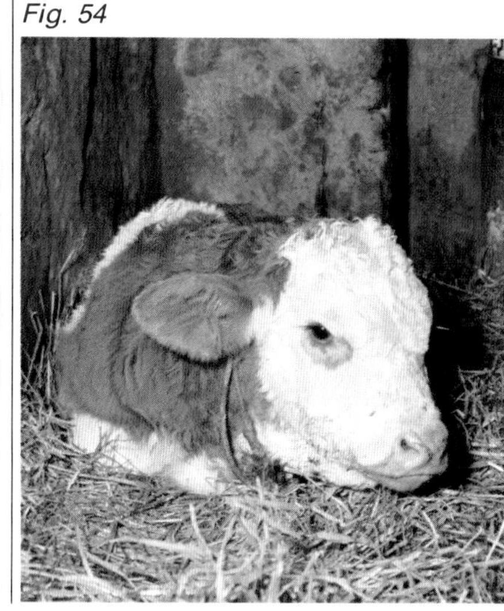

Fig. 55

**Term**

Pneumonia of sucking calves, also called pneumococcosis, is a generalised bacterial infection which takes a very rapid course and affects mainly the respiratory organs.

**Incidence**

The disease occurs particularly in the 3rd week of life, mainly during the winter months and if the animals are permanently kept in the cattle house.

**Pathogen**

The causative organism is diplococcus pneumoniae, several types of which occur in man and animals.

**Importation / Route of infection**

The types occurring in man are also pathogenic to the calf.

The disease is transmitted by droplet infection (cough). In many cases the pathogens are introduced by staff working in the cattle house who have a latent infection.

**Symptoms and Course of the Disease**

The very rapid course of the disease (highly acute) usually leads to the death of the animal within a few hours. The body temperature rises to 41.5° C. Inflammation of the large airways (bronchi) and focal changes in the lungs are observed. With highly acute forms (septicaemia) these signs may not be present.

Fig. 56

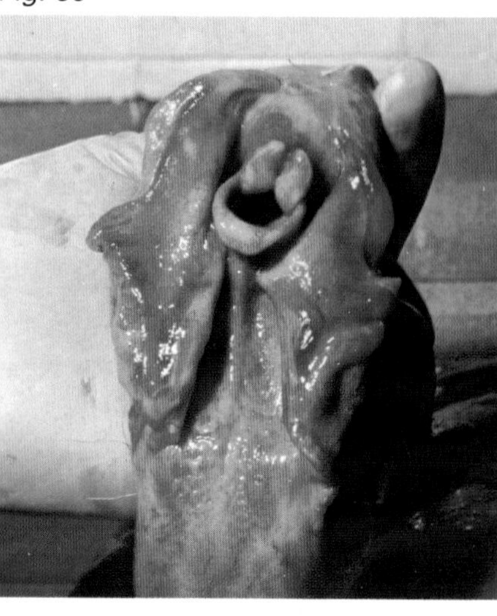

Fig. 57

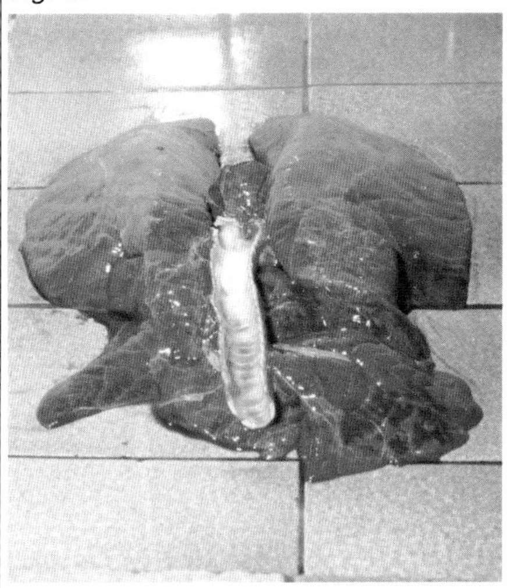

In dead animals an enlarged, firmly elastic spleen (rubber-like spleen) is found in more than half the cases.

**Similar symptoms**

The rapidly progressing acute form of salmonellosis and of E. coli infection is indistinguishable from the highly acute form of pneumococcal infection. The cause of the disease can only be established by bacteriological investigation.

**Treatment**

Treatment must be started immediately at the first sign of the disease. Penicillin is the drug of choice.
In order to maintain adequate tissue levels, a further half-dose is given 12 hours after the initial dose.
For follow-up treatment of affected calves and for prevention in neighbouring animals of the same age, treatment with penicillin-containing medicated feed over a period of one week has proved of value.

Fig. 58

| | | |
|---|---|---|
| 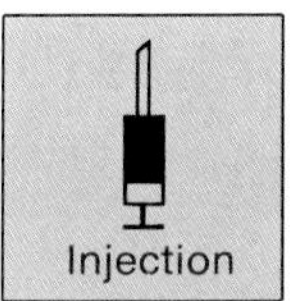 Injection | **Affected calf:** 3 ml FORAPEN/10 kg body-weight intramuscularly as soon as possible; follow up with half dose after 12 and 24 hours. | immediately and after 12 and 24 h |
| 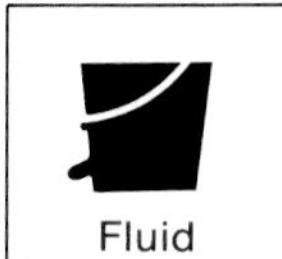 Fluid | **Affected calf and neighbouring calves:** 4 g of BUSAL/10 kg body-weight daily for 7 days via the drinking fluid. | 1st to 7th day |
| 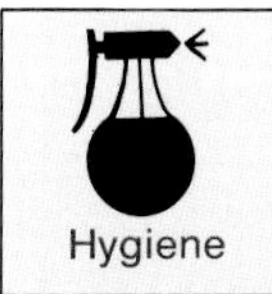 Hygiene | **Place in cattle house or calf pen:** Muck out, clean, disinfect with 2% CHEVI 45 solution. | 2nd day |

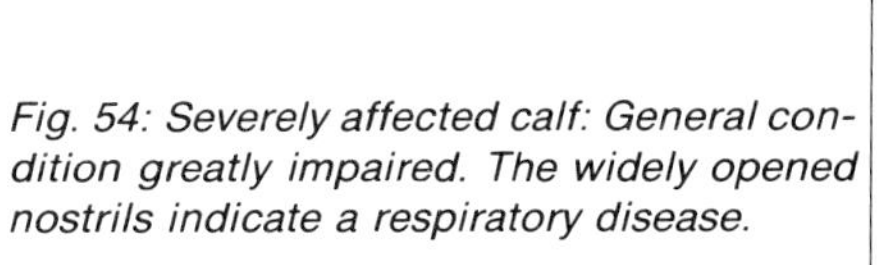

*Fig. 54: Severely affected calf: General condition greatly impaired. The widely opened nostrils indicate a respiratory disease.*

*Fig. 55: Pneumonia: Both lungs and the pulmonary pleura are severely inflamed and changed.*

*Fig. 56: Inflammation and swelling of pharynx and larynx.*

*Fig. 57: Pneumonia with accumulation of foam in the bronchi and windpipe. With pneumococcosis, focal lung changes are seen only in cases of protracted disease.*

*Fig. 58: Treatment schedule for pneumonia.*

# Salmonellosis of calves

Fig. 59

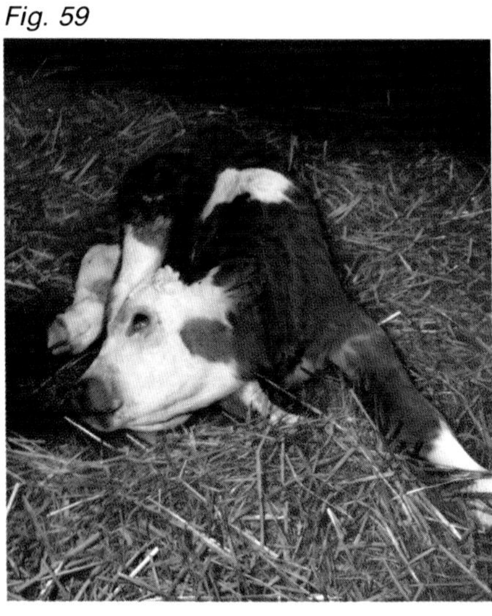

Fig. 60

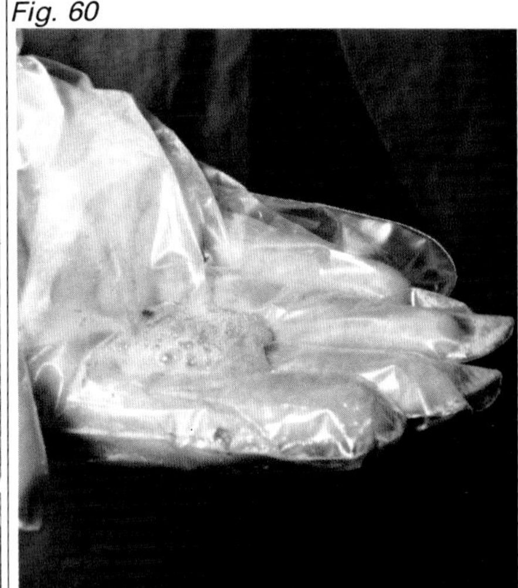

**Term**

Salmonellosis is an epidemic with a high mortality rate, which causes substantial losses. The pathogens, salmonella bacteria, initially multiply in the intestine where they cause severe inflammation and diarrhoea.

**Incidence**

The disease occurs throughout the world. All animal species and man may contract salmonellosis. Not only warm-blooded mammals and birds, but also cold-blooded animals (e. g. reptiles, fish) are salmonella carriers.

In calves salmonellosis usually appears in epidemic form at the age of 2 to 6 weeks, causing heavy losses. Calves surviving the disease often become carriers. These are animals which have survived the infection in the intestine and continue to excrete salmonellae without showing signs of the disease. They continually infect other animals.

**Pathogen**

Salmonellae are 1 to 3 $\mu$ long, rod-shaped bacteria capable of ciliary movement. Several hundred types are known. In cattle, **salmonella enteritidis** and **salmonella typhi murium** are of particular importance. These two salmonella types can also cause disease in other animal species and in man, whilst other types are host-specific, that is they cannot be transmitted to certain animal species or to man.

Salmonellae are very resistant. In dried-out faeces they retain their infectivity for several years, on infected pastures for several months, and in hay obtained from these pastures they remain infective for up to 11 weeks.

*Fig. 59: Septicaemic forms of salmonellosis also produce disorders of the central nervous system: Animal unable to rise, cramped posture, rolling of eyes and twisting of head.*

*Fig. 60: Bubbly mucoid faeces in salmonellosis.*

*Fig. 61: As a result of the destruction of the intestinal mucosa, the faces become mucoid with admixtures of whitish-grey flakes (Fibrin).*

*Fig. 62: Salmonellae also invade the vascular intestinal wall causing severe bleeding inflammation of the intestine.*

Fig. 61

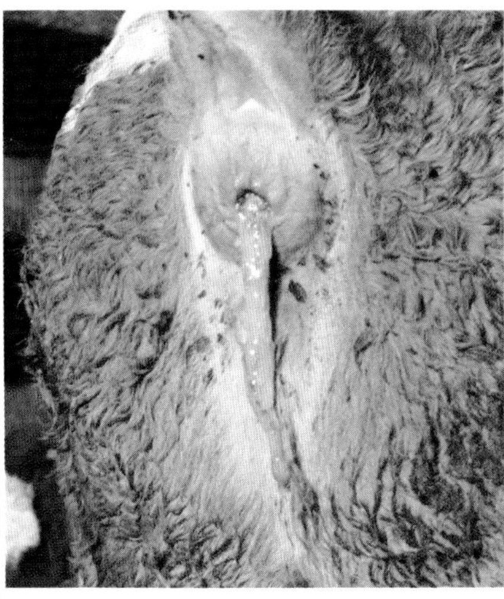

Fig. 62

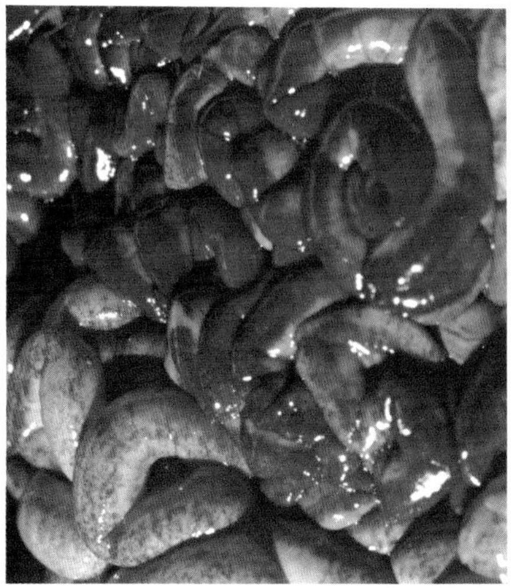

Salmonella infection may be imported into livestock by many routes.

**Importation / Route of infection**

- Purchase of calves is the main source. The danger is particularly acute if the animals purchased originated from several different stocks (dealers' cattle houses) or have passed through cattle markets, have contracted the infection there and thus introduce salmonellosis into the purchaser's livestock. Healthy animals contract the infection by direct contact with salmonella-contaminated faeces or by contact with faeces-contaminated fodder, drinking fluid or objects. The outbreak of the infection is further promoted by the stress of transport, re-housing and change of feed.

- Man must be regarded as a further source of infection. Salmonellosis is introduced by persons moving from cattle house to cattle house in the course of their work (i.e. veterinary surgeons, artificial inseminators, drivers of cattle transport vehicles and cattle dealers) by the transmission of salmonella-containing faeces adhering to the rubber profile soles of wellington boots.

  Since man is attacked by the same types of the causative organism, he is himself a possible source of infection. A particular danger arises where a person has recovered from the infection and has become a carrier. Persons excreting salmonella pathogens do not notice the disease. This is why – when salmonellosis has been officially diagnosed in calves – the persons looking after the animals are also examined.

- Domestic and wild animals (dogs, cats, mice, rats, deer, rabbits, birds, particularly sea-gulls and ducks) may also transmit the disease.

- Salmonella pathogens may also be introduced by the purchase of contaminated feedstuffs.

- During the grazing period waterways, ponds and lakes also constitute a danger. Protein-containing impurities (blood, waste materials) sink to the bottom where they offer the salmonellae an ideal growth medium. If the bottom of the waterway, pond or lake is disturbed (ducks, high water, flooding), the pathogens rise to the surface of the water. If the animals drink the water, they infect themselves directly. In the event of flooding the pasture is contaminated and the cattle contract the infection by eating the grass.

Fig. 63

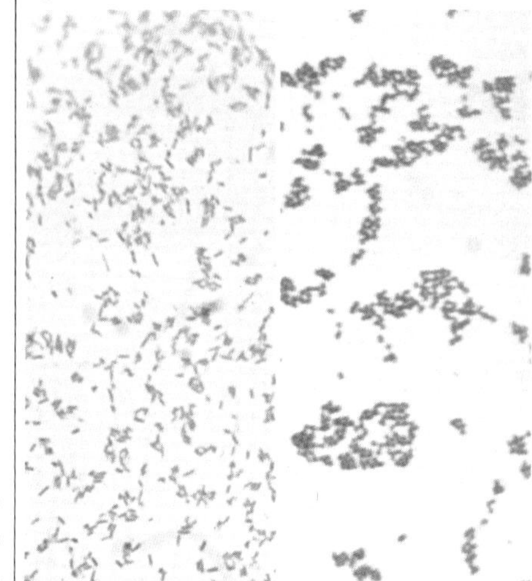

After the salmonellae have been taken up by mouth, they pass into the intestine where they multiply profusely and damage the intestinal mucosa. From there the pathogens and their toxic breakdown products (toxins) reach the blood stream and can thus invade any organ.

**Symptoms**

The pathogens taken up by mouth multiply profusely in the small intestine. This results in intestinal inflammation giving rise to diarrhoea with yellow, fluid and malodorous faeces. The faeces increasingly change colour, become greyish-green and contain mucosal fragments. With the further progress of the inflammation the entire intestinal tract is affected and haemorrhages appear in the large intestine and rectum. The faeces become dark brown or black, contain traces of fresh blood (unchanged blood from the rectum) and remain fluid. The salmonellae provoke a defence reaction in the intestine of the calf whereby blood components (fibrin) are released. This fibrin and fragments of the mucosa appear as off-white mucoid flakes in the faeces.

Right at the start of the intestinal disorder the calf shows dullness and a raised temperature. However, the animals continue to accept drink since they are very thirsty as a result of the high temperature and diarrhoea.

Fig. 64

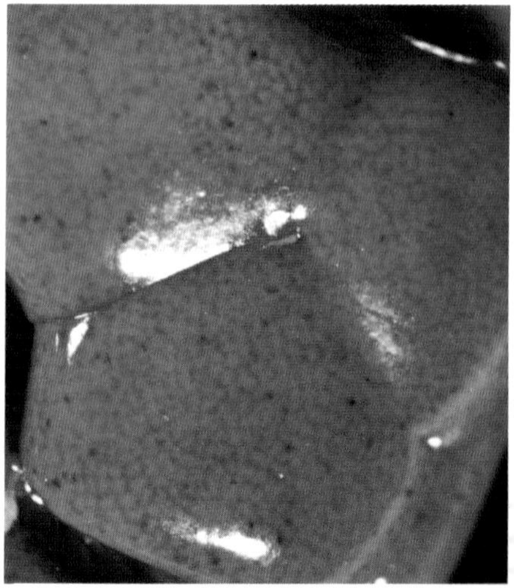

The salmonella infection is not confined to the intestine. As a result of the rapid multiplication of the pathogens in the intestine and the damage to the mucosa, the salmonellae and their toxic breakdown products (toxins) get into the blood stream (bacteraemia, septicaemia) and can therefore settle in all organs of the body. Inflammations of the joints, meninges and lungs are common.

The severe, bloody intestinal inflammation alone can lead to the animal's death within a few days. If the pathogens are present in the blood (septicaemic form), death ensues very quickly as a result of damage to the brain and the spinal cord, and paralysis.

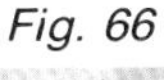

*Fig. 63: Gram-stained bacteria under the microscope.*
*Left: Salmonellae appear reddish.*
*Right: Cocci have a violet shade of colour.*
*Microscopic examination alone does not enable a definitive differentiation between salmonella and other intestinal bacteria.*

*Figs. 64 and 65: The toxins of salmonellae damage the walls of the fine terminal ramifications of the blood vessels, causing punctiform as well as extensive haemorrhages in organs like the kidneys (left) and heart (right).*

*Fig. 66: Intestine with extensive haemorrhages: This section of the intestine shows pronounced fibrinous deposits.*

*Fig. 66*

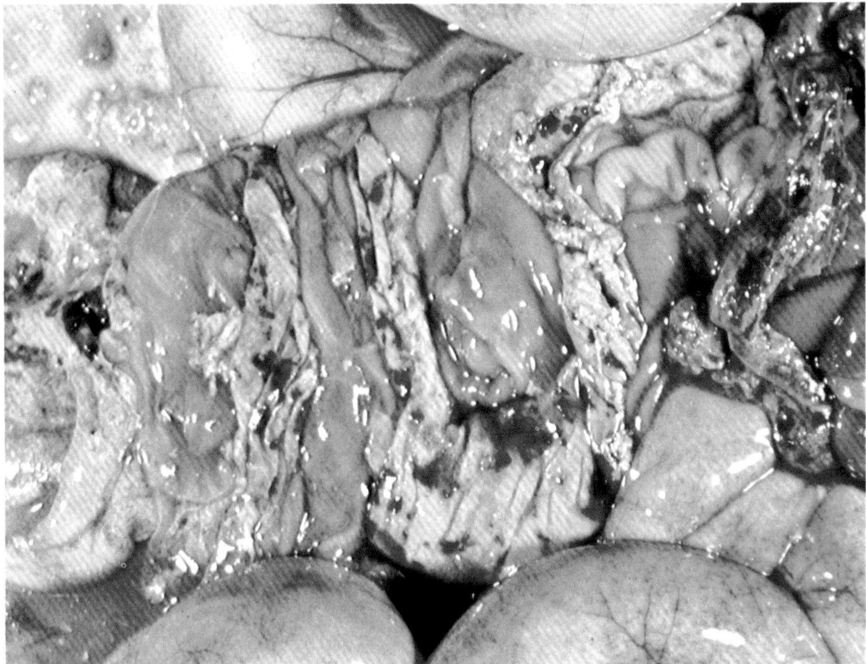

**Symptoms**

This severe form of the infection which carries a high mortality rate (30 to 50%), is found particularly in calves from the 2nd to 6th week of life.

If older calves contract the disease, the losses are much smaller. In such cases we frequently observe diarrhoea which abates after a few days. With these animals, some of the pathogens remain in the intestine without causing further symptoms, although they continue to multiply and are continually excreted in the faeces. Since such calves show no visible symptoms, they cannot be identified when they are brought to market.

The stress suffered on re-housing promotes the multiplication of the salmonellae and increases the danger of infection. Other calves purchased at the same time are then particularly at risk. The change in feed which brings about a shift in acidity (pH value) and a change in the intestinal flora, favours the infection. For this reason medicinal preventive treatment should be carried out on re-housing (cf. pages 262 and 270).

*Fig. 65*

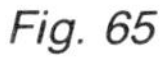

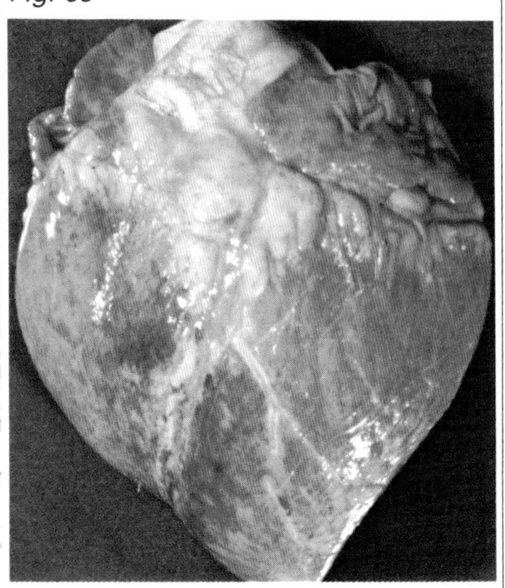

Fig. 67

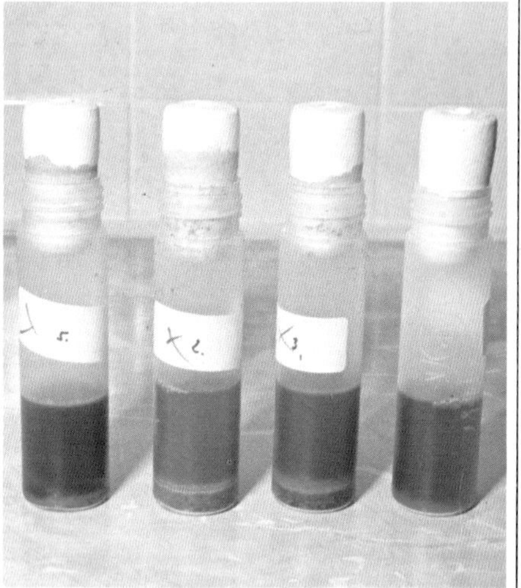

Fig. 68

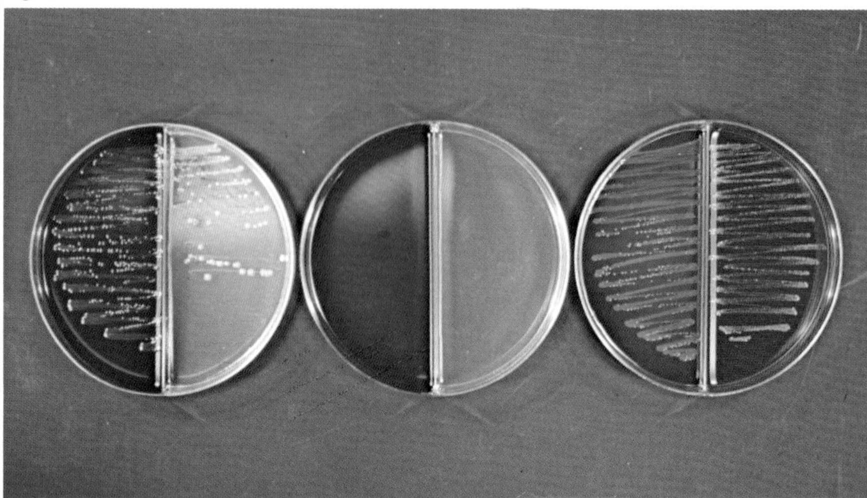

In the living animal a definitive demonstration of the pathogen can only be achieved by an examination of faecal samples in the laboratory. For this purpose the so-called "enrichment method" is employed, using culture media which promote the multiplication of salmonellae and at the same time inhibit the growth of other intestinal bacteria (e. g. E. coli). If salmonellae are present, a characteristic change in colour is observed. By means of further examinations it is then possible to distinguish salmonellae from other bacteria occurring in the intestine and to determine individual types of salmonella.

The pathogens are not continuously excreted in the faeces. If the faecal examination reveals salmonellae, it is certain that an infection is present. If the finding is negative, i. e. if no salmonellae are excreted, this does not necessarily mean that there is no infection, since the pathogens are often excreted intermittently.

Autopsy of animals that have died or have been slaughtered reveals an inflammation of the intestine and an enlargement of the spleen. Typical small, punctiform, greyish-white or yellowish tissue changes are found in the intestine, liver, spleen, kidneys and lungs.

Fig. 70

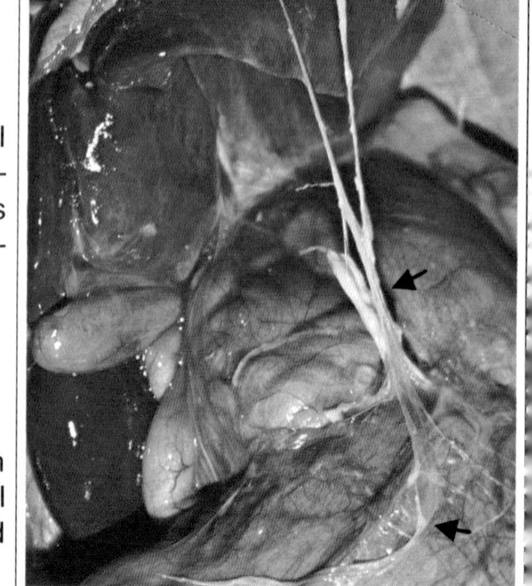

*Figs. 67 and 68: Bacteriological examination: Approx. 3 to 5 g of material suspected of containing salmonellae is placed in the enrichment bouillon. Three tubes have been inoculated, the tube on the right serves as an uninoculated control. After incubating for 18 to 24 hours at 37° C, a smear is taken and placed on two-colour selective culture media which contain a colour indicator which shows a characteristic colour change if salmonellae are present.*
*Left disc – coli bacteria; right disc – salmonellae; middle disc – uninoculated control.*

*Fig. 69: To differentiate between the numerous salmonella species and types, the so-called "mixed series" is used. For this purpose the economical "enterotube" test by Roche can be employed.*
*8 chambers of a test tube contain special culture media which, following inoculation with the suspected pathogen and incubation, enable the simultaneous demonstration of 11 different biochemical properties.*

*Fig. 70: Peritonitis with fibrin exudation. In chronic salmonellosis, this causes adhesion of the organs (arrows).*

*Fig. 69*

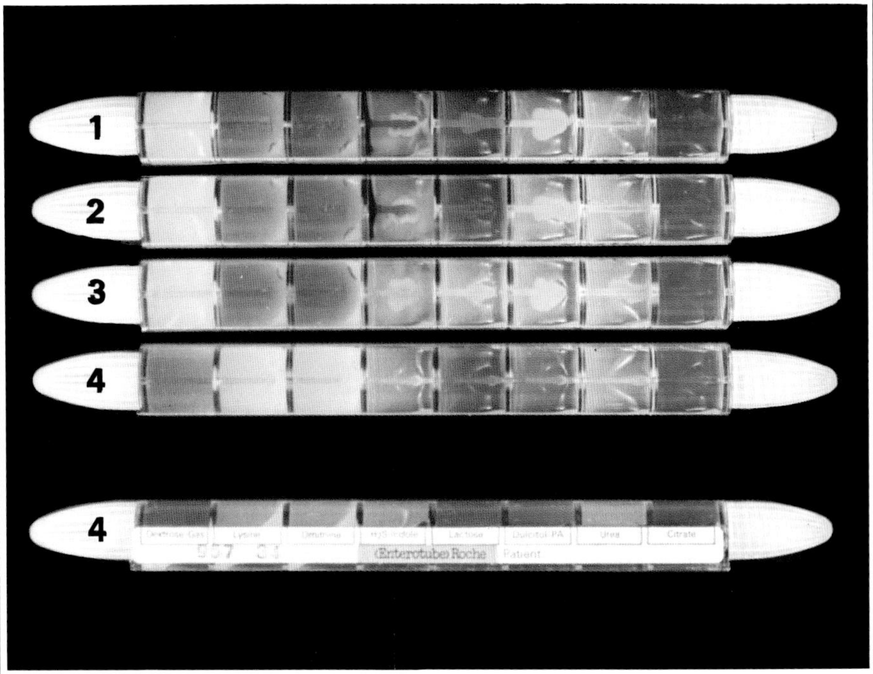

*Fig. 71*

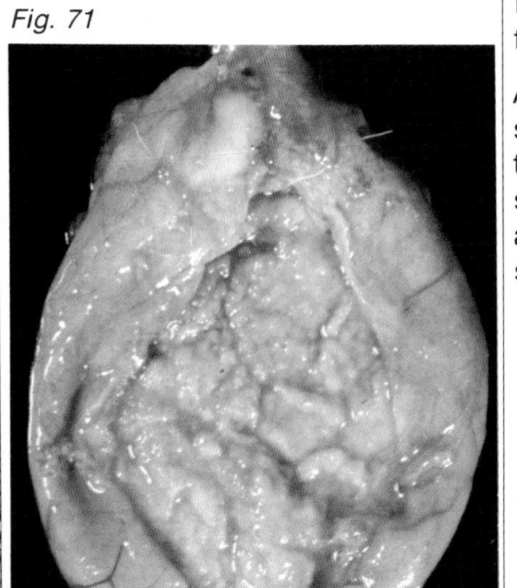

**Diagnosis**

The cultivation of pathogens from the organs of animals that have died is carried out on similar lines to the bacteriological examination of faecal samples.

A further aid in diagnosis is the serological blood test which demonstrates the antibodies formed as a result of the infection. However, this test only shows that the animal has been in contact with the infection at some time. The serological blood test does not become significant until a high level of antibodies is found in the blood or until repeated tests show a rising antibody level (rising positive titre).

**Similar symptoms**

All diseases associated with diarrhoea and/or articular inflammation show a clinical picture that is similar to that of salmonellosis.

Similar symptoms

| Disease | Scours of sucking calves | Salmonellosis |
|---|---|---|
| Cause | Rota and corona viruses; coli bacteria. | Salmonella bacteria. |
| Time of appearance of disease | 1st or 2nd week of life, usually 3rd to 5th day. | Usually 2nd to 6th week of life. |
| Type of farm/system of keeping animals.<br>Provisional report/observation | Mainly cows. Frequent calving aggravates the condition from calf to calf. Calves contract the disease successively, at approximately the same age. | Calf fattening and rearing, particularly with purchase of calves. Epidemic outbreak of the disease. Calves of different ages contract the disease simultaneously. The older the animal, the milder the course of the disease. |
| Symptoms | High temperature, occasionally abnormally low temperature. Abdomen drawn in. Drugs have practically no effect on the diarrhoea. Animal strains to defaecate. Faeces are forcefully ejected. | Moderate to high temperature. Diarrhoea. Swelling of joints in some animals. |
| Consistency of faeces | Aqueous with undigested coagulated milk constituents.<br>*Fig. 72* 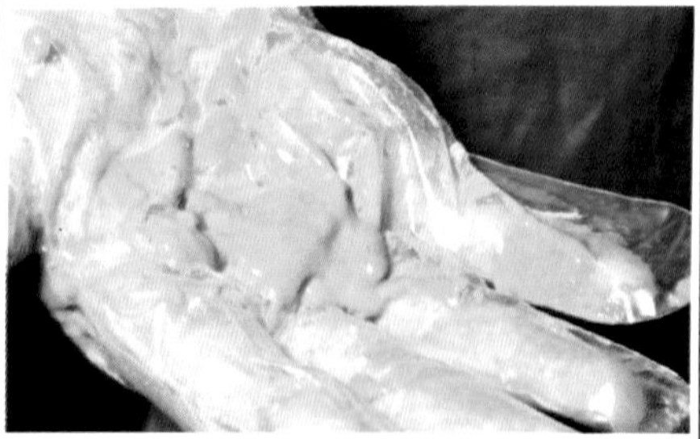 | Mucoid, fluid and pappy, malodorous, admixtures of blood, colour grey to dark green; off-white mucoid flakes (fibrin).<br>*Fig. 73* 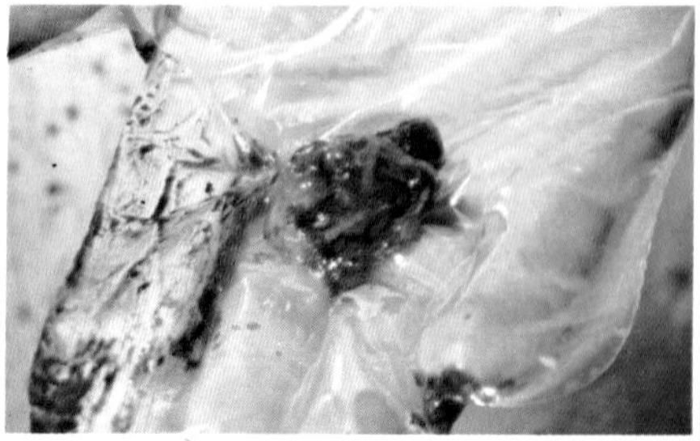 |
| Demonstration of pathogen: Examination in laboratory | Demonstration of virus very difficult and possible only at the start of the infection. | Bacteriological examination of faeces. Serological blood tests. Autopsy of animals that have died. |
| Read up | Page 26 | Page 36 |

| Poisoning | Nutrition-induced diarrhoea |
|---|---|
| Furazolidone or poisons which inhibit blood coagulation. | Incorrect use and composition of feed. |
| All age groups, usually from the 3rd week of life. | All age groups. |
| All systems of keeping animals; individual animals, groups. Overdosage (too high and/or for too long) of furazolidone-containing drugs. Take-up of mouldy clover hay (coumarin), rat poison (coumarin, warfarin). | All systems of keeping animals; individual animals, groups. Deteriorated feed, change of feed, inappropriate temperature of drinking fluid, irregular feeding times; incorrect feeding. |
| Temperature often raised; haemorrhages on conjunctiva and all visible mucosae. Paralysis and convulsions possible. Bleeding following injury very difficult to stop. | Flatulence, diarrhoea; temperature normal or below normal. |
| Soft faeces with fresh blood. | Fermentative diarrhoea: Fluid/pappy, yellow to dark brown, bubbly with unpleasant sweetish odour, acid pH. Putrescent diarrhoea: Fluid/pappy, yellowish to grey, putrid odour; alkaline pH. |
| *Fig. 74* 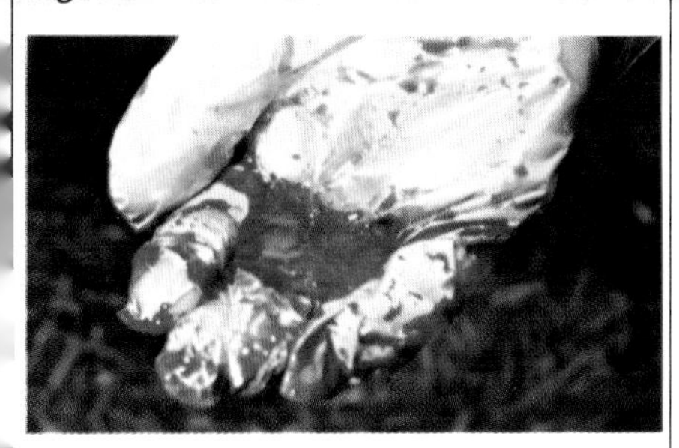 | *Fig. 75* 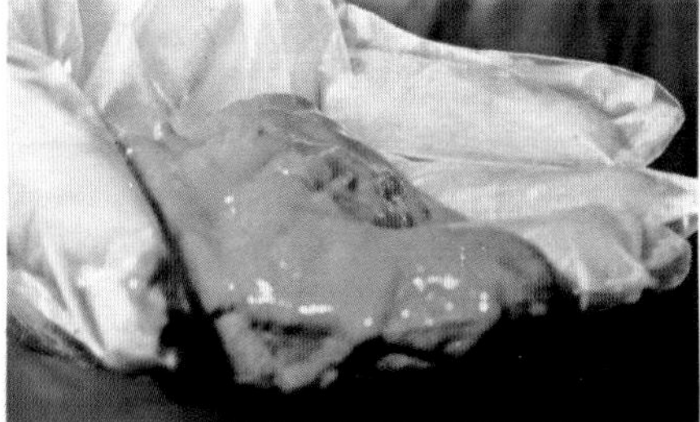 |
| Examination of feed. Check drugs for active ingredient content and duration of administration. | Bacteriological examination of faeces negative. Later secondary bacterial infection. Check pH. |
| Page 121 | Page 48 |

*Fig. 71: Inflammation of the bladder associated with salmonellosis of the urinary tract.*

*Figs. 72 to 75: Summary of the most common diseases associated with scours in sucking calves.*

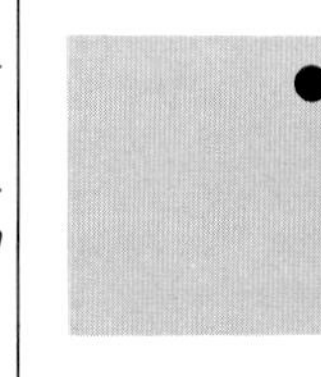

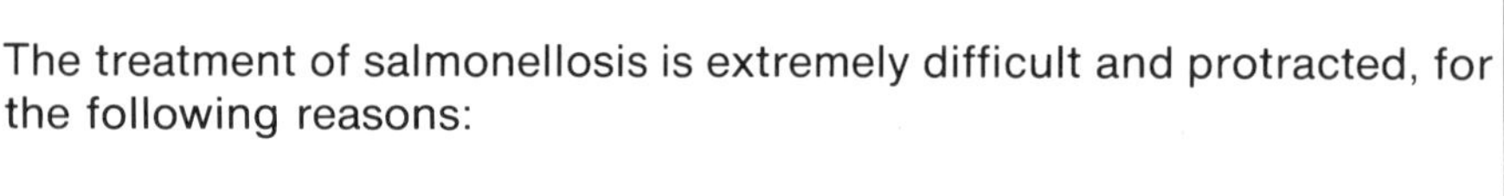

The treatment of salmonellosis is extremely difficult and protracted, for the following reasons:

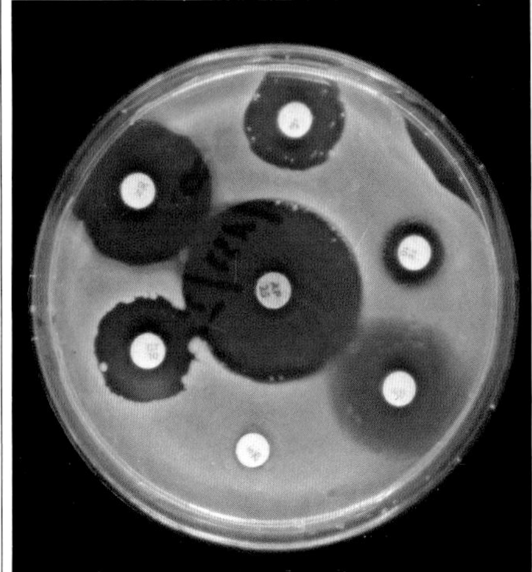

*Fig. 76*

- There is a large number of different salmonella strains with differing pathogenic properties.
- The great adaptability of salmonellae quickly leads to resistance. After a short time of treatment the drugs used are no longer sufficiently effective or fail altogether. This applies particularly if the dosage was inadequate and the duration of use too short (cf. page 236).
- After the initial intestinal infection, salmonellae may settle in all parts of the body. It is difficult to combat the abscess-like encapsulated foci in the organs and the high salmonella concentrations in the synovial fluid with antibiotics. They can provoke a fresh infection at any time.
- Because of the possibility of carriers, the infection may recur again and again. It is only by repeated bacteriological examination of faecal samples from every animal of the stock that carriers can be identified.

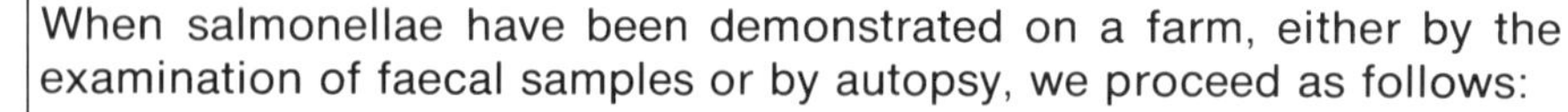

When salmonellae have been demonstrated on a farm, either by the examination of faecal samples or by autopsy, we proceed as follows:

1. Notification of the local veterinary officer.*
2. Immediate treatment of all animals at risk via the drinking fluid. Since the legally prescribed official tests* for salmonellae and the resistance test take several days, a water-soluble medicament containing chloramphenicol is used immediately. Although this antibiotic is not free from side-effects, particularly on the intestinal flora of sucking calves, it is nevertheless highly effective in salmonellosis. Administered intramuscularly to affected animals, chloramphenicol is the drug of choice in the first instance.

---

* Valid in W. Germany

Fig. 77

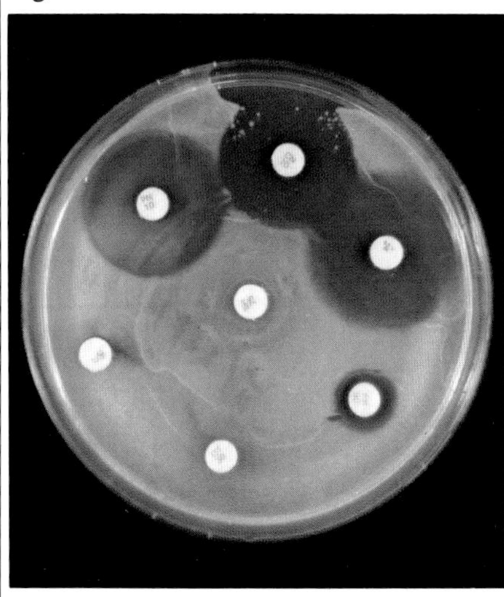

*Figs. 76 and 77: The sensitivity of bacteria against chemotherapeutic agents and antibiotics is determined by means of an antibiogram.*
*Before starting antibacterial therapy, a sensitivity test is carried out, because the pathogen may be insensitive to some of the antibacterial products being considered for treatment.*
*In the resistance test carried out in the laboratory the bacterial pathogen is first cultivated from the material available for testing. The strain obtained is then inoculated onto a special culture medium. Round paper discs impregnated with different antibiotic substances are placed on the inoculated medium.*
*After incubating overnight, the zones of inhibition of varying extent indicate whether the bacterial strain is highly sensitive, shows little sensitivity or is resistant. The absence of a zone of inhibition indicates resistance and provides an answer to the question as to which substance should not be used for treatment.*



These immediate measures are supported by an appropriate hygiene programme. Here the following points should be considered:

- Best possible separation of different parts of cattle houses and entire cattle houses.
- Laying down disinfection mats impregnated with CHEVI 45 (3%).
- If possible, allocate separate attendant for affected stock/cattle house.
- Separate clothing for cattle house (rubber boots, overall).
- Improve cleanliness.
- Mucking out, thorough cleaning and disinfection after treatment.

These immediate hygienic measures should be carried out until the authorities intervene. The veterinary authorities will then determine further measures.*

On receipt of the result of the resistance test, the treatment already started is continued or modified in accordance with the test result. The antibiotics or sulphonamides found to be effective in the resistance test are selected according to the following criteria:

Efficacy, tolerance (side-effects of the products), absorbability and price.

* Valid in W. Germany

Treatment

*Fig. 78*

| | | |
|---|---|---|
| 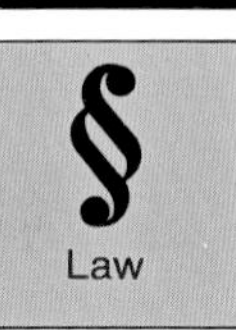 Law | **Notification** of salmonellosis to local veterinary officer. Purchase and sale of animals prohibited.* | Immediately |
| 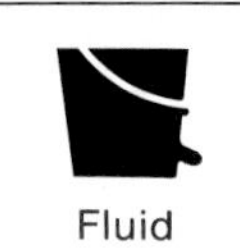 Fluid | **Immediate treatment of all animals at risk:** Via the drinking fluid, 4 g CANIV/10 kg body-weight, distributed over 3 feeds. Adapt to result of resistance test. | For at least 5 days |
| 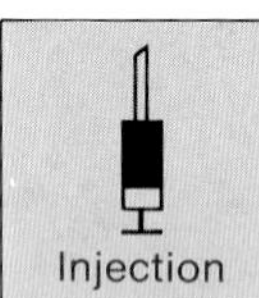 Injection | **Immediate treatment of all affected animals:** In addition to CANIV, intramuscular injection of 1 ml FORACOL/10 kg body-weight 2 or 3 times at intervals of 12 h. | 3 times at intervals of 12 hours |
| 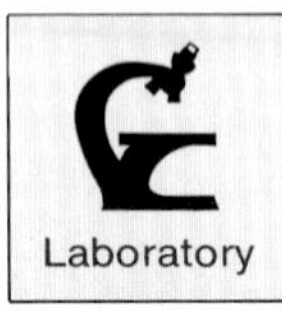 Laboratory | **Resistance test of pathogen:** Collect faecal sample **before** starting treatment. Adapt treatment to result of resistance test. | Immediately |
| 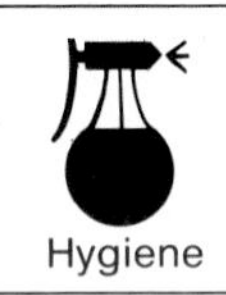 Hygiene | **Hygienic measures:** Isolate affected animals. Separate attendants, disinfection mats, special clothing and shoes. Further measures determined by the authorities.* | Immediately |
| 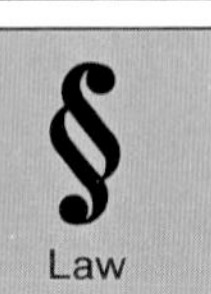 Law | Authorities place stock in quarantine. Quarantine is lifted, if faecal samples are negative. During quarantine, only emergency slaughter possible. | |

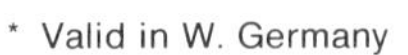

* Valid in W. Germany

*Fig. 79*

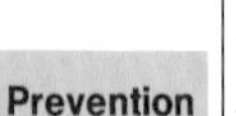

Prevention

Specific measures for the prevention of salmonella infection, such as vaccination, are not possible. If the presence of the infection is suspected, treatment of the calves is inappropriate for the following reasons:

Fig. 80

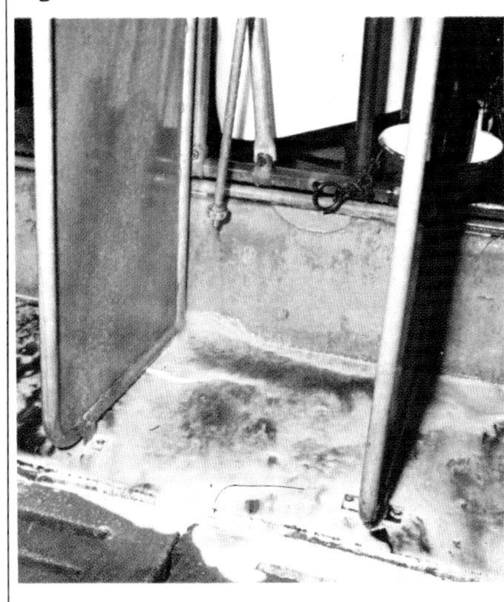

For the treatment of salmonella infection, antibiotics must be given in high dosage. However, such treatment also destroys bacteria which are required for digestion. Loss of appetite and intestinal disorders may thus be caused unnecessarily.

**Prevention**

Since stress also favours the outbreak of salmonella infections, prophylaxis should be adapted to the animals' age and the form of management. These preventive measures are described in detail in part 5 of this book.

**Danger to livestock farmer**

Man usually contracts the infection by eating food contaminated with the pathogens. Even a small number of pathogens (smear infection) is sufficient to poison food, since salmonellae multiply very rapidly in protein-containing substances at room temperature.

Approx. 24 hours after ingesting the pathogen, the disease manifests itself in man in the form of fever, vomiting and diarrhoea and gastrointestinal inflammation.

**Legal provisions***

If salmonellosis is suspected and diagnosed, the local veterinary officer should be notified. The requirement of notification is confined to the veterinary surgeon who has diagnosed the disease.

The veterinary authorities then place the livestock in quarantine and determine measures of treatment and disinfection.

After treatment, several faecal samples are collected which must all be negative before the quarantine is lifted. During the quarantine period, no animals may be purchased or sold.

After the official diagnosis of salmonellosis has been established, the veterinary authorities may order immediate slaughter without any treatment being carried out. In this case compensation amounts to 100%. Full compensation is also paid for losses of animals occurring after notification. For animals dying before notification of the authorities and where salmonellosis can be shown as the cause of death, compensation amounting to 50% of the value of the animals is paid.

*Fig. 78: Measures to be taken at the first sign of salmonellosis.*

*Figs. 79 and 80: Most important measure in infectious diseases: Clear out animal houses, thorough cleaning and disinfection. Heavily soiled areas must be soaked with detergents, followed by cleaning with high-pressure hose or brush. All parts of the house to be sprayed with disinfectant in adequate concentration until droplets form. The duration of action varies with different products. Manufacturers' directions for use should therefore be followed.*

---

* Valid in W. Germany

# Nutrition-induced diarrhoea

Fig. 81

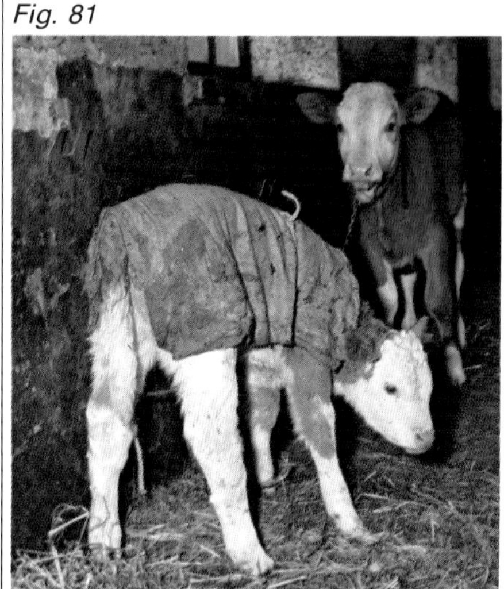

Fig. 82

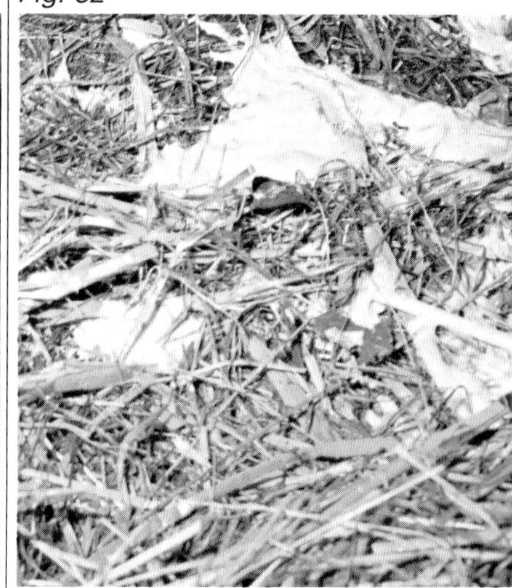

**Term**

Calves often suffer from diarrhoea which is not caused by an infection, but is due to incorrect feeding.

**Cause**

Calves should be fed with great care since they react with great sensitivity to any error and to any irregularity. At the time of birth the first three stomachs of the sucking calf are not yet able to function. They develop in the course of the next few weeks through mechanical and chemical stimulation. For this reason colostrum and the right milk substitute are the only appropriate feed for calves during the initial period. Thus, at the age of 1 to 3 weeks, feeds like maize silage, dairy cattle fodder, whole meal or green forage cannot yet be given to calves. Such fodder has a detrimental effect on coagulation by chymosin. The change in acidity causes a shift of the intestinal flora in favour of proteolytic or saccharolytic bacteria. If there is an abundance of proteolytic bacteria, we speak of a digestive disorder caused by putrefaction. If saccharolytic bacteria predominate, we refer to a digestive disorder produced by fermentation.

*Fig. 81: Intestinal disorder caused by licking the cattle house wall. Sweat and nitrate salts are taken up and cause diarrhoea.*

*Fig. 82: Fluid whitish-grey faeces with undigested milk constituents.*

*Figs. 83 and 84: Fermentative diarrhoea: Fluid/pappy, yellowish brown to dark brown faeces, bubbly with unpleasant sweetish odour.*

*Fig. 85: Summary of the most common causes of nutrition-induced diarrhoea.*

Fig. 83

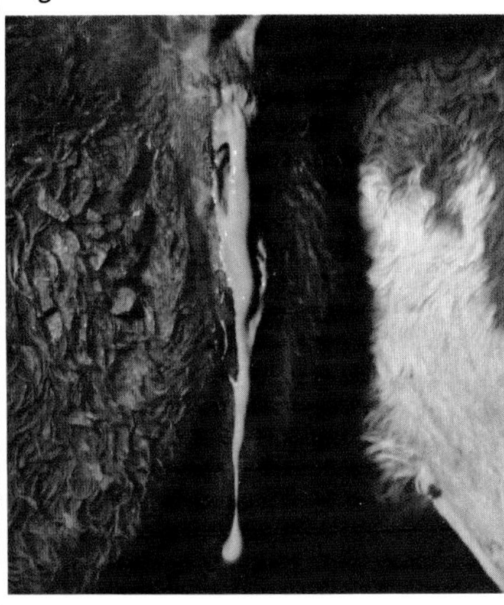

Fig. 84

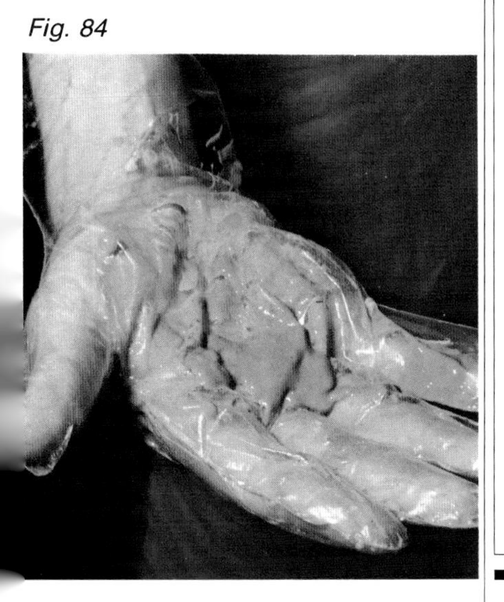

Errors in the feeding methods may also cause digestive disorders. These are summarised in Fig. 85

Cause

Fig. 85

| Errors in nature and composition of feed | Errors in preparing the feed |
|---|---|
| ■ Milk substitute not appropriate to age (e. g. fat content too high)<br>■ Feed deteriorated due to inappropriate storage, e. g. rancid fat, mouldy calf starter feed.<br>■ Inappropriate feed because of wrong components. (unsuitable fats)<br>■ Feed not appropriate to age, e. g. maize silage, dairy cattle fodder. | ■ Incorrect stirring. Lumps in drink.<br>■ Wrong temperature of drink. Above 39 °C or below 35 °C.<br>■ Wrong concentration of drink: More than 125 g or less than 100 g of milk substitute powder per litre of drinking fluid.<br>■ Stirring whole meal or calf starter feed into the drink.<br>■ Varying concentration of drink.<br>■ Excessive volume of drink. For normal volumes, see page 259.<br>■ Sudden change-over from milk to milk substitute.<br>■ Sudden change of milk substitute, e. g. make, type.<br>■ Drinking vessels soiled with milk residues; take-up of acid milk drips. |

Fig. 86

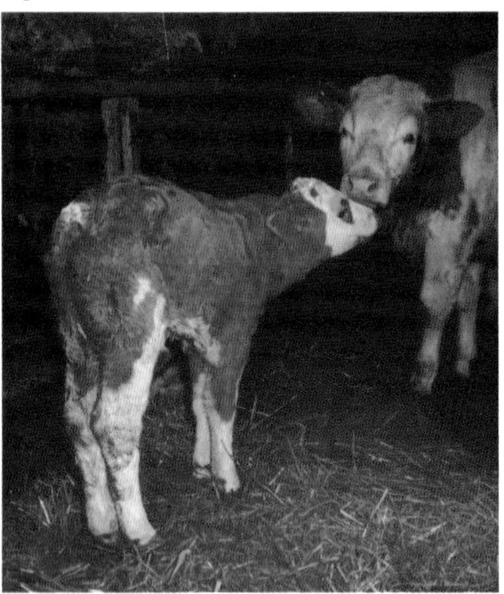

Fig. 87

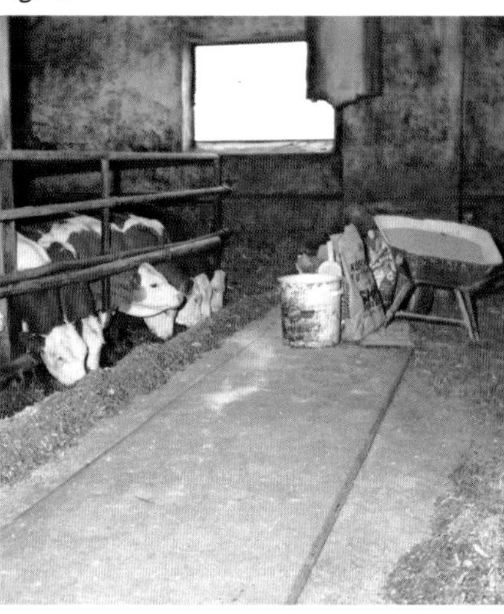

Fig. 88

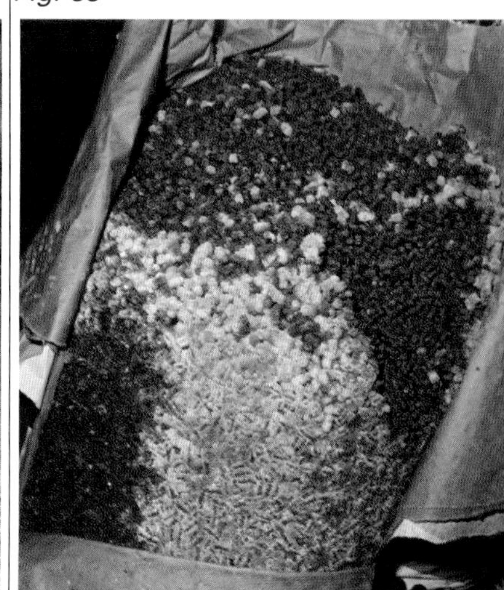

**Cause**

Under natural conditions (e. g. keeping with suckling cow) the calf receives its milk in the right composition, in small quantities and at the cow's body temperature (39 °C). In order to simulate natural conditions as far as possible, 4 drinking periods, a temperature of the drink of 38 °C to 39 °C and, for milk substitute, an appropriate concentration should be adhered to at least during the initial period. If this is not done, coagulation by chymosin is disturbed. The enzyme is either diluted too much or is not present in sufficient quantity. Similarly, if the fluid volumes taken up are too large or if lumps form in the drink, the time during which the milk remains in the abomasum is reduced. If the temperature of the drink is too low (under 35 °C), this delays the effect of chymosin. Uncoagulated, partly acid milk will then pass from the abomasum into the small intestine and will cause digestive disorders.

**Symptoms**

Nutrition-induced diarrhoea manifests itself by putrescence in the form of fluid or pappy, yellowish to grey, malodorous faeces. Fermentative diarrhoea is characterised by bubbly, fluid or pappy, yellowish brown to dark brown faeces of acid smell.
Since the calf is weakened by the diarrhoea, bacterial infection can easily supervene. As with all other forms of diarrhoea in calves, the animals show deep-set eyes, reduced elasticity of the skin and a dull shaggy coat if the condition persists.

*Fig. 89*

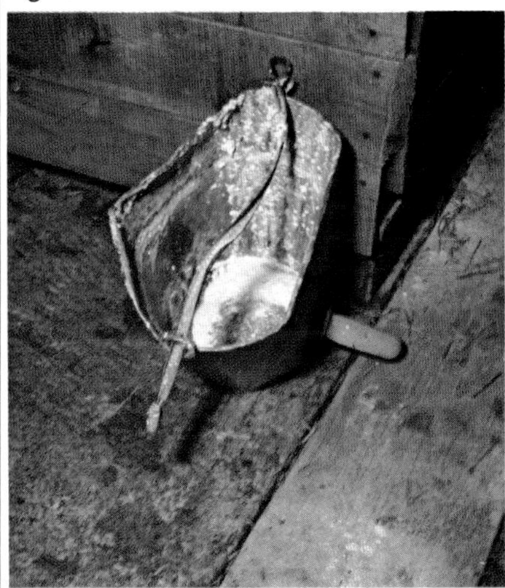

**Diagnosis**

Purely nutritional diarrhoea is rare. After the condition has existed for a short time, a bacterial infection usually supervenes. The difference between nutritional diarrhoea and a bacterial infection is then no longer clearly discernible. Other causes can be excluded by appropriate tests. (cf. page 42).
The provisional report and errors in the method of feeding provide the first indications of an initially nutrition-induced digestive disorder. Part 5 of this book deals with the most important criteria for avoiding nutritional diarrhoea.

**Treatment**

The first step in the treatment of nutrition-induced intestinal disorders is to eliminate errors in feeding. Since milk or milk substitute provides an ideal growth medium for bacteria, only electrolyte solution with the addition of medicated feed that is well tolerated by the intestine, is given for two days.

*Fig. 90*

| | | |
|---|---|---|
| Provisional Report | Check feeds used and feeding method. **Observe** calf: Licking of wall, eating from trough of older neighbouring animal (silage) | 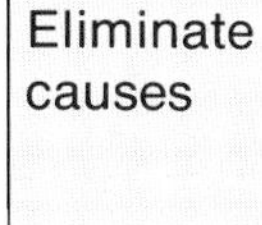 Eliminate causes |
| 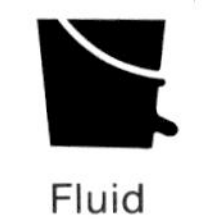 Fluid | **Replacement of milk substitute or milk** by electrolyte solution (90 g ELRISAL + 15 g CHEVICALF in 2 litres of water, twice daily. Plus 1 litre of tea twice daily. | 1st and 2nd day |
| Fluid | **Change-over to milk:** 1 litre of milk substitute with 1 litre of electrolyte solution (45 g ELRISAL + 15 g CHEVICALF in 1 litre of water, twice daily). | 3rd day |
| 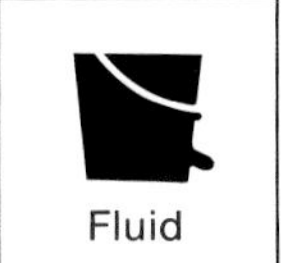 Fluid | **Follow-up treatment:** Milk or milk substitute with 10 g CHEVICALF twice daily. | From 4th to 10th day |

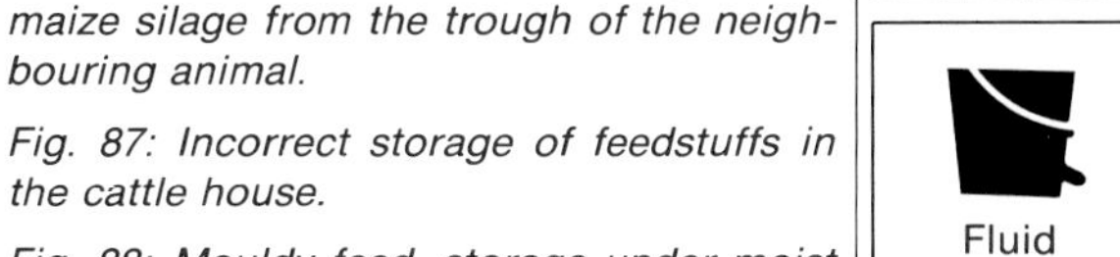

*Fig. 86: Sucking calf with diarrhoea. Abdomen drawn in; faeces-soiled rear. In this case the condition was caused by eating maize silage from the trough of the neighbouring animal.*

*Fig. 87: Incorrect storage of feedstuffs in the cattle house.*

*Fig. 88: Mouldy feed, storage under moist conditions. The toxins of moulds cause severe digestive disorders and generalised conditions (poisoning).*

*Fig. 89: Dirty drinking bucket. Deteriorated milk residues cause digestive disorders.*

*Fig. 90: Treatment schedule for nutrition-induced diarrhoea.*

# Navel-ill of calves

Fig. 91

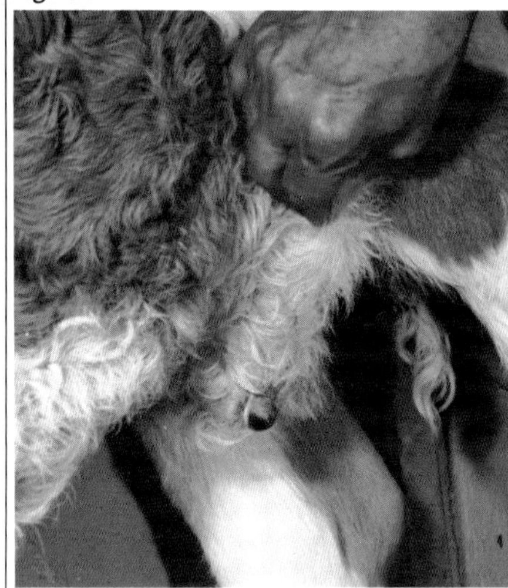

Fig. 92

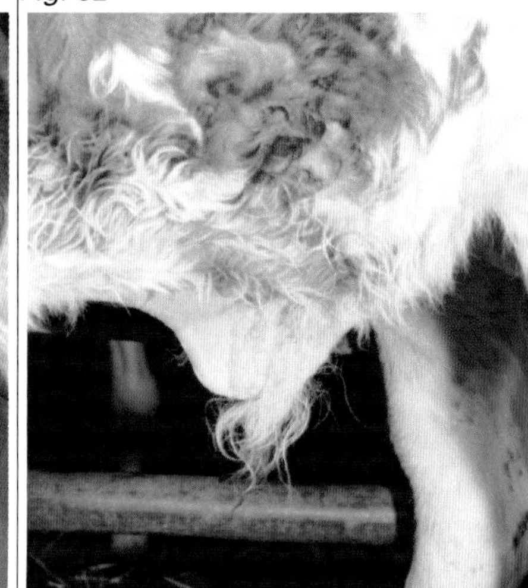

**Term**

Navel-ill of calves is caused by bacterial contamination of the umbilical cord during or shortly after birth. The infection may be confined to the navel or may develop into a generalised condition.

**Cause**

At birth the umbilical cord contains residual blood which forms an ideal medium for the growth of bacteria. Inadequate dressing of the navel enables bacteria (which occur everywhere in the cattle house) to invade the navel. The bacteria involved are pus-forming pathogens, particularly corynebacteria, streptococci and staphylococci. Sucking of the navel whereby it cannot dry out and is irritated, also enables the invasion of bacteria. Since, at birth, the navel is still connected to the blood stream, the pathogens may also penetrate into the blood circulation and cause a generalised infection.

**Symptoms and course of the disease**

In cases of **fresh, acute** inflammation of the navel, the calves stand with their abdomens drawn in and their backs arched. They show little appetite, and their body temperature is increased. Inspection of the navel usually reveals swelling and redness, and the hairs may stick together as a result of pus secretion. On palpation the calf shows severe pain (kicking out, defensive movement) and the navel feels hot.

Fig. 93

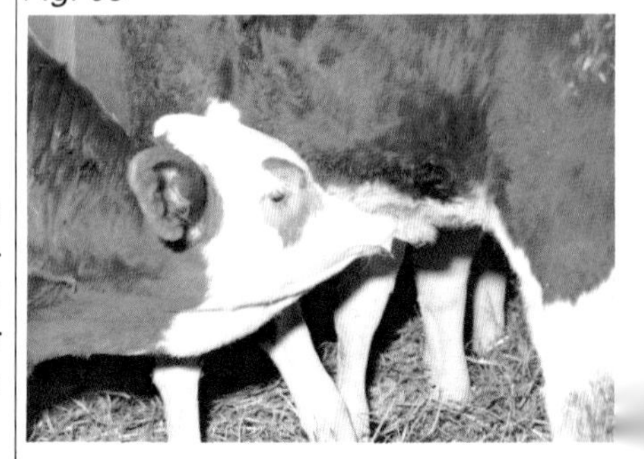

Fig. 94

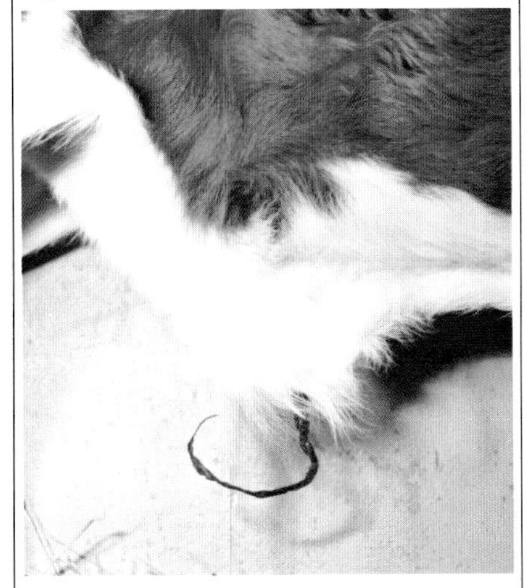

Fig. 95

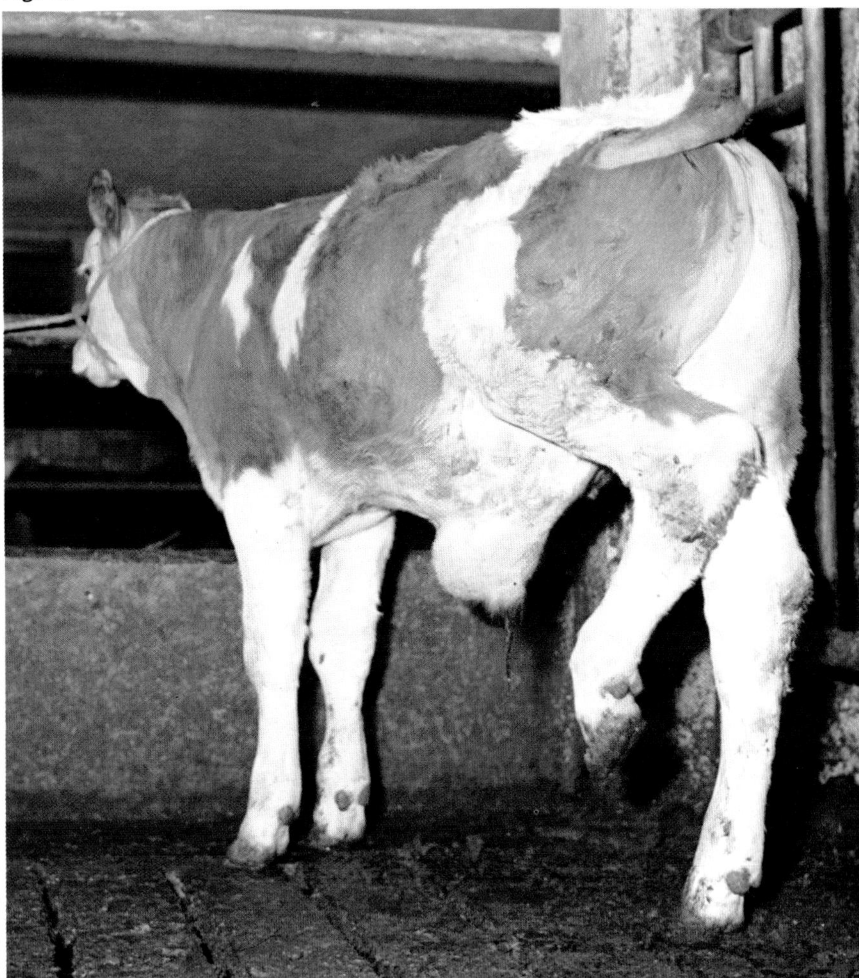

*Fig. 91: Inflammation of the navel: Firmly elastic navel stump swollen to the thickness of a thumb.*

*Fig. 92: Sucked navel. Constant sucking of the navel leads to navel inflammation and substantial enlargement of the umbilical fold.*

*Fig. 93. Sucking of the navel occurs particularly in early weaning without feeding rack.*

*Fig. 94: Healthy navel. Remainder of umbilical cord well dried out.*

*Fig. 95: Umbilical abscess: Painful ball-shaped swelling, the size of a child's head. The animal shows the pain by kicking out with its hindlegs.*

**Symptoms and course of the disease**

Starting from a local inflammation, the pathogens may spread throughout the body (septicaemia). In this way they reach all organs, causing changes there. They frequently provoke inflammations in one or more joints.

*Fig. 96*

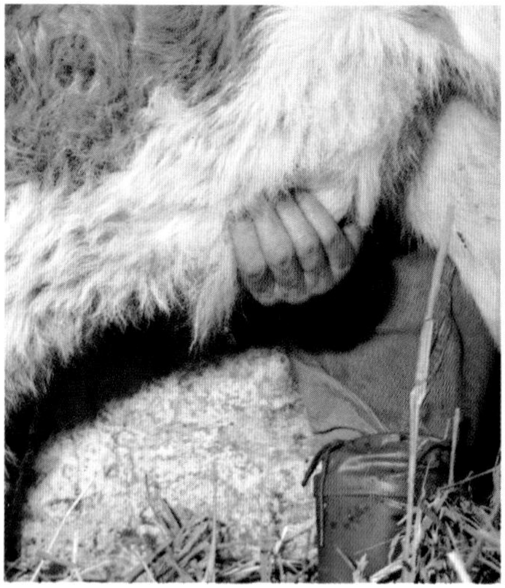

*Fig. 97*

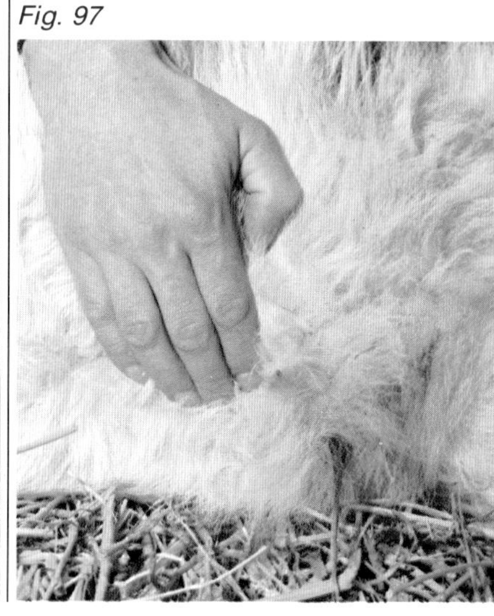

*Fig. 98*

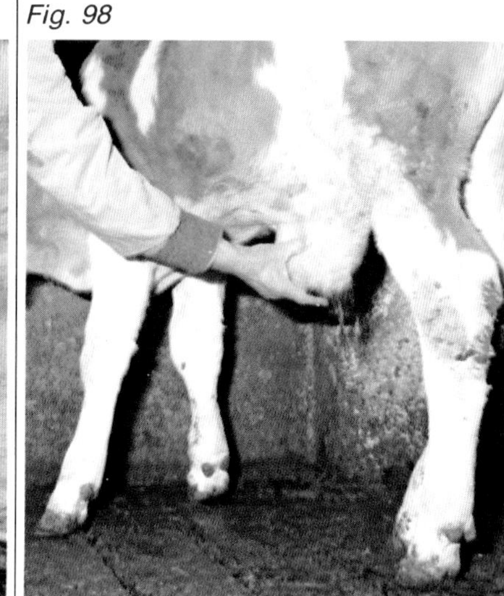

**Symptoms and course of the disease**

These very painful inflammations of the joints produce the symptoms of "septicaemia". The animals are reluctant to stand up and lie down even for drinking. Eventually they are unable to rise. A **neglected** umbilical inflammation is often found in apparently healthy, but listless and dull calves. The navel is swollen to thumb size and firmly elastic.

If the pus formed as a result of the umbilical inflammation cannot drain off, an **umbilical abscess** develops, swelling to the size of a fist or a child's head. In rare cases the abscess develops in the umbilical cord within the abdominal wall, so that it is not visible or palpable from the outside.

**Diagnosis**

The proper examination of an affected calf should always include a manual examination of the navel (see illustration).

**Similar symptoms**

The external appearance of an umbilical abscess is difficult to distinguish from that of an umbilical hernia. In umbilical hernia, an orifice in the abdominal wall is palpable. Whilst a uniform, evenly distributed accumulation of fluid (as if it were contained in a rubber sac) is palpable

*Fig. 99*

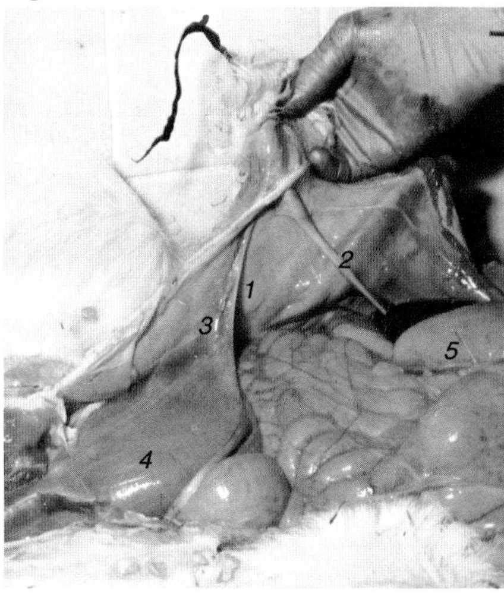


*Fig. 100*

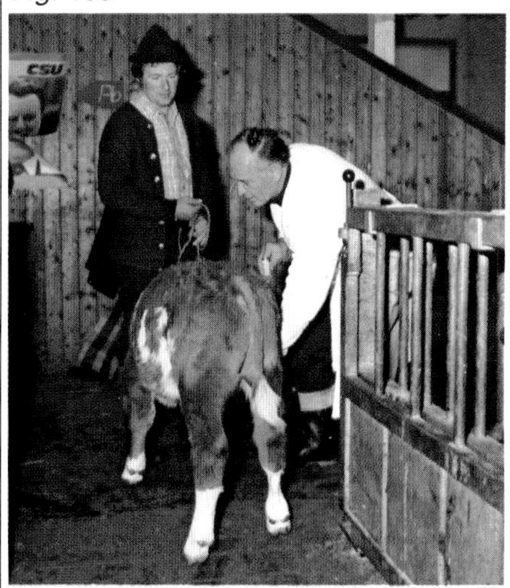

*Fig. 101*

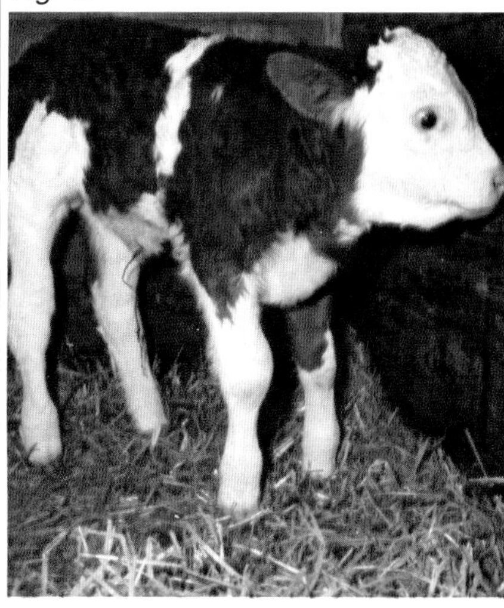

*Fig. 96: Manual examination of the navel whereby the umbilical cord is allowed to slide through the fingers.*

*Fig. 97: Palpation of the abdominal wall in the umbilical region. With umbilical hernia, the orifice of the hernia is palpable.*

*Fig. 98: Umbilical abscess: A uniform, evenly distributed accumulation of fluid (as if it were contained in a rubber sac) is palpable.*

*Fig. 99: Course of umbilical vessels in the newborn calf:*
*1 Urachus: Connection of urinary bladder to amniotic sac.*
*2 Umbilical vein: Blood supply from the placenta to the vena cava and liver.*
*3 Umbilical arteries: Blood flow from the aorta to the placenta.*
*4 Urinary bladder*
*5 Liver*

*Fig. 100: Examination of the navel at the cattle market before auction.*

*Fig. 101: Swollen joints. Late sequel of an umbilical infection where bacteria have invaded the joints.*

**Similar symptoms**

with an umbilical abscess, displaceable parts of differing constitution (intestinal loops) can be felt in umbilical hernia.
The intestinal loops usually slip back into the abdominal cavity when the calf is laid on its back (see under "umbilical hernia").

Lameness due to articular inflammation (septicaemia) is also seen in salmonellosis (cf. page 36) and in coli infections (cf. page 26). Examination of the navel will clarify whether the infection started from the navel.

**Treatment**

In **fresh, acute umbilical inflammation,** treatment by injection of antibiotics or sulphonamides is likely to be successful. We use a mixture of penicillin and streptomycin since it is well tolerated by the sucking calf and has a rapid effect on the putrefactive pathogens mentioned.

**Neglected umbilical inflammation.** In addition to the above-mentioned injection treatment, 25% camphor ointment is applied daily to the navel and rubbed in.

An **umbilical abscess** should be lanced when it has come to a head. Simultaneous injection treatment is necessary if the calf's general well-being is affected (raised body-temperature, loss of appetite).
In all three conditions follow-up treatment with a medicated feed (penicillin/streptomycin) via the drinking fluid is necessary.

Fig. 102

| | | |
|---|---|---|
| 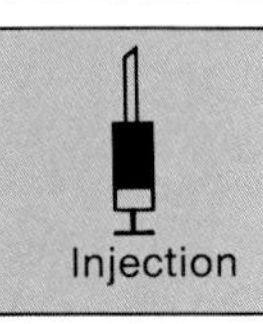 Injection | **Fresh and neglected umbilical infection:** 3 ml FORAPEN/10 kg for at least 3 days. **Umbilical abscess:** Injections in cases of increased body temp., loss of appetite. | 1 injection daily |
|  Local application | **Neglected umbilical inflammation and abscess:** Rub in PHLEGMALON ointment twice daily. Lance **mature abscess.** | Twice daily until abscess is mature |
| 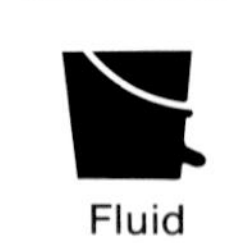 Fluid | **Follow-up treatment via the drinking fluid:** 20 g BUSAL per calf/day for one week. | 1st to 7th day |
| 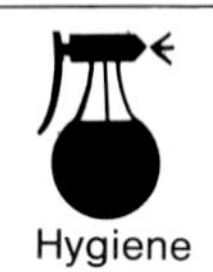 Hygiene | **After completion of treatment:** Cleaning and disinfection of the site in the cattle house or calf pen with 2% CHEVI 45 solution. | |

*Fig. 102: Treatment schedule for umbilical inflammation and abscess.*

*Figs. 103–106: Treatment of a burst umbilical abscess:*

Fig. 103

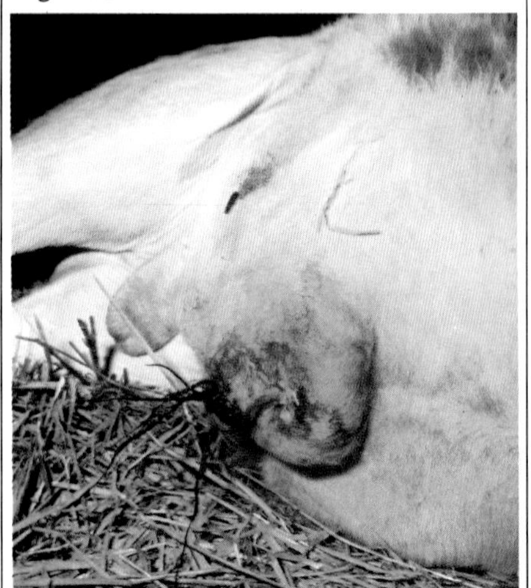

*Cleaning and shaving abscess site*

Fig. 104

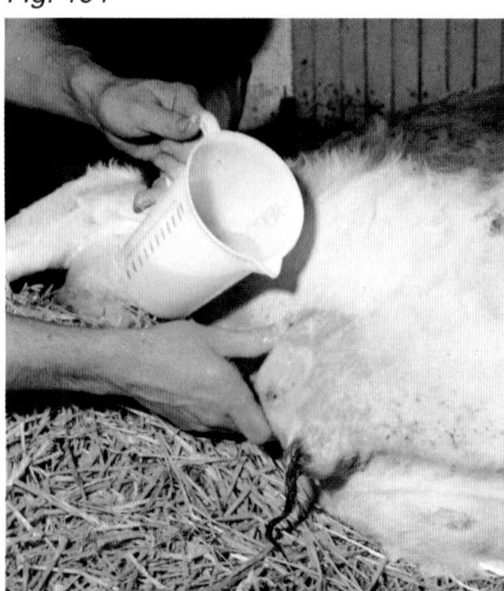

*Applying disinfectant spray*

Fig. 105

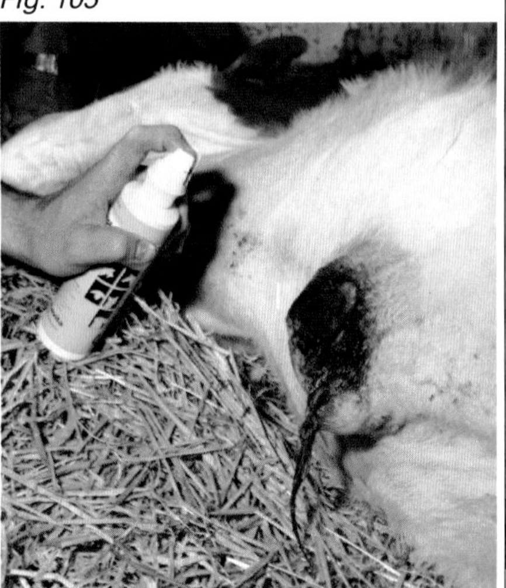

Figs. 107 und 108: Cord dressing after birth. Wiping umbilical cord with haematoxylon-soaked gauze swab. Opening the cord and spraying inside.

*Fig. 107*

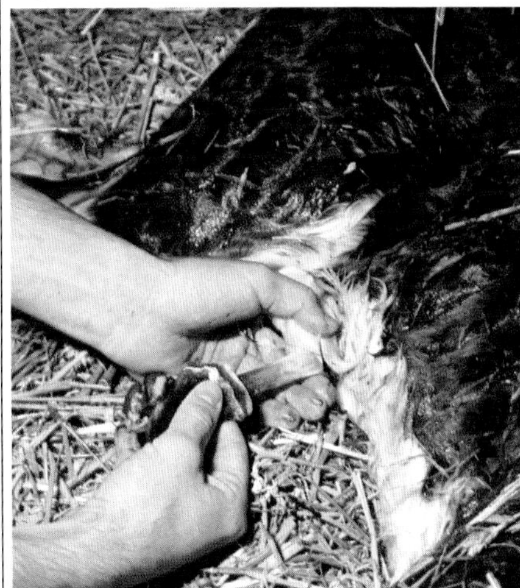

*Fig. 108*

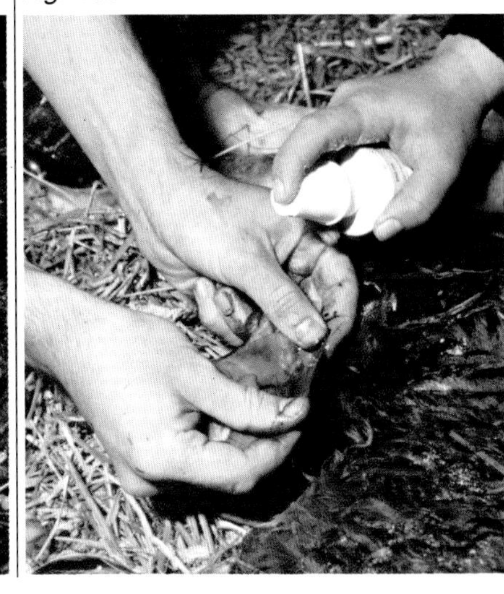

**Prevention**

An umbilical inflammation can be prevented by appropriate accommodation (individual pens, dry litter, calving shed) and also by adequate navel care immediately after birth. Here the following points should be considered:

- Touch navel only with clean and disinfected hands.
- If necessary, detach umbilical cord approx. one hand-breadth below the point of exit and gently squeeze out residual blood.
- Spray in LOGWOOD TINCTURE to achieve rapid drying and disinfection of the cord. The umbilical cord should not only be sprayed externally. In addition, the stump of the cord is opened and LOGWOOD TINCTURE is sprayed inside.
- The navel should be checked several times during the first week of life. If painful swelling occurs, treatment should be initiated.

*Blunt extension and checking of abscess cavity*

*Fig. 106*

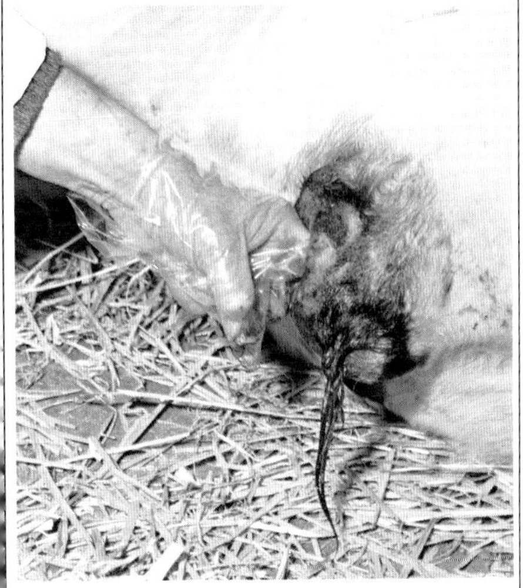

# Umbilical hernia in calves

Fig. 109

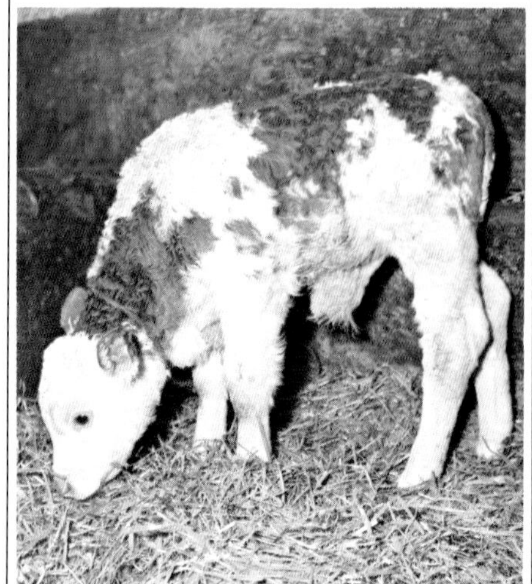

Figs. 110/111

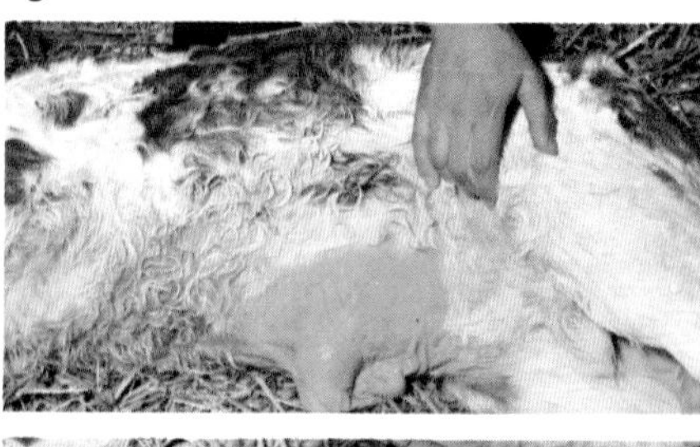

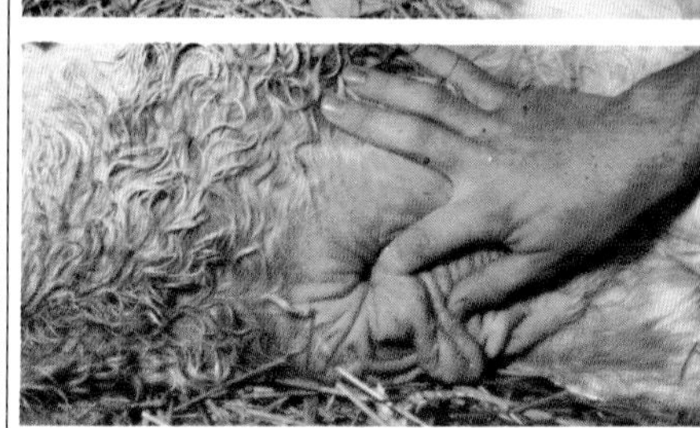

*Fig. 111: With the calf lying on its back, the contents of the hernia can easily be pushed back into the abdominal cavity.*

**Term**

Like an umbilical abscess, umbilical hernia is characterised by an enlargement in the umbilical region, which may range in size from a hen's egg to a child's head.

**Cause**

Umbilical hernia is often hereditary, but may also be caused by softening, overdistention or injury to the abdominal wall. In predisposed animals, a sudden increase in abdominal pressure leads to a distention of the abdominal wall at the umbilical orifice and finally to a visceral prolapse. The abdominal wall and outer skin form the hernial sac, abdominal muscles the hernial orifice.

**Diagnosis**

In umbilical hernia, the prolapsed visceral parts should be palpated. The swelling can be eliminated by gently pushing the contents of the hernia back into the abdomen. This is best achieved with the calf lying on its back. On palpation the hernial orifice should be felt with the fingers. This does not usually cause any pain.

By contrast, a constricted hernia which is caused by congestion of the viscera or contraction of the hernial orifice, causes severe pain. In this case the animal's general condition deteriorates rapidly and speedy action is necessary.

*Fig. 109: Calf with umbilical hernia.*

*Figs. 110–114: Operation on umbilical hernia. Umbilical region prepared for surgery.*

*Fig. 115: Diagram of anatomical conditions in umbilical hernia.*

Fig. 112

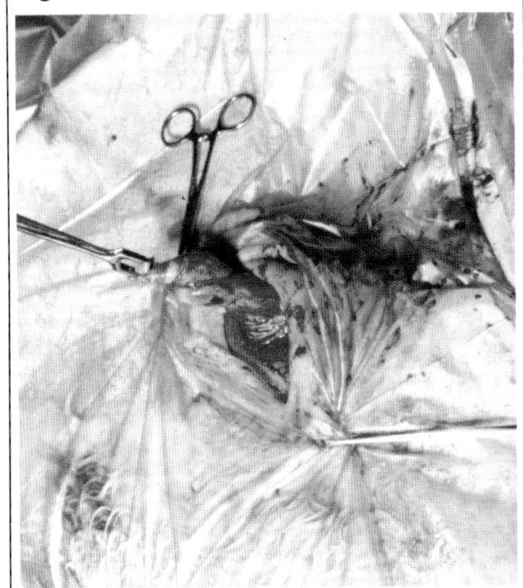

*Fig. 112: The hernial sac is exposed. By turning the hernial sac, the intestinal loops are pushed back into the abdominal cavity.*

Fig. 113

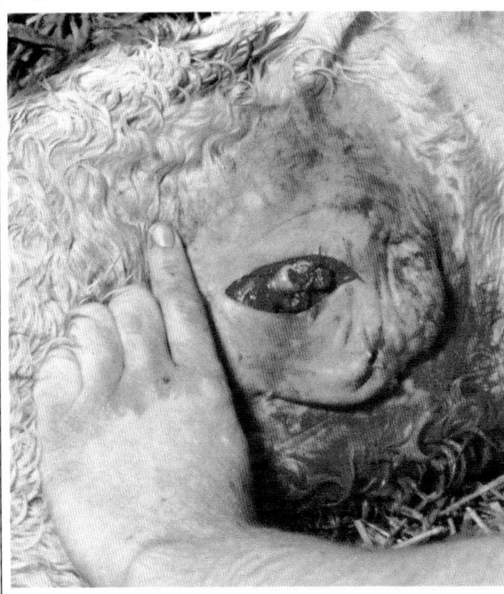

*Fig. 113: The hernial sac is severed and sutured, followed by suture of the outer skin.*

Fig. 114

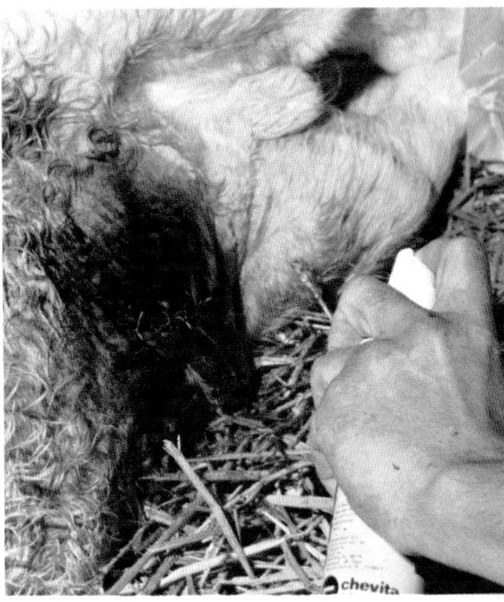


*Fig. 114: The skin suture is sprayed with a disinfectant solution.*

Fig. 115

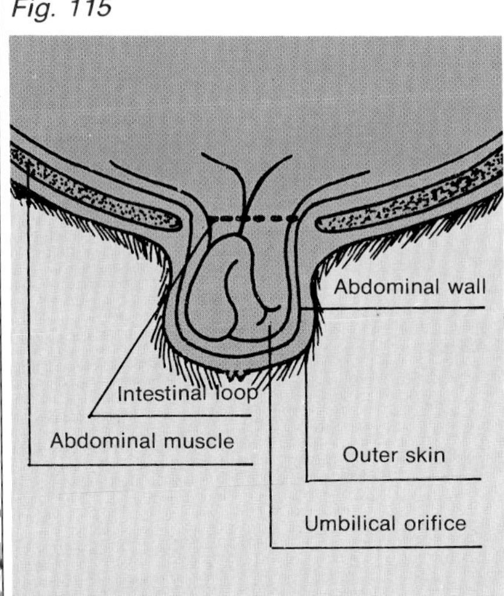


**Similar symptoms**

Umbilical hernia can be differentiated from an umbilical abscess by palpation of the protrusion. If an umbilical abscess is present, an evenly distributed accumulation of fluid is felt, which cannot be pushed back into the abdominal cavity.

**Treatment**

Even if the protrusion reaches the size of a child's head, the prospects for a successful treatment of umbilical hernia are good, provided that the hernia is not constricted. In calves with a **small** hernia, it is often sufficient to apply a hernia bandage for three weeks. If the hernia is **large,** surgery is required.
However, treatment by rubbing in an irritating ointment is not advisable, since this may cause uncontrollable inflammation and adhesions.

# Septicaemia of newborn calves

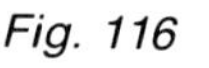

Fig. 116

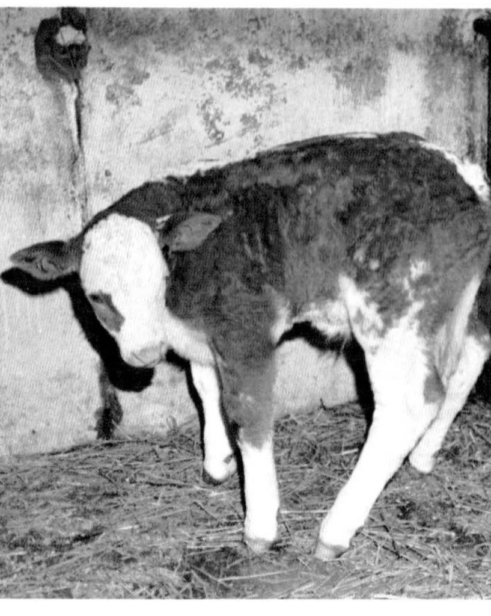

*Fig. 116: Calf septicaemia in the acute initial stage. The joints affected are very painful, but not noticeably swollen. The calf is reluctant to walk and stands up only for brief periods.*

*Figs. 117 and 118: Calf septicaemia, advanced stage: Decubitus of the highly inflamed and swollen joints.*

*Fig. 119: Diagrams of joints.*
*1 Normal joint.*
*2 Inflamed joint: Articular capsule increasingly filled with Products of inflammation and swollen.*
*3 Rachitic joint: Bones tumefied at the ends. Articular capsule not enlarged.*

*Fig. 120: Treatment schedule for calf septicaemia.*

**Term**

Septicaemia in calves is a disease caused by bacteria and associated with signs of lameness and articular inflammation.

**Incidence**

This disease occurs quite frequently on farms with poor hygienic conditions, lack of navel care and poor housing of the calves.

**Pathogens**

Putrefactive bacteria like corynebacteria, streptococci and staphylococci as well as salmonellae and E. coli cause the disease. Mixed infections occur in most cases. Re-infection is rarely observed. In periods in which many calves are born, the pathogenic effect (virulence) of the causative organisms increases.

**Importation / Route of infection**

The navel and the intestinal tract are the main points of entry of the infection. Following an inflammation of the navel or intestine, the bacteria pass into the blood stream and spread throughout the body. The joints are particularly affected.

**Symptoms**

Since the pathogens are carried in the blood stream to all parts of the body, changes may occur in any organ. Reduced appetite, listlessness and prolonged periods of lying down are the first signs. The joints are increasingly filled with products of inflammation, are hot to the touch and painful.

*Fig. 117*

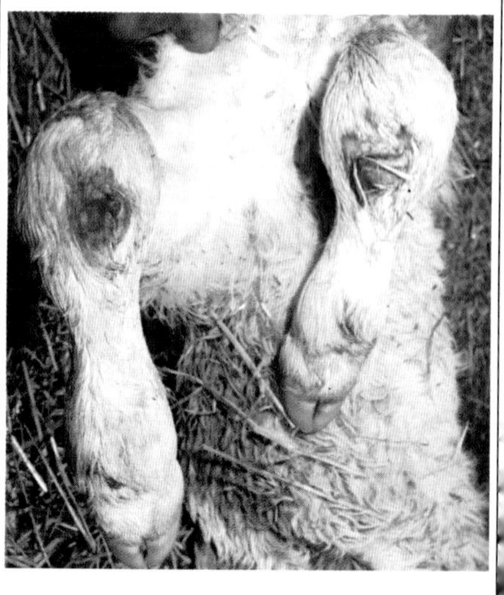

Fig. 119

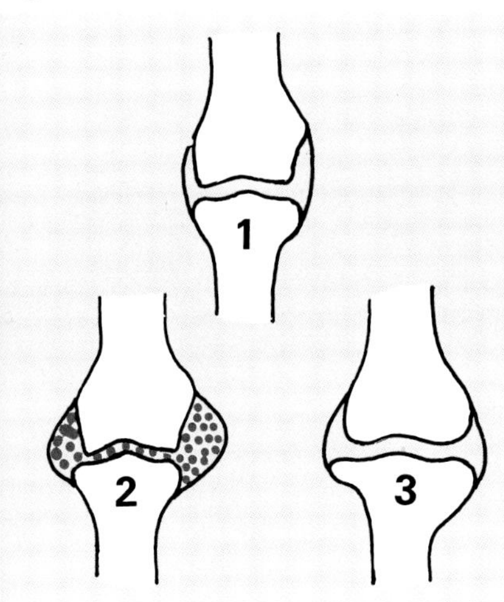


At a later stage, the calves are reluctant to rise or fail to get up at all. Diarrhoea and pneumonia may supervene.

**Similar symptoms**

Calves with rickets (impaired calcium/phosphorus metabolism, vitamin D deficiency) show tumefaction of the bones at the joints, whilst joints with inflammatory changes are filled with synovial fluid (cf. Fig. 119).

**Treatment**

Like umbilical inflammation, calf septicaemia is treated with high doses of antibiotics or sulphonamides. Local treatment of the navel and the affected joints with salicylic camphor ointment is indicated.

| | | |
|---|---|---|
| 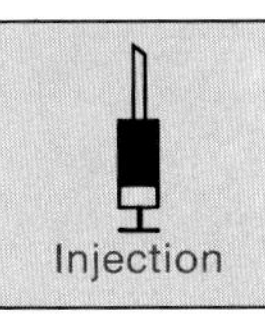 Injection | **Injection treatment:** 3 ml FORAPEN/10 kg bodyweight, given intramuscularly at least 3 times at intervals of 24 hours. 10 ml PHENYLARTHRIT FORTE per calf. | 1st, 2nd and 3rd day |
| 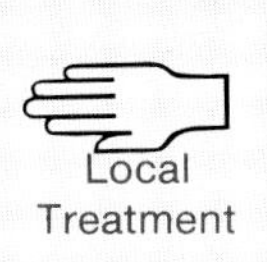 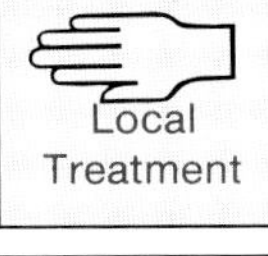 Local Treatment | Joints and possibly navel: Apply and rub in PHLEGMALON Ointment twice daily. | Twice daily |
| 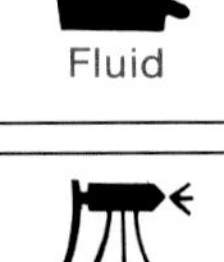 Fluid | **Additional treatment via the drinking fluid:** 20 g BUSAL per calf/day for 1 week. | 1st to 7th day |
| 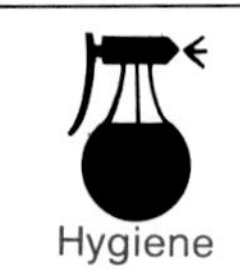 Hygiene | **Hygienic measures:** Cleaning and disinfection of place in cattle house or calf pen with 2% CHEVI 45 solution. | 3rd and 4th day |

Fig. 120

Fig. 118

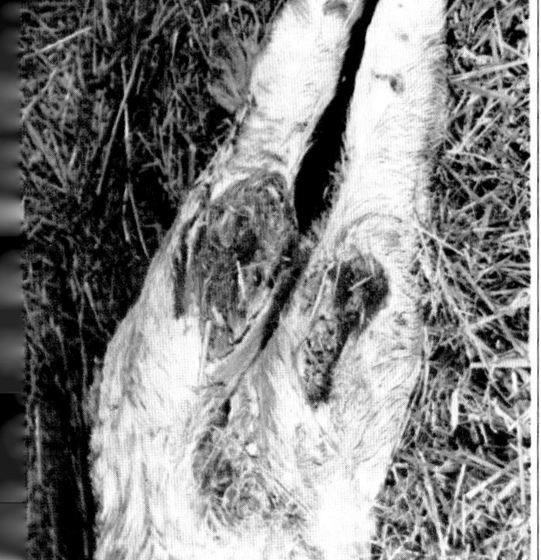

**Prevention**

If calf septicaemia occurs repeatedly, the cow stock needs to be examined for the presence of salmonellae (cf. salmonellosis, page 36). Read up navel care at birth on page 57. Calf septicaemia is also prevented by prophylactic measures against coli infections (page 32) and by appropriate housing (cf. page 258).

# Worm infestation of sucking calves

Fig. 121

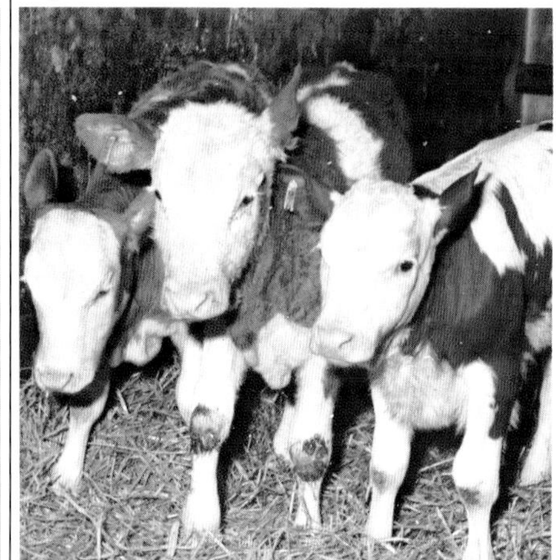

Fig. 122

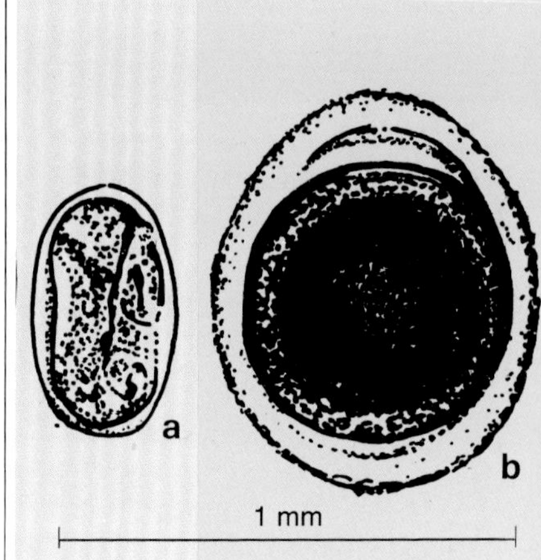


**Term**

Roundworms (Toxocara vitulorum) and threadworms (strongyloides papillosus) infest calves particularly in the first few weeks of life.

**Pathogen / Development**

If cows ingest the eggs of roundworms or threadworms, their larvae are hatched in the intestine. The larvae migrate through various organs, finally reaching the subcutaneous connective tissue and the udder where they lie dormant until the next calf is born. Some of the larvae perish. As a result of hormonal changes at the time of birth, the dormant larvae regain their activity, migrate into the milk ducts and are excreted in the colostrum and milk for up to 3 weeks after birth. The calves thus become infected via the milk (galactogenic infection) during the first few hours of life. Strongyloides larvae may in addition penetrate the skin (percutaneous infection) and develop in the small intestine into mature worms the eggs of which are excreted in the faeces. Roundworm eggs become infective after maturing in the outside world. The cattle ingest the worm eggs, and the larvae are hatched in the intestine. In older cattle – from 6 months upwards – no mature roundworms and strongyloides are found in the intestine.

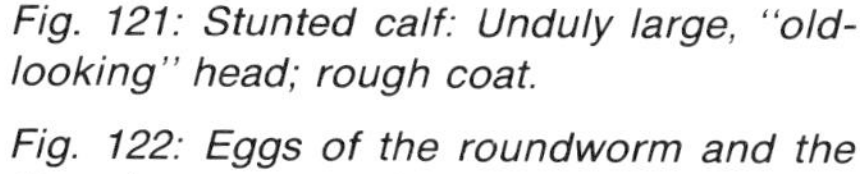

*Fig. 121: Stunted calf: Unduly large, "old-looking" head; rough coat.*

*Fig. 122: Eggs of the roundworm and the threadworm occurring in calves. The eggs can be demonstrated by parasitological examination of faecal samples (cf. page 194).*
*a strongyloides egg*
*b roundworm egg*

*Fig. 123: Life cycle of roundworms in calves: Cows ingest roundworm eggs from the faeces of calves. The larvae are then transmitted to the calf via the milk.*

*Fig. 123*

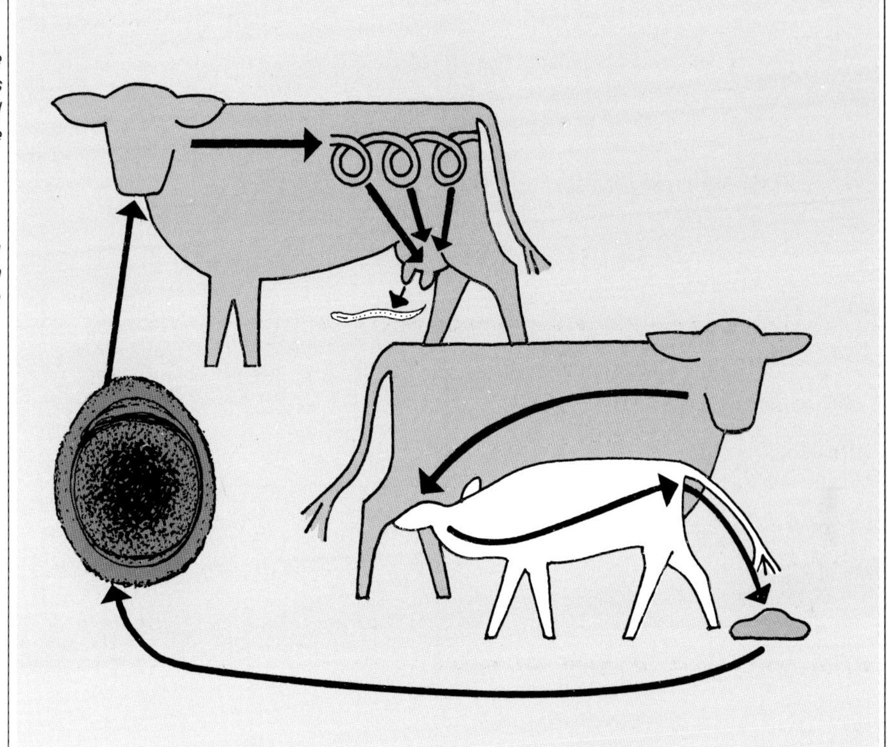

**Symptoms**

In severe infestation the calves show varying appetite, constipation and diarrhoea. Their coats become rough. The migration of the larvae (organ migration) produces minute lesions in the tissue which may become points of entry for bacterial infections. With stunted animals, worm infestation should always be considered. Serious damage to the calf's health will only occur in severe roundworm or threadworm infestation.
The meat hygiene inspection of calf gut infested with roundworm larvae and used in sausage manufacture (boiling rings), highlights an entirely different aspect. If such sausages are heated, an unpleasant odour of butyric acid appears which makes the sausages unpalatable.

**Diagnosis**

Worm infestation of sucking calves is confirmed by microscopic examination of faecal samples for worm eggs (cf. page 194).

In order to interrupt the life cycle of roundworms and threadworms and to clear the affected stock from infestation, each calf is de-wormed at the age of 10 to 14 days. This treatment must be carried out by the 20th day at the latest, since calves start to eliminate worm eggs at that stage. By de-worming calves at the age of 14 days, re-infestation of cows is prevented. Since all cows of the stock harbour larvae, it is necessary to carry out de-worming treatment in all calves which are born in one year.

**Treatment**

*Fig. 124*

| | | |
|---|---|---|
| 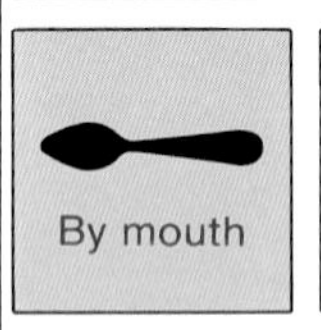 By mouth | **Addition to drinking fluid or oral administration:** 5 g TIPI/10 kg body-weight, one dose only. | approx. 14th day of life |
| 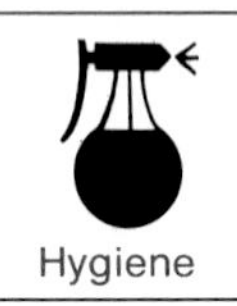 Hygiene | **Hygienic measures:** Remove litter, faeces, dirt. Clean with water, allow to dry. Disinfection with 5% CHEVI 75 solution | 1 day after de-worming treatment |

*Fig. 124: Treatment schedule for worm infestation in calves.*

*Fig. 125: Calf with malocclusion.*

**Disinfection**

After de-worming the calves, their place in the cattle house or the calf pen is thoroughly cleared of litter and dirt and then washed using brush, high-pressure hose or steam jet cleaner. Allow thoroughly cleaned areas and equipment to dry and then apply a 5% solution of CHEVI 75 (1 litre of solution to 10 square metres of surface). Allow to take effect for at least $2^1/_2$ hours. Do not rinse.

*Fig. 125*

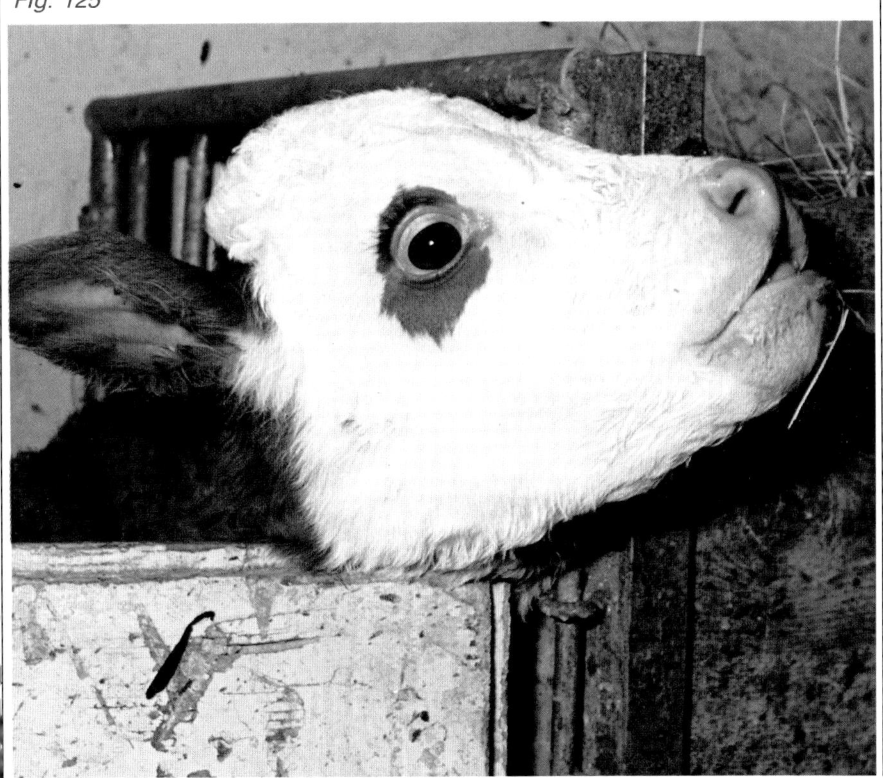

# Congenital Malformations

## Shortening of the Upper or Lower Jaw

**Term**

If the incisors of the lower jaw are out of alignment and meet the upper jaw in front of the toothless plate, this condition is referred to as "undershot". If the lower jaw is too short and the incisors meet the upper jaw behind the toothless plate, this anomaly is called "overshot". The causes of these anomalies have not yet been established.

**Symptoms**

The drinking fluid is taken up slowly and noisily. Because of the congenital anomaly the calves swallow air when drinking, which results in flatulence and diarrhoea.

**Treatment**

Treatment is not possible. Calves with pronounced malformations of this nature can only be used for fattening with milk.

# Congenital Malformations

## Overextension or hyperflexion of joints

Fig. 126

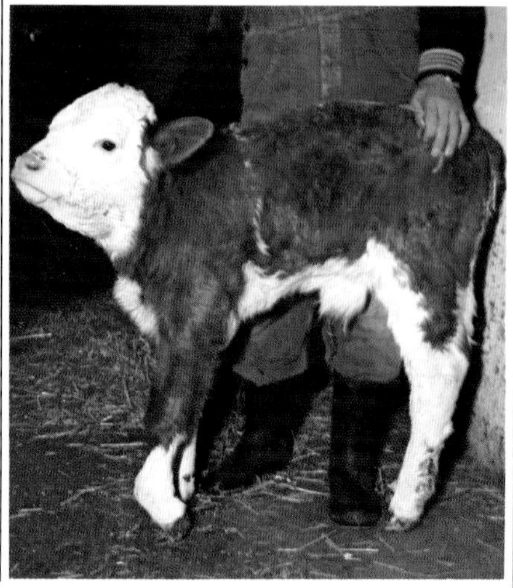

Fig. 127

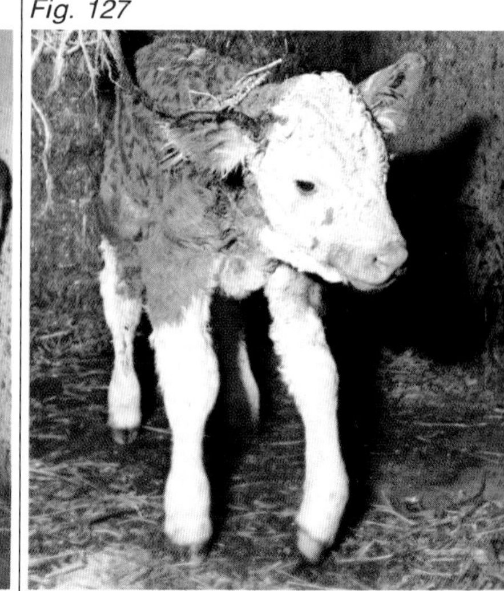

**Term**

Excessive bending or stretching of one or more joints considerably impairs the animal's ability to stand up. In some cases the calves are unable to rise, particularly on the forelegs.

**Cause**

This condition is due to underdevelopment of individual muscles, leading to an apparent or actual shortening of some tendons. Anomalies of the spinal cord or certain nerves are the cause of underdeveloped muscles.

**Symptoms**

The calves stand on the tip of the hoof or even on the head of the pastern. Overextension usually leads to injuries to the skin at the coronal and fetlock joints.

**Treatment**

In the calf, extreme shortening of the flexor tendon leads to decubitus on the joints. Soft litter is therefore required. Supportive extension bandages and padded splints may help to achieve an improvement in these postural anomalies.
Surgery whereby the shortened tendons are severed, often enables an extension of severely affected joints to be obtained.

Fig. 128

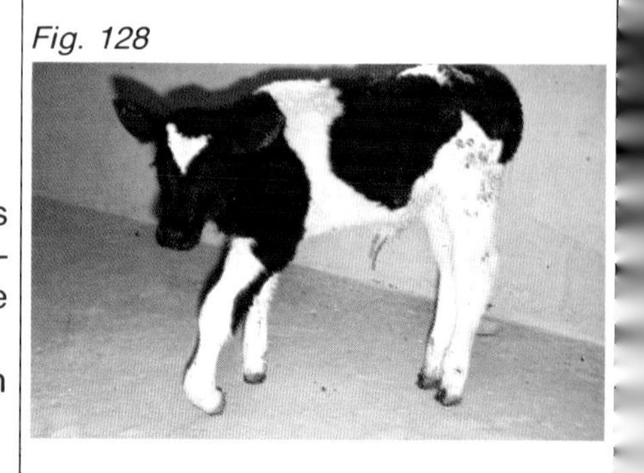

Fig. 129

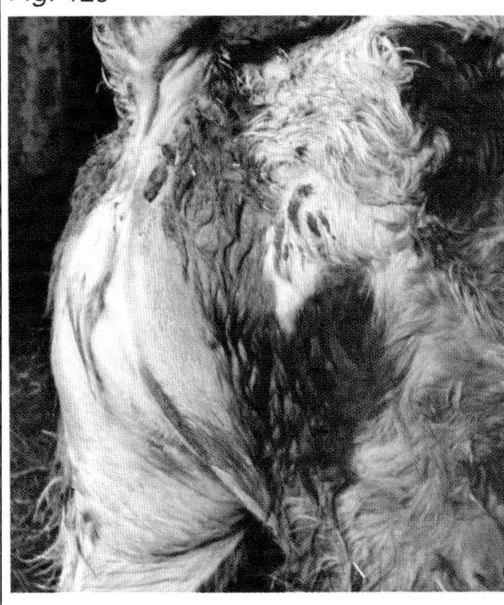

Fig. 130

# Congenital Malformations

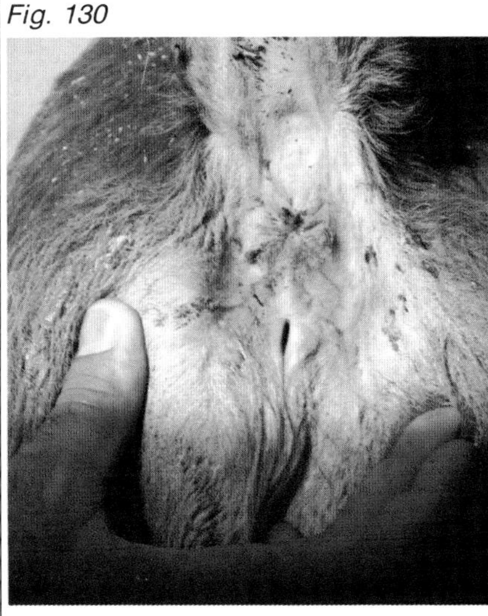

## Hermaphroditism

**Term**

Hermaphroditism or bisexuality manifests itself in a mixture of male and female sexual characteristics.

**Incidence**

Hermaphroditism in cattle is not uncommon. It is seen quite often in twins of different sex.

**Cause**

Bisexuality is due to an accidental genetic defect.

**Symptoms**

Ovaries and testes may occur in the same animal. There may be an ovary on one side and testes on the other. Depending on the preponderance of male or female sex hormones, the foetus may already develop hermaphroditic primary sex characteristics.

**Assessment**

Hermaphrodites should be excluded from breeding. They can best be used as fattening calves, since their further development is uncertain. Hermaphrodites may cause restlessness if kept with bull calves for fattening.

*Figs. 126 to 128: Congenital overextension or hyperflexion of joints in calves aged up to 14 days.*

*Fig. 129: Excessive development of vulva and clitoris in a hermaphroditic calf. The abdominal cavity contained an ovary and testes.*

*Fig. 130: Underdevelopment of primary sex characteristics due to hormonal disorder.*

## Important characteristics of healthy calves

### 5th to 12th week of life

### General behaviour

Size and development corresponding to age; lively, alert and inquisitive behaviour; upright posture, lively facial expression, alert eye and ear movements; shining short coat.
Calves readily approach visitors and are alert to what is happening around them.

### Body temperature

38.5 to 39.0 °C

### Pulse

Rate 72 to 92, strong and regular.

### Breathing

Calm, regular, even. Respiratory rate: 20 to 40 per minute.

### Elasticity of the skin

Raised skin folds immediately level out again.

### Urine

Thin clear amber fluid.
Daily volume: 1–2$^{1}/_{2}$ litres.
pH value: 6.8 to 8.0
Specific gravity: 1,010 to 1,040

### Faeces

Pappy or formed. Colour brown to olive green, depending on feed used. Daily quantity: 500 to 1,500 g.

### Blood volume

Approx. 80 ml blood per kg body-weight.

### Digestive system

Digestion has partly changed over to multi-compartment stomach system (except for calves fattened with milk). Rumination.

*Fig. 131*

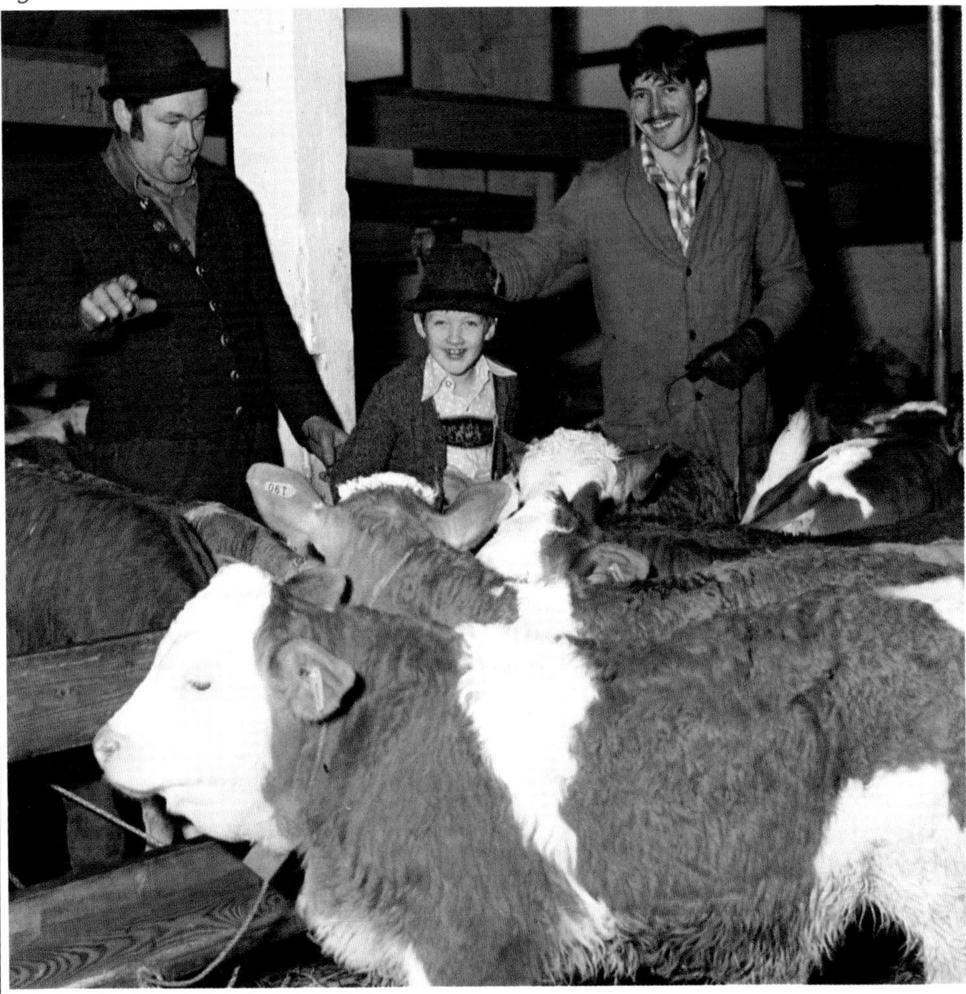

*Purchase of calves at the market: A thorough routine examination of the calves for present or past diseases is very important (cf. examination at the time of purchase, part 5, Fig. 510 and subsequent summary).*

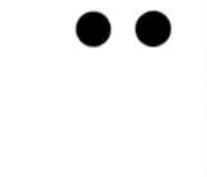

# Part 2

## The most important diseases 5th to 12th week of life

## Summary of important signs in sick calves

### 5th to 12th week of life

| | *Fig. 132* | *Fig. 133* |
|---|---|---|
| | 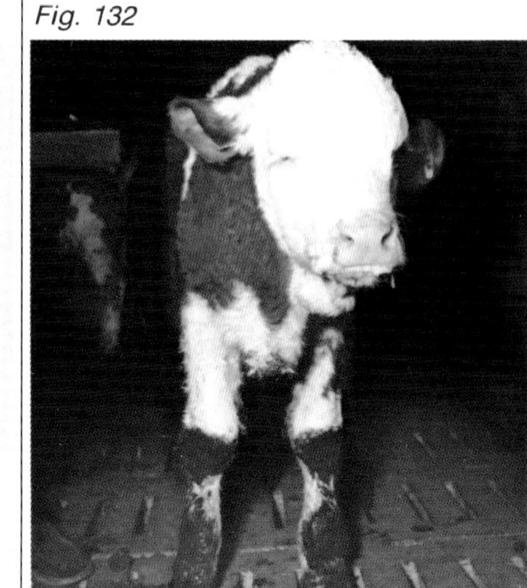 | 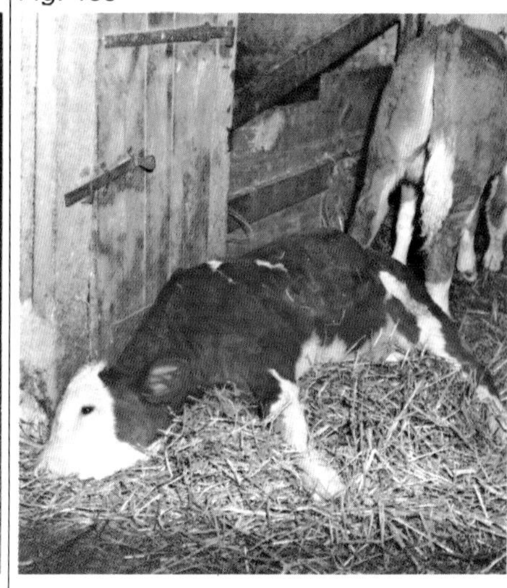 |
| Outwardly visible symptoms | Nostrils opened wide; stretched head and neck posture; the calf is audibly fighting for breath; breathing with open mouth; sometimes formation of froth. | Severe disorder of the central nervous system; cramped posture; typical retroversion of the neck. |
| Diagnosis by examination | Temperature raised to above 41° C. Inhalation and exhalation supported by abdominal muscles (beating of flanks). | Temperature: normal in vitamin $B_1$ deficiency, raised in infections. Reflexes usually increased. Refusal of drink. |
| Read up diseases that may be involved | Crowding disease, pages 138 and 140<br>IBR, pages 138 and 155<br>Malignant catarrhal fever, pages 147, 160 and 168. | Vitamin $B_1$ deficiency, page 102<br>Rabies, page 176<br>ISTME, page 172<br>Listeriosis, pages 104, 147 and 174. |

*Fig. 134*

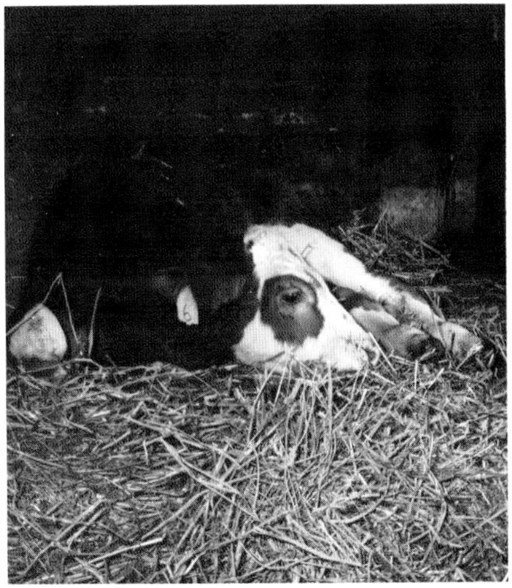

*Fig. 135*

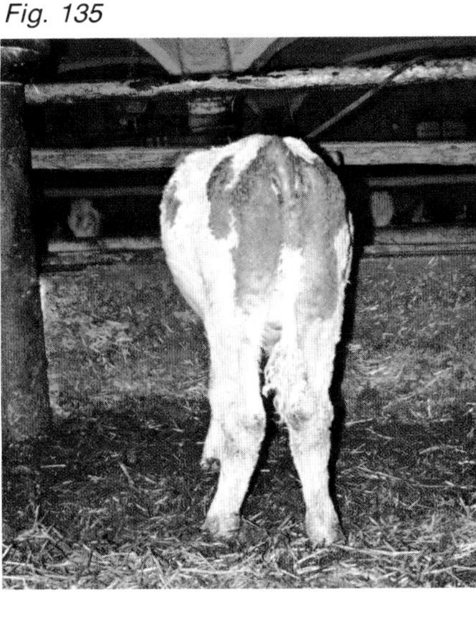

*Fig. 136*

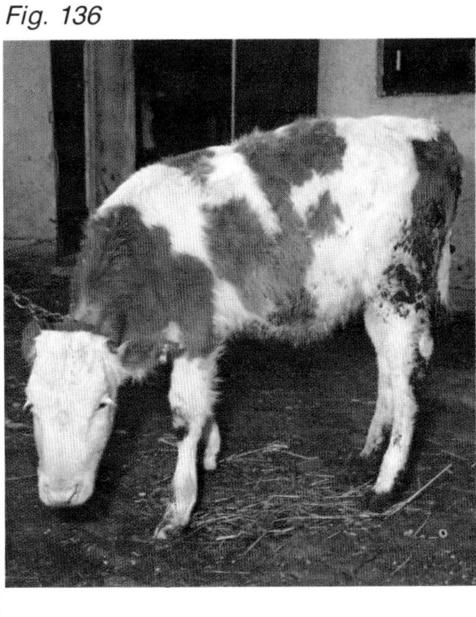

| Fig. 134 | Fig. 135 | Fig. 136 | |
|---|---|---|---|
| Severe disorder of the central nervous system; cramped posture (see also Fig. 133) | Abdomen distended and hard, frightened look, restlessness; kicking with the legs against the abdomen. | Unduly large, "old-looking" head; size and development not corresponding to age; rough coat. | **Symptoms** |
| Look for: animal easily frightened; frequent urination and defaecation in small quantities; muscle twitching, possibly salivation. | Palpation of bulging abdominal wall: loud hollow sound; abomasum on the right; first three stomach compartments on the left. Check urination. Examine filling of bladder rectally. Rumination? | Check feed and water intake. Bacteriological and parasitological examination of faeces. | **Examination** |
| Poisoning with:<br>Furazolidone, page 121<br>Phosphoric acid ester, page 212<br>Heavy metals, page 43. | Bloat, page 92<br>Disturbed micturition, page 178. | Dehydration, see part 5<br>Worm infestation, pages 62 and 192.<br>Congenital malformation, page 65<br>Chronic bloat, page 94<br>Not completely cured diseases, see chapter on treatment, part 4. | **Reap up** |

*Fig. 137*

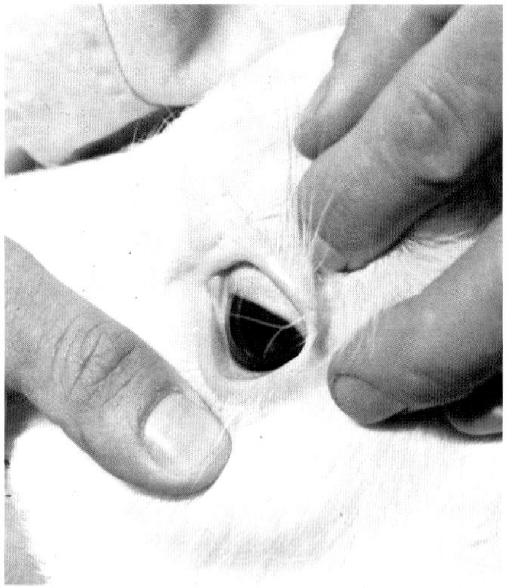

**Symptoms:** Healthy eye; frank look; regular ciliary movement; no discharge, no swelling of the eyelid, no changes around the eye.

**Examination:** Opening eyelid: Pale pink, well moistened palpebral conjunctiva.

*Fig. 138*

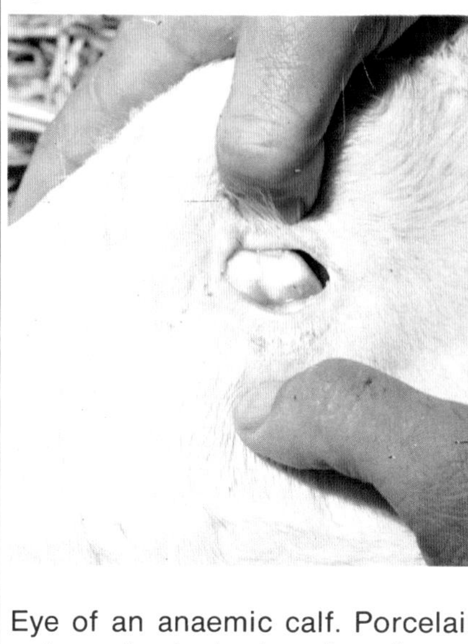

**Symptoms:** Eye of an anaemic calf. Porcelain colour of palpebral conjunctiva; no discharge.

**Examination:** Buccal mucosa also pale. On exertion (rounding up animals) the respiratory rate increases immediately.

**Read up:** Anaemia due to iron deficiency, frequently seen in calf fattening, cf. part 5. Coccidiosis, page 108.

*Fig. 139*

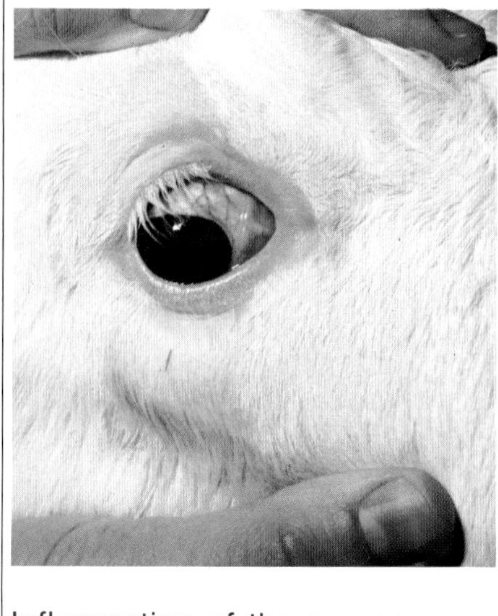

**Symptoms:** Inflammation of the eye: aqueous discharge, lacrimation, swelling of eyelid; later adhesion of eye lashes, shunning light and squeezing eyelids together.

**Examination:** Reddening and inflammation of the palpebral conjunctiva; protruding blood vessels on the sclera. Take temperature!

**Read up:** Infectious bronchopneumonia, page 82
Inflammation of the eyes due to chill (draughty cattle house, transport)
Mucosal disease, page 162

*Fig. 140*

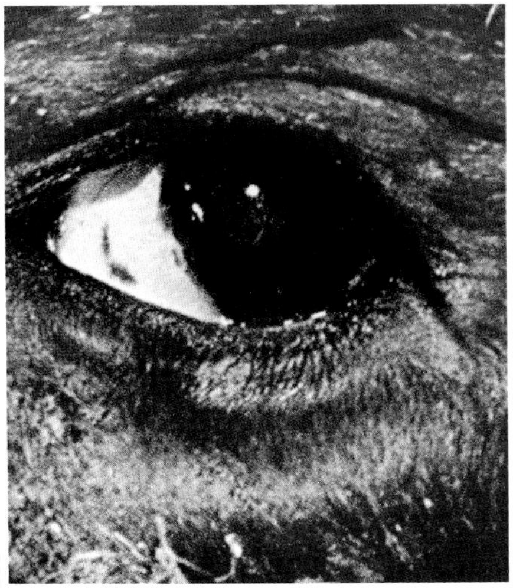

**Symptoms:** Haemorrhage in sclera

**Examination:** Look for punctiform haemorrhages in other visible mucosae. Admixture of blood in faeces?

**Read up:**
Furazolidone poisoning, page 121
Disorder of blood coagulation (coumarin poisoning, page 43)

*Fig. 141*

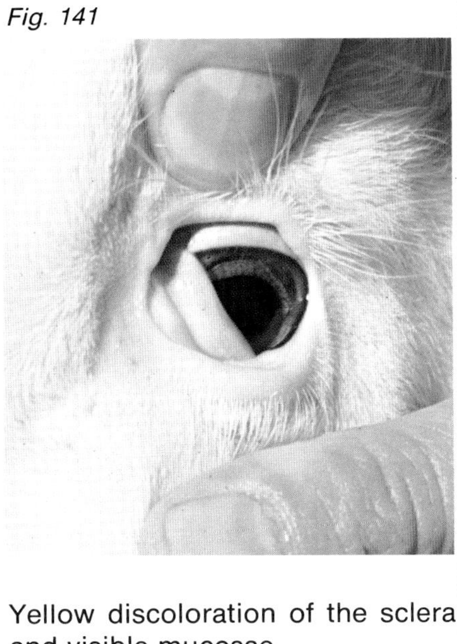

**Symptoms:** Yellow discoloration of the sclera and visible mucosae.

**Examination:** Mucosae show yellow colour. Urine often has a reddish glow. In the terminal stage, increase in heart rate and respiratory rate.

**Read up:**
Copper poisoning, page 119
Liver fluke infestation, page 187

*Fig. 142*

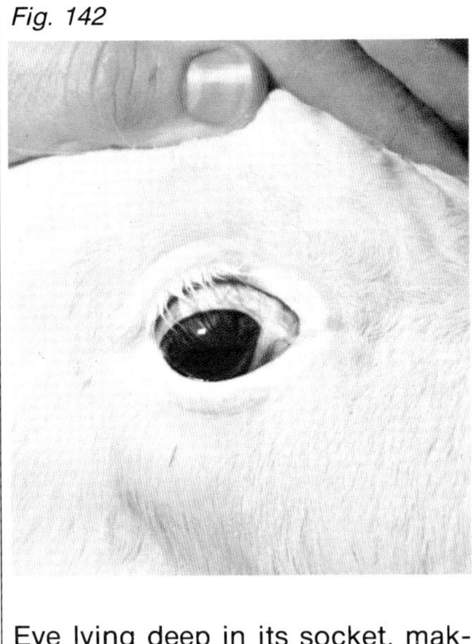

**Symptoms:** Eye lying deep in its socket, making the orbit stand out and giving the impression that the eye is getting smaller.

**Examination:** Desiccation of the connective tissue due to loss of fluid. Skin tension reduced (cf. illustration No. 42). Take temperature! Diarrhoea?

**Read up:**
Coccidiosis, page 108
Mucosal disease, page 162
Salmonellosis, page 36

| | Fig. 143 | Fig. 144 | Fig. 145 |
|---|---|---|---|
| **Symptoms** | Healthy calf: Muzzle pale pink, well moistened; clean nostrils. | Aqueous nasal discharge: Outflow of clear colourless fluid. | Mucopurulent nasal discharge. Viscous mucoid yellowish secretion. |
| **Examination** | Buccal mucosa: Pale pink, well moistened. Sublingual region: No changes. | Temperature above 39.0° C. Husk, possibly accelerated breathing; listlessness; standing away from group of animals. | Difficulty in breathing. Temperature varies, usually above 39.0° C. Strained facial expression. Poor feed intake. |
| **Read up** | | Infectious bronchopneumonia, page 82<br>IBR, page 155<br>Malignant catarrh, page 160 | Advanced stage of infectious bronchopneumonia, page 87 |

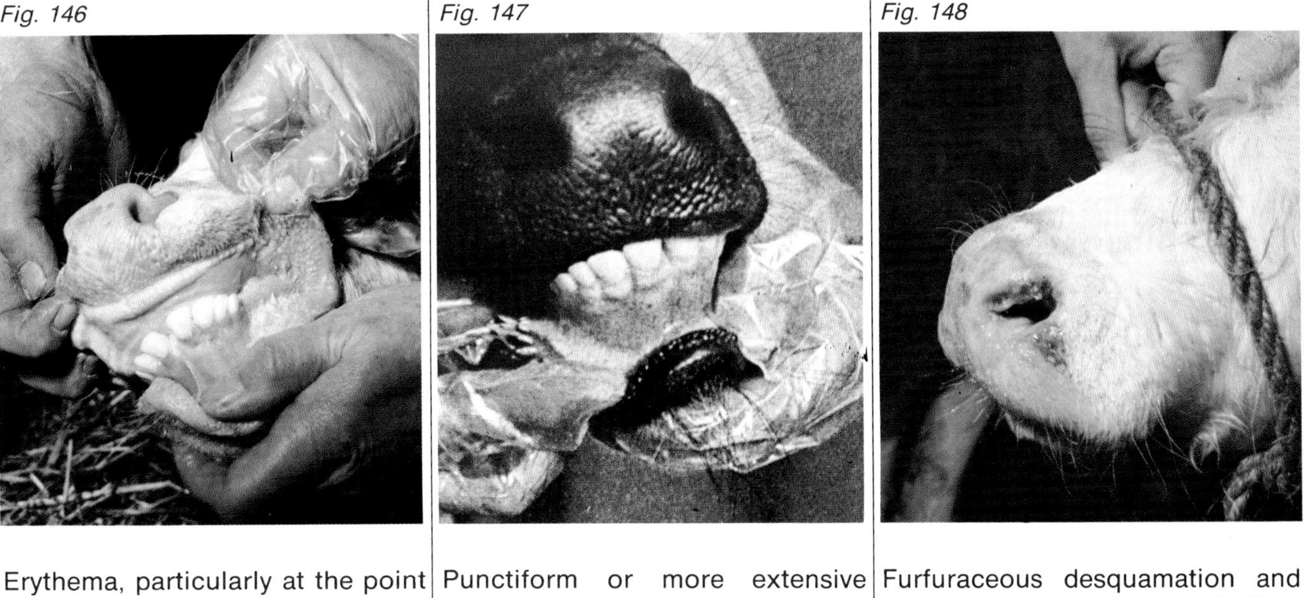

*Fig. 146*

**Symptoms:** Erythema, particularly at the point of transition from the haired skin to the muzzle. Cheek pouch and gum margin inflamed.

**Examination:** Raised temperature (above 41° C), with aqueous intractable diarrhoea in mucosal disease.

**Read up:** IBR, pages 138 and 155
Mucosal disease, pages 138 and 162

*Fig. 147*

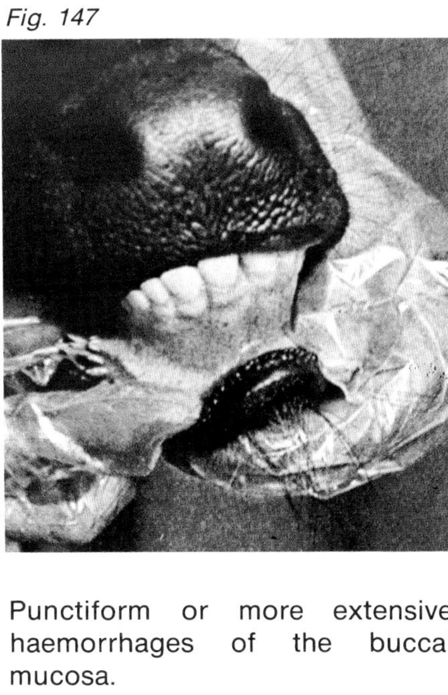

**Symptoms:** Punctiform or more extensive haemorrhages of the buccal mucosa.

**Examination:** Temperature normal; admixture of blood in the faeces. Other visible mucosae also show haemorrhages.

**Read up:** Furazolidone poisoning, page 121
Coumarin poisoning, page 43

*Fig. 148*

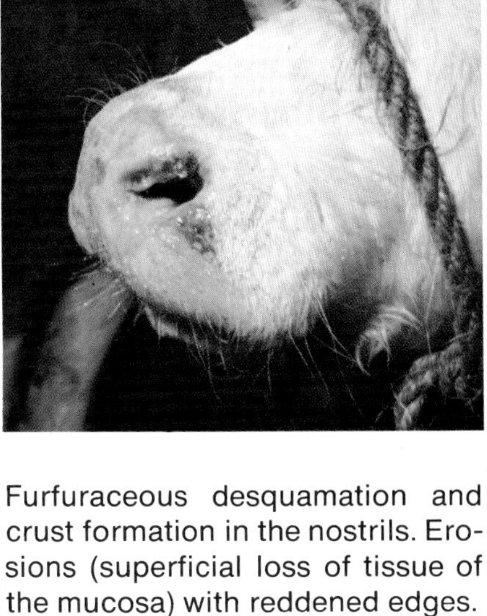

**Symptoms:** Furfuraceous desquamation and crust formation in the nostrils. Erosions (superficial loss of tissue of the mucosa) with reddened edges.

**Examination:** Temperature greatly increased; possibly the same changes on the teats, the coronal edge and in the space between the claws.

**Read up:** Foot-and-mouth disease, page 170
Mucosal disease, page 162

| | *Fig. 149* | *Fig. 150* | *Fig. 151* |
|---|---|---|---|
| **Symptoms** | Faeces of normal calf with fully developed stomach compartments: Pappy to slightly formed. Colour olive green to brown, depending on feed. | Faeces aqueous, very fluid, yellowish brown to greyish green. In the advanced stage, the animal strains, but does not pass faeces. | Faeces fluid, greyish brown, bubbly. Admixtures of blood in the advanced stage. |
| **Examination** | | Check muzzle, nostrils and oral cavity for changes. Temperature often below normal. | Take temperature. Parasitological and bacteriological examination of faeces. Check feeding. |
| **Read up** | | Mucosal disease, page 162<br>Nutrition-induced diarrhoea, page 48<br>Coccidiosis, page 108 | Coccidiosis, page 108<br>Nutrition-induced diarrhoea, page 48<br>Salmonellosis, page 36 |

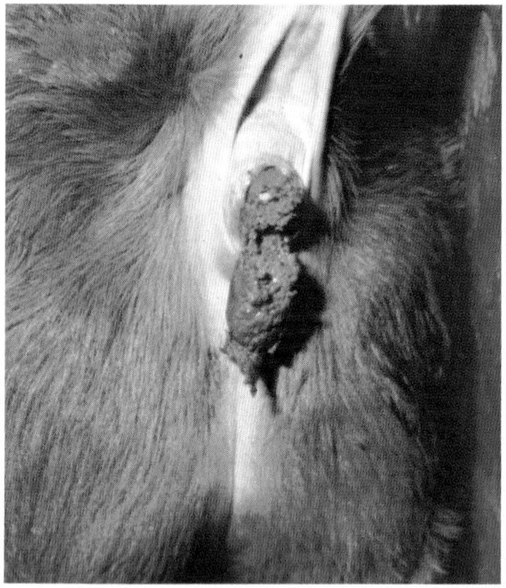

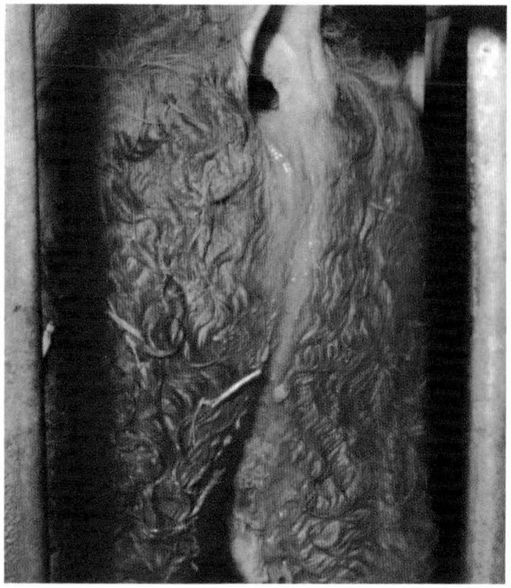

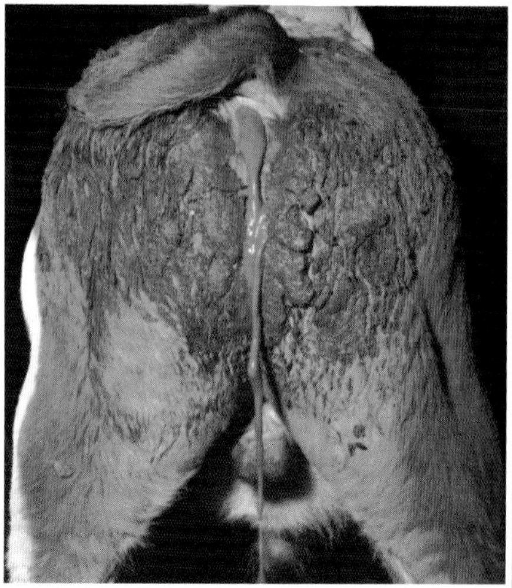

*Fig. 152*

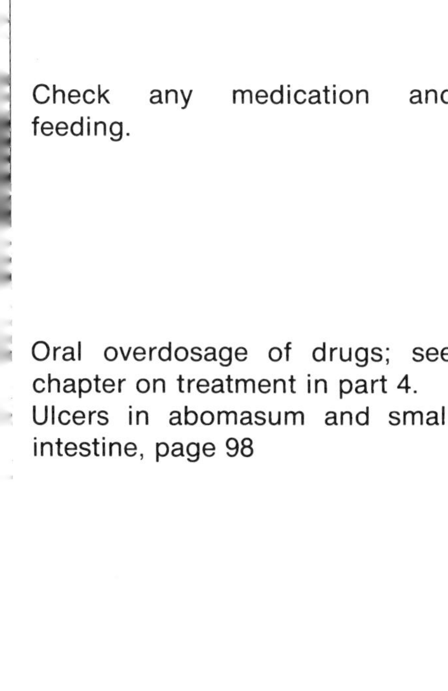

**Symptoms:** Faeces aqueous, dark brown or black; putrid smell

**Examination:** Check any medication and feeding.

**Read up:** Oral overdosage of drugs; see chapter on treatment in part 4.
Ulcers in abomasum and small intestine, page 98

*Fig. 153*

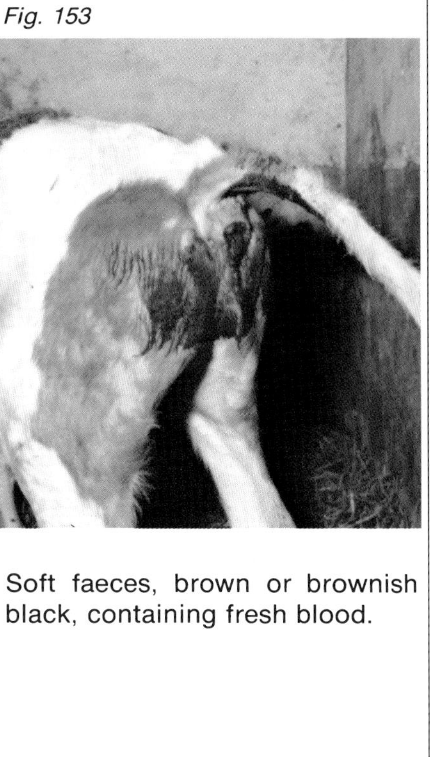

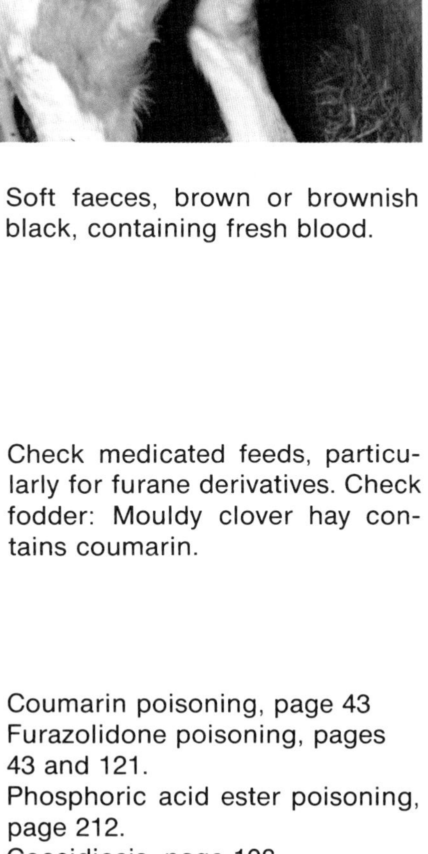

**Symptoms:** Soft faeces, brown or brownish black, containing fresh blood.

**Examination:** Check medicated feeds, particularly for furane derivatives. Check fodder: Mouldy clover hay contains coumarin.

**Read up:** Coumarin poisoning, page 43
Furazolidone poisoning, pages 43 and 121.
Phosphoric acid ester poisoning, page 212.
Coccidiosis, page 108

*Fig. 154*

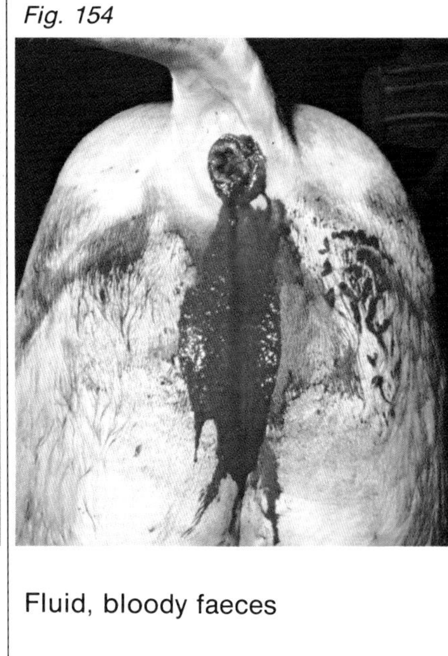

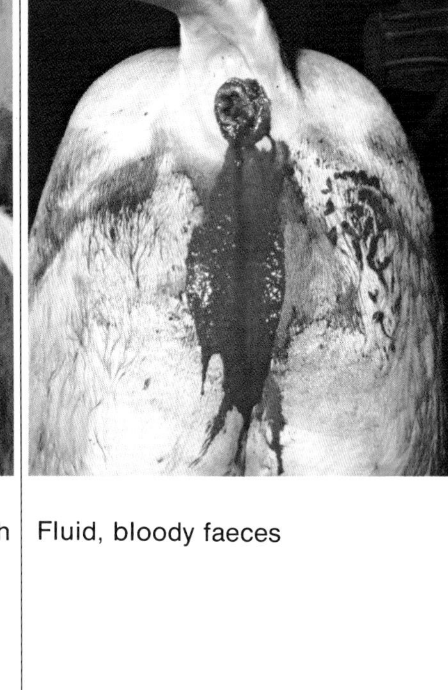

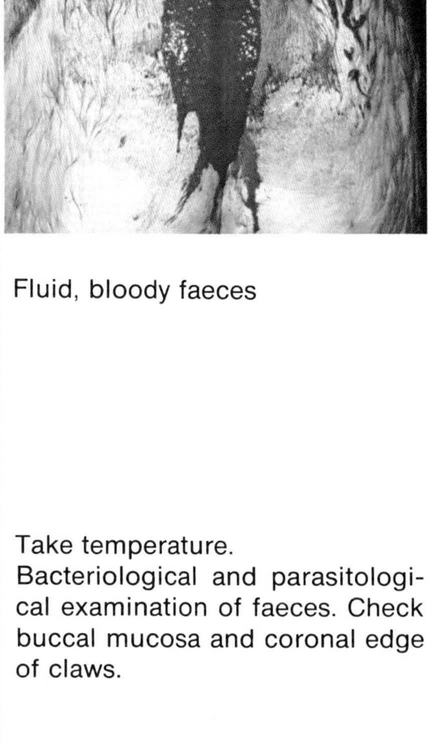

**Symptoms:** Fluid, bloody faeces

**Examination:** Take temperature.
Bacteriological and parasitological examination of faeces. Check buccal mucosa and coronal edge of claws.

**Read up:** Coccidiosis, page 108
Poisoning, pages 43, 121 and 212
Mucosal disease, page 162

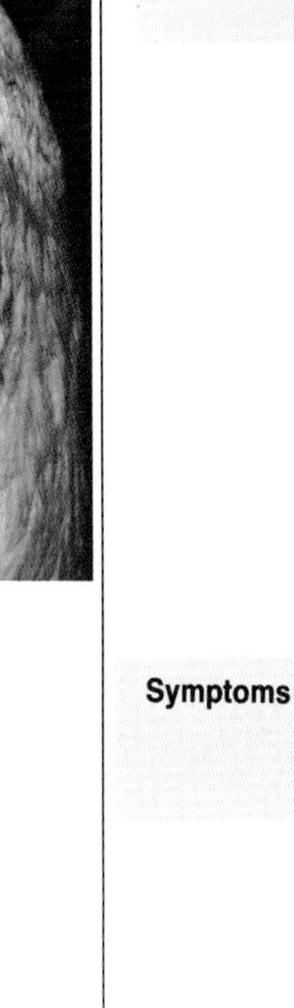

| | *Fig. 155* | *Fig. 156* | *Fig. 157* |
|---|---|---|---|
| | 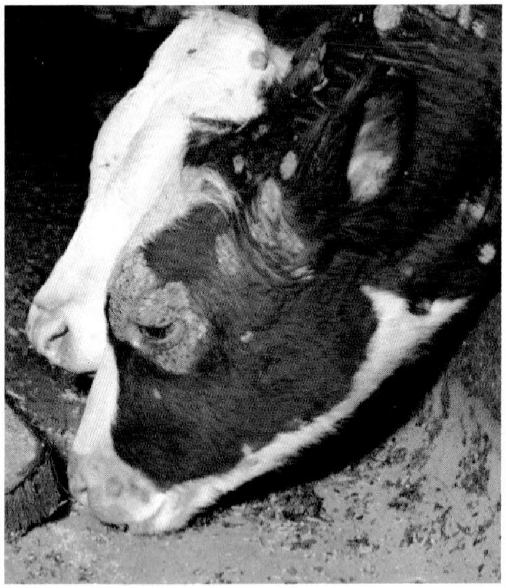 | 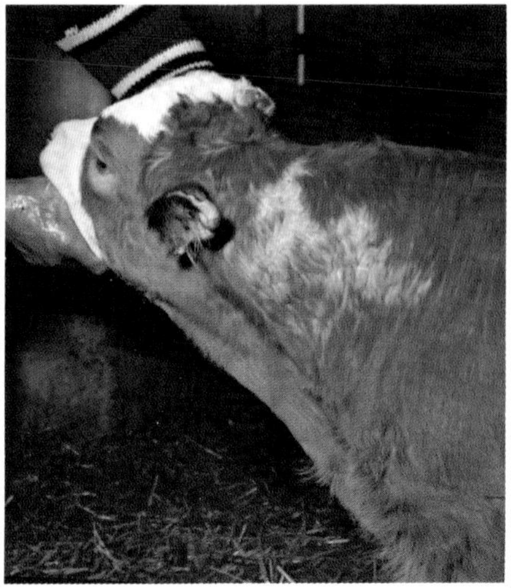 | 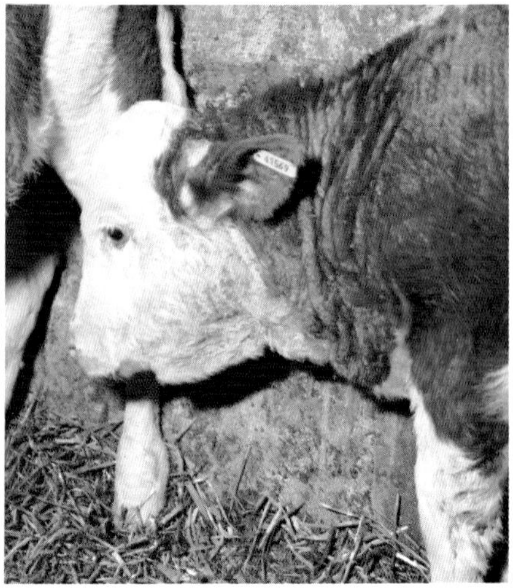 |
| **Symptoms** | Trichophytosis, ringworm: Round bald patches, initially reddened, later asbestos-like crusts. | Infestation with lice: Bald areas. | Incipient mange: Irregular bald, raised areas with scab and crust formation. |
| **Examination** | No itching.<br>Fungus can be demonstrated in the laboratory. | Itching, restlessness; sucking sites visible. Collect hairs for examination for lice and nits under a magnifying glass. | Itching. Examine skin scrapings under the microscope to confirm presence of mites. |
| **Read up** | Trichophytosis, ringworm, page 112 | Infestation with lice, page 208 | Mange, page 200 |

*Fig. 158*

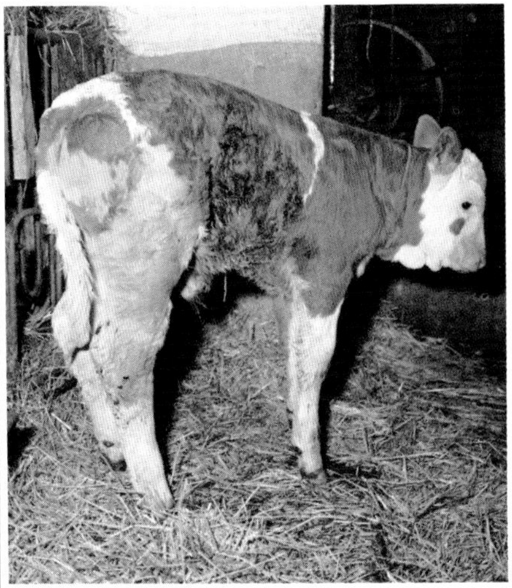

**Symptoms:** Bald patches, starting on the head and in the region between the thighs. The skin shows no changes.

**Examination:** Hair can be pulled out in tufts. Examination of milk substitute for fat composition.

**Read up:** Nutrition-induced loss of hair, page 100

*Fig. 159*

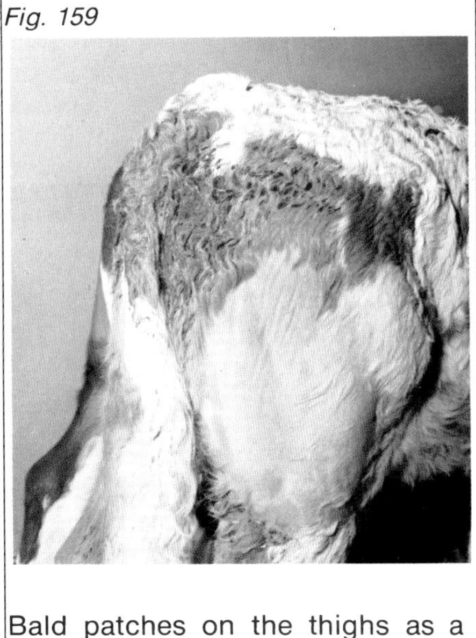

**Symptoms:** Bald patches on the thighs as a result of protracted diarrhoea or lying on wet litter.

**Examination:** Check consistency of faeces. Bacteriological and parasitological examination of faeces for salmonellae and parasites.

**Read up:**
Coccidiosis, page 108
Late sequelae of salmonellosis, page 36
Nutrition-induced diarrhoea, page 48
Worm infestation, pages 62 and 192

*Fig. 160*

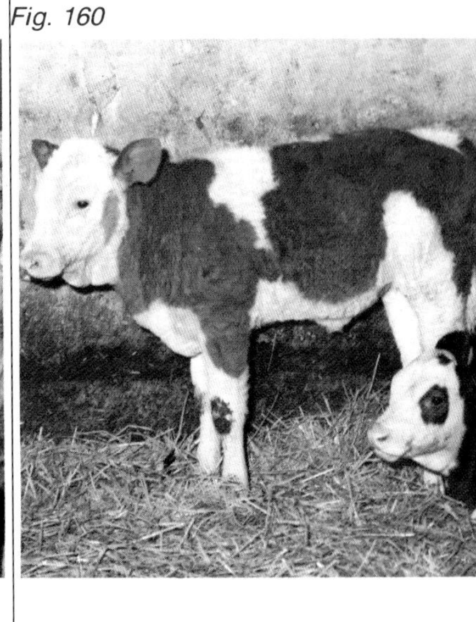

**Symptoms:** Dull rough, long hair.

**Examination:** Bacteriological and parasitological examination of faeces. Check feeding and water intake.

**Read up:**
Incomplete recovery from earlier disease; see chapter on treatment in part 4.
Worm infestation, pages 62 and 192.
Tympany, page 92
Incorrect weaning, pages 260 to 269.

Fig. 161

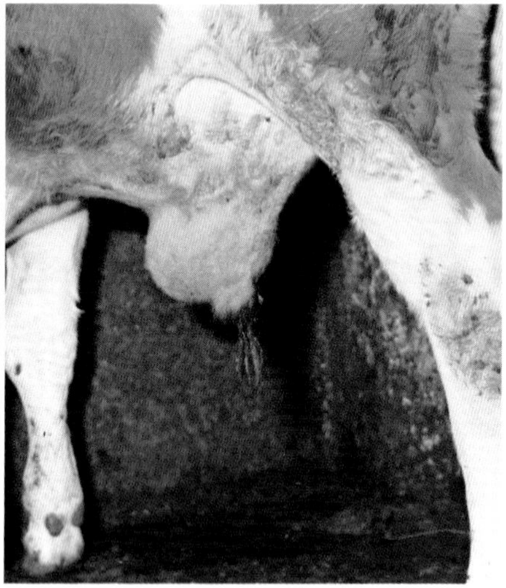

**Symptoms**
Umbilical abscess, umbilical hernia: In both conditions there is a sac-like extension of the skin above the navel.

**Examination**
Check abdominal wall.
Umbilical hernia: Hole in abdominal wall, intestinal loops palpable.
Umbilical abscess: hot, painful.

**Read up**
Umbilical abscess, page 52
Umbilical hernia, page 58

Fig. 162

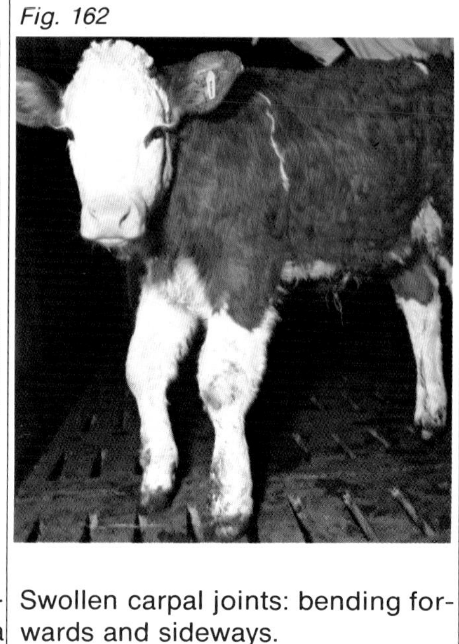

**Symptoms**
Swollen carpal joints: bending forwards and sideways.

**Examination**
Rickets: Palpation reveals bone-hard tumefactions.
Joint inflammation: Articular capsule increasingly filled with fluid; painful.

**Read up**
Rickets, page 225
Calf septicaemia, page 60
Salmonellosis, page 36
Infectious bronchopneumonia, page 82

Fig. 163

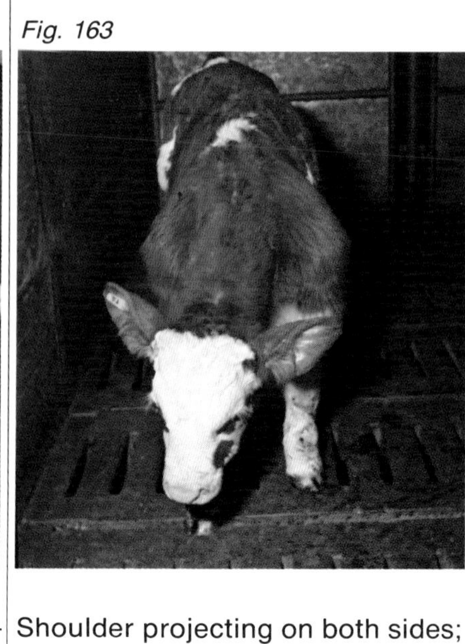

**Symptoms**
Shoulder projecting on both sides; "loose shoulder".

**Examination**
Check shoulder and lymph nodes of shoulder for swelling.

**Read up**
Nerve lesions following infectious bronchopneumonia in calves and cattle; pages 82, 94 and 140.
Genetic weakness of the muscles of the pectoral girdle.

*Fig. 164*

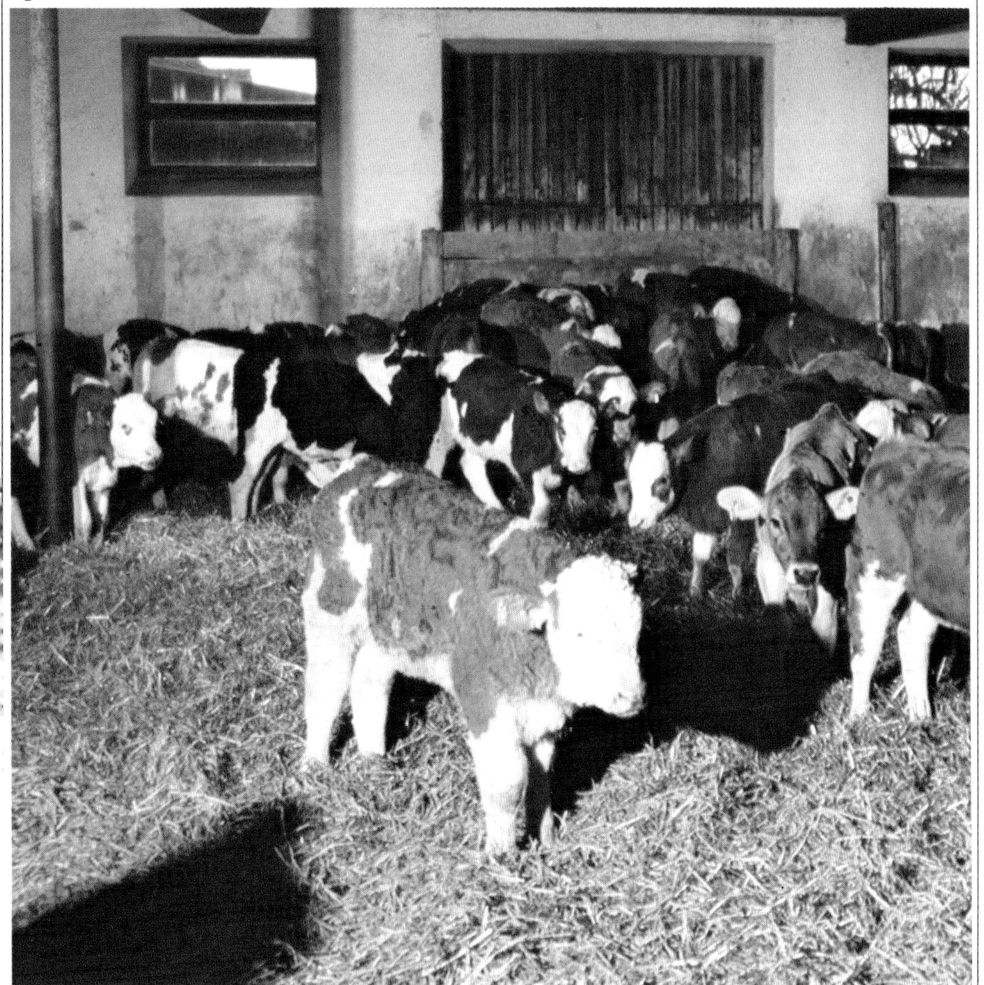

*First signs of generalised disease: Listless and inattentive behaviour, languid posture. The calf does not make way for the visitor.*

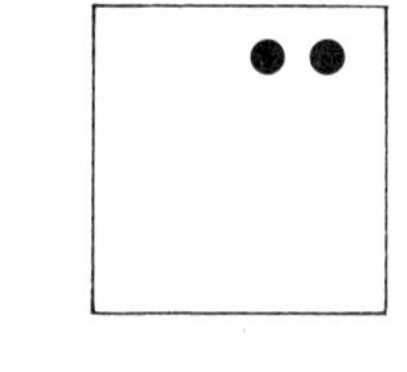

# The most important diaseases 5th to 12th week of life

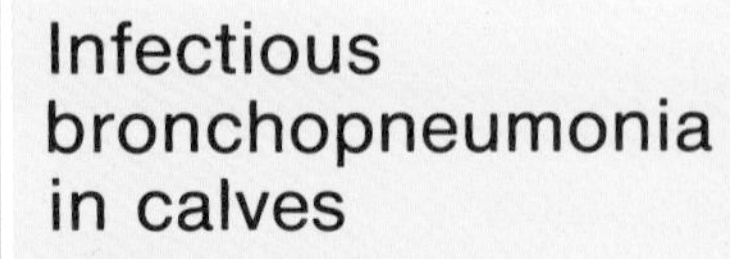

# Infectious bronchopneumonia in calves

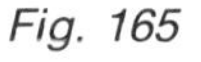

*Fig. 165*

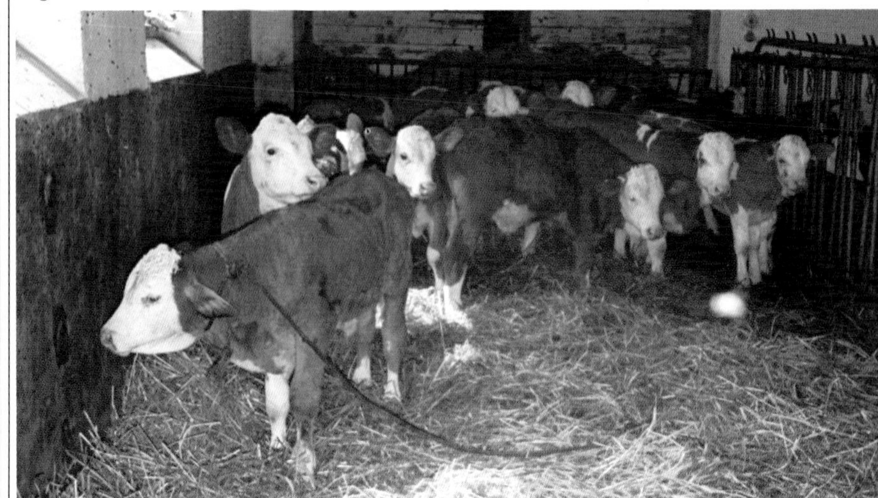

**Term**

The general term infectious bronchopneumonia covers diseases of the respiratory organs which have different causes, but show similar symptoms. For an outbreak of the disease, stress factors need to be present which reduce the resistance of the calves, enabling viruses and, at a later stage, bacteria to multiply in the animal organism.

**Incidence**

As a result of enlarged animal stocks, high-density housing and intensive feeding, infectious bronchopneumonia in calves has appeared as a new disease complex. It has long been known and used to be regarded as harmless. However, in today's intensive livestock farming it can reach epidemic proportions, causing heavy losses. Livestock farms purchasing animals and having as a result a large number of animals of the same age, are particularly affected.

In the 4th to the 6th week of life, the calf has only a limited resistance to infection, which it originally received via the colostral milk. This immunity acquired via the colostral milk (passive immunity), steadliy decreases and has lost its effect by the age of 5 weeks. However, at that point the animal organism has not been sufficiently exposed to pathogens. Its own (active) immunity is still in the process of being built up. At the age of 4 to 6 weeks the calf is particularly susceptible, because its passive immunity is disappearing and its active immunity is as yet insufficient.

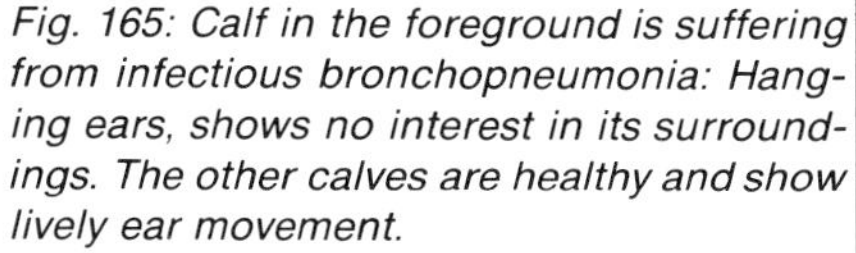

*Fig. 165: Calf in the foreground is suffering from infectious bronchopneumonia: Hanging ears, shows no interest in its surroundings. The other calves are healthy and show lively ear movement.*

*Fig. 166: Mucopurulent nasal discharge, increased salivation: start of a secondary bacterial infection.*

*Fig. 166*

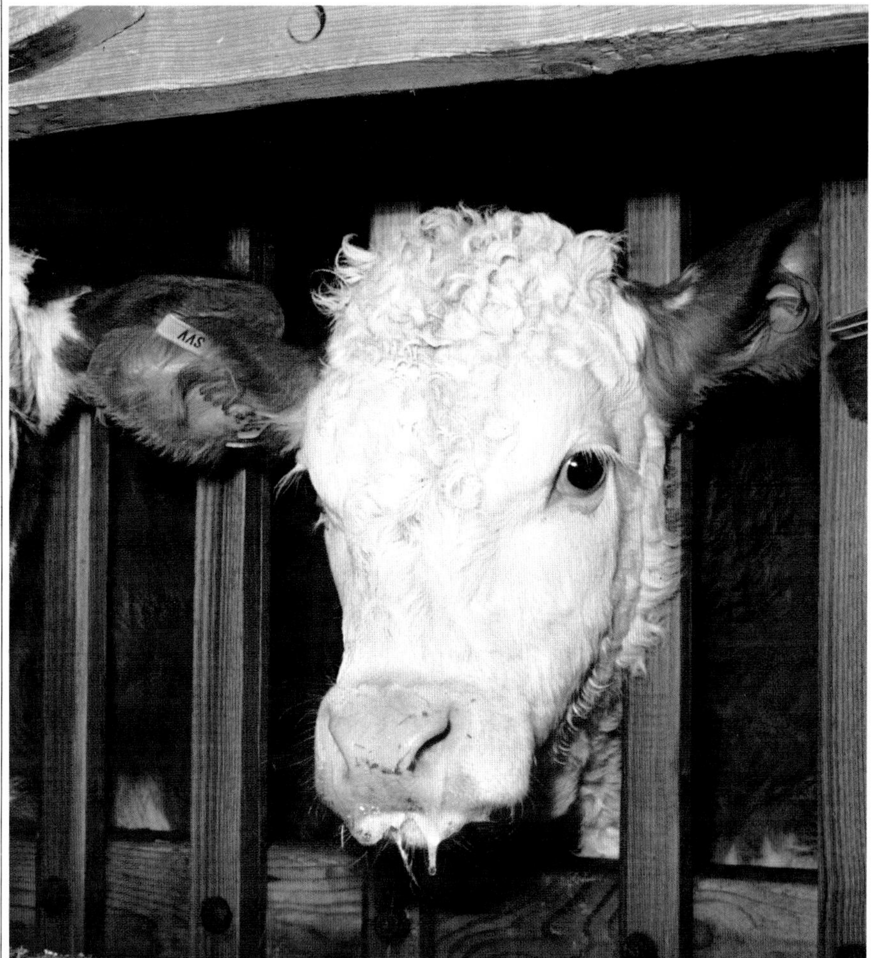

**Incidence**

It is usually at this stage in their lives that calves are marketed and housed on calf or bull calf fattening farms. Marketing, subsequent transport and re-housing cause much additional stress to the calf and contribute to the increased appearance of infectious bronchopneumonia during this period.
Changes in the environment, such as re-housing, change-over from straw litter to slatted floor, high-density housing as well as changes in attending personnel and fodder must be regarded as precipitating factors. In particular, poor controlled environment and abrupt changes in weather conditions weaken the non-specific defence mechanisms of the animal organism.

Fig. 167

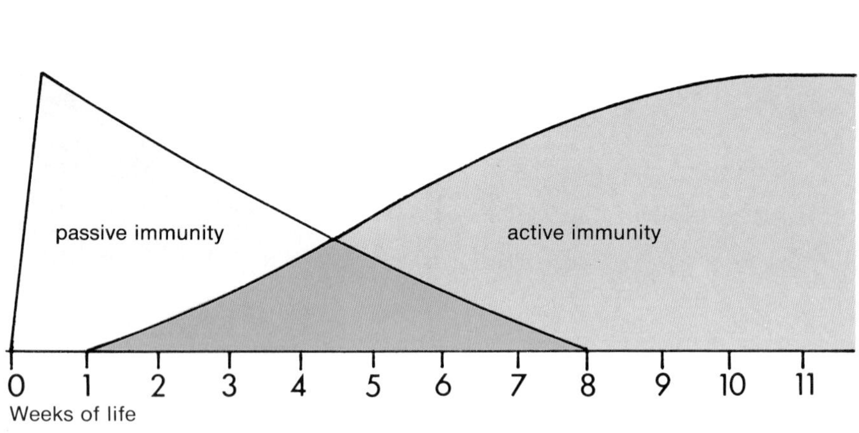


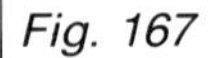

*Fig. 167: Development of immunity in the calf: Via the colostral milk, the calf receives protective substances against infective pathogens to which the mother animal has been exposed. This protection gradually loses its effect and ceases altogether in approx. the 8th week. However, under cover of the maternal protective substances, the calf starts to develop its own defence mechanism from the first week onwards. During the 4th and 5th weeks of life the calf is particularly susceptible.*

*Fig. 168: Summary of the stress factors which reduce the calf's resistance and enable the spread of viral and bacterial infections in bronchopneumonia.*

**Incidence**

A high concentration of noxious gas (ammonia) reduces the activity of the cilia in the windpipe and of the mucigenous glands in the upper respiratory tract. This enables viruses to adhere to the mucosa where they settle and multiply rapidly. The damage to the animal organism caused by the viruses favours the development of bacteria which cause a secondary infection and thus greatly aggravate the disease.

The pathogenic effect of viruses and bacteria differs from stock to stock. In every case, several factors and different viruses and bacteria combine in their effect to cause "infectious bronchopneumonia".

**Importation / Route of infection**

The purchase of calves from different farms favours the spread of the disease. The calves show a varying immune status, since they have only been exposed to viruses occurring on the farm where they were born. They have no protection against pathogens from other farms. Each calf brings with it the pathogens present in the stock of origin. The calf itself is protected against these pathogens. A calf from another stock may not have this immunity. Given normal health and optimal environmental conditions, it builds up its own defences when it is exposed to pathogens. In the event of excessive exposure and severe stress, the calf will develop infectious bronchopneumonia. As a result of the weakening of the animal's defences through stress factors (cf. Figs. 168 and 499), the viruses multiply at enormous speed.

Fig. 168

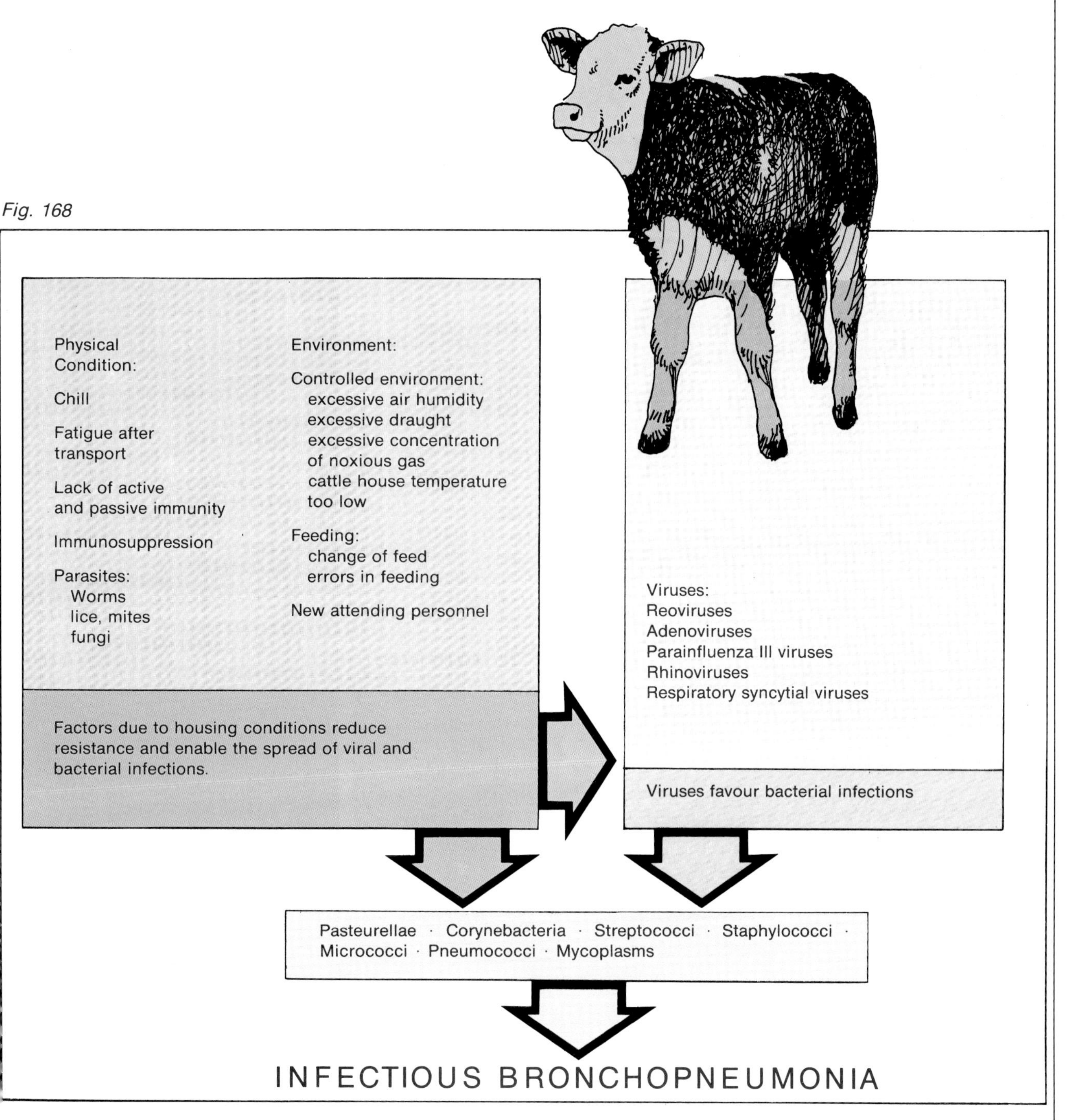
Physical
Condition:
Chill
Fatigue after
transport
Lack of active
and passive immunity
Immunosuppression
Parasites:
Worms
lice, mites
fungi
Environment:
Controlled environment:
excessive air humidity
excessive draught
excessive concentration
of noxious gas
cattle house temperature
too low
Feeding:
change of feed
errors in feeding
New attending personnel
Factors due to housing conditions reduce
resistance and enable the spread of viral and
bacterial infections.
Viruses:
Reoviruses
Adenoviruses
Parainfluenza III viruses
Rhinoviruses
Respiratory syncytial viruses
Viruses favour bacterial infections
Pasteurellae · Corynebacteria · Streptococci · Staphylococci ·
Micrococci · Pneumococci · Mycoplasms
INFECTIOUS BRONCHOPNEUMONIA

Fig. 169

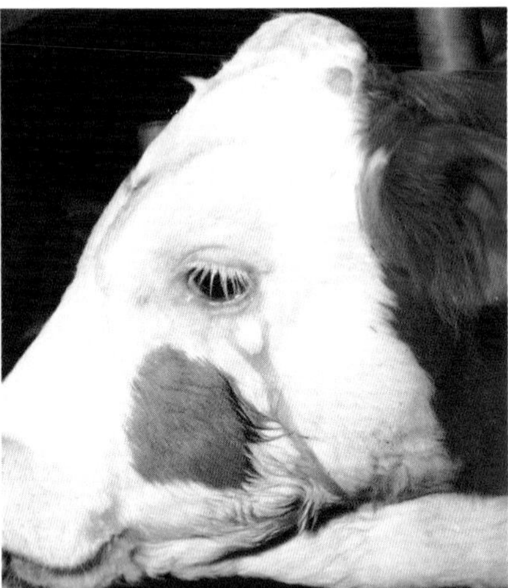

Fig. 170

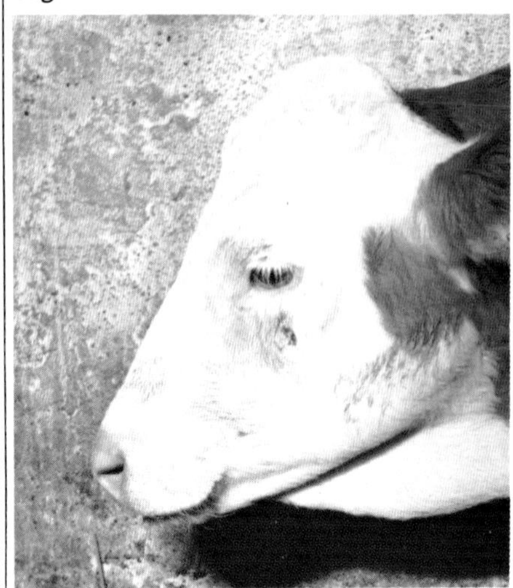

Fig. 171

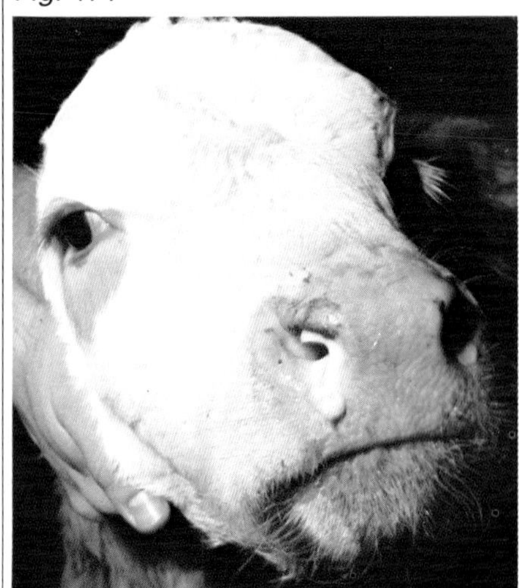

Symptoms

Although infectious bronchopneumonia depends on a great variety of environmental factors and pathogens, the condition presents a uniform clinical picture. The course of the disease is characterised in principle by two attacks of fever.

The viruses settle mainly on the mucosae where they multiply. At the end of the incubation period the pathogens are intermittently distributed throughout the body. This stage of the infection which manifests itself by a brief attack of high fever (41° C) and a slight aqueous discharge from the eyes and the nose, is usually overlooked by attending staff. After this brief period of fever, the body temperature returns to normal.

Fig. 172

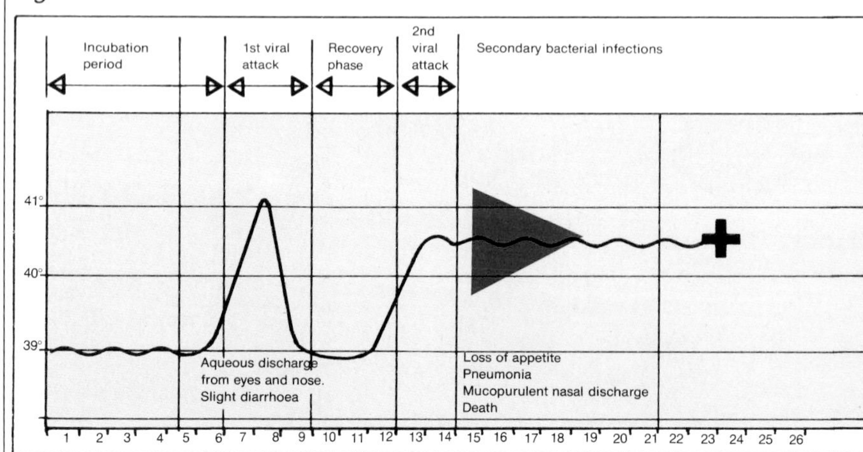

Fig. 173

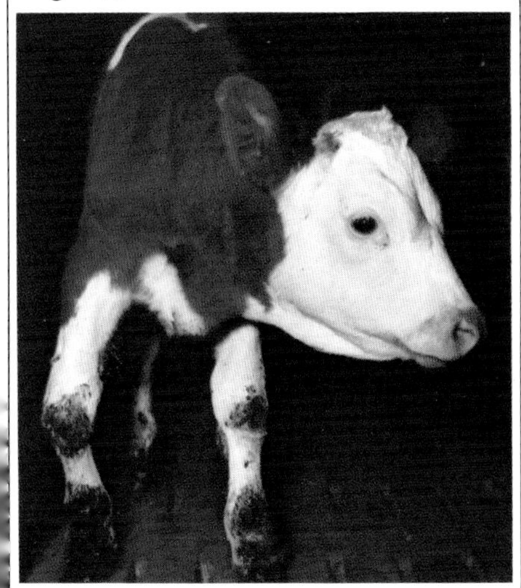

Fig. 174

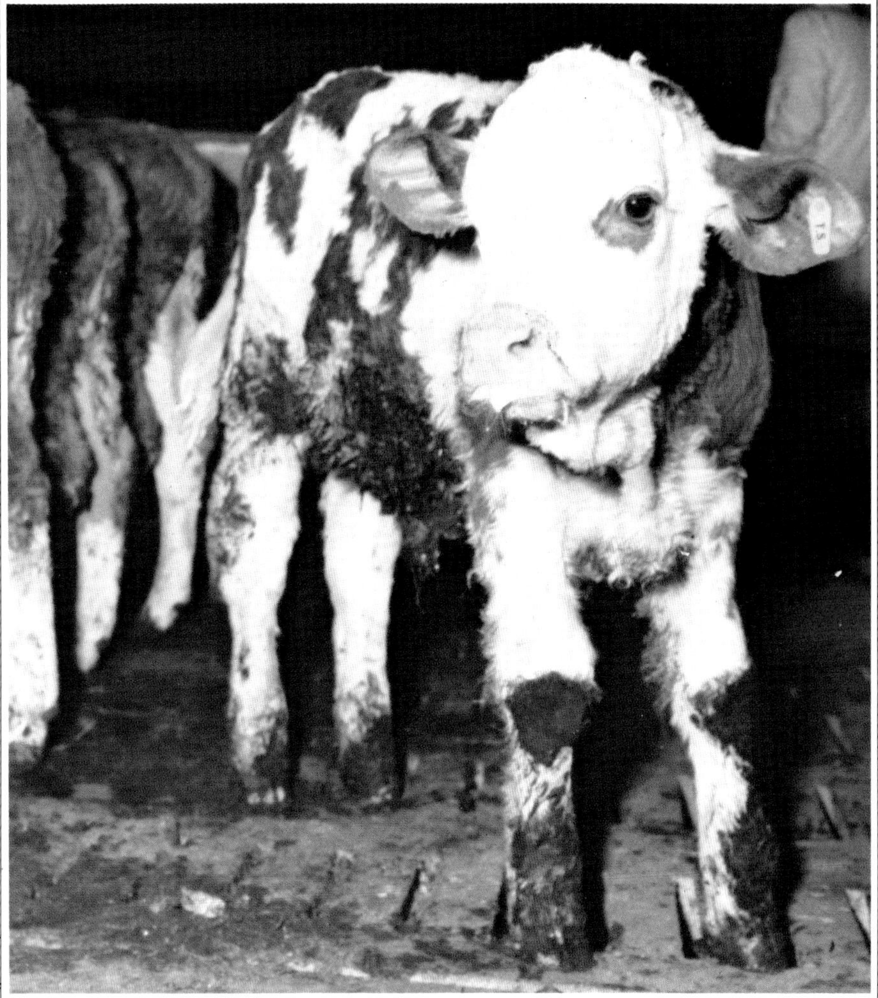

*Fig. 169: Start of infectious bronchopneumonia in calves. Aqueous discharge from the eyes during the first viral attack.*

*Figs. 170 and 171: Advanced stage: The purulent discharge from the eyes and the nose is a sign of a secondary bacterial infection.*

*Fig. 172: After the incubation period, the initially purely viral infection leads to the first attack of fever. This stage is usually overlooked by the animal attendant. After a brief recovery phase in which the temperature returns to normal, the second virus-induced increase in temperature occurs which is then maintained by secondary infections. These secondary infections are usually responsible for the death of the animals.*

*Fig. 173: Rickets-like symptoms: Result of partial neuroparalysis in infectious bronchopneumonia.*

*Fig. 174: Dull calf with severe difficulty in breathing; nasal discharge, foaming at the mouth.*



Several days later a second viral attack produces a further increase in body temperature. But now the calves show loss of appetite, listlessness and an aqueous or mucoid discharge from the eyes and the nose. Unless treatment is started at this stage, bacteria will aggravate the condition.

Pasteurellae and putrefactive pathogens produce severe pneumonia. The animals affected stand or lie listlessly in the pen. They refuse to feed, splay their forefeet and are audibly fighting for breath. Death ensues in many cases.

Fig. 175

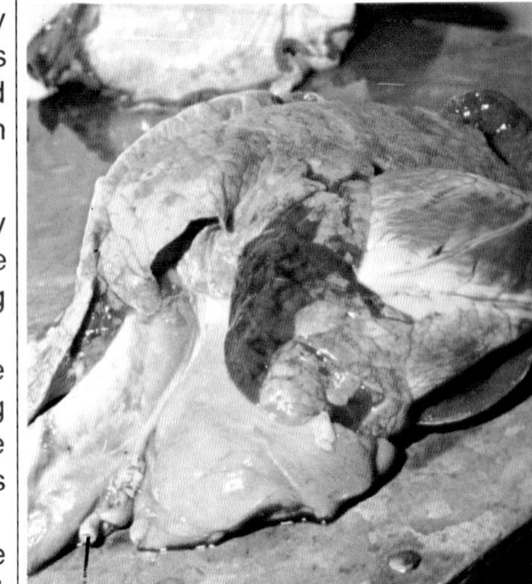

The characteristic course with two attacks of fever and the outwardly visible signs of a respiratory disease point to the presence of infectious bronchopneumonia. It is particularly the discharge from the eyes and the nose and the high body temperature that indicate an infection with viruses and bacteria.

**Diagnosis**

The demonstration of the viruses involved serves a useful purpose only on farms where this condition occurs regularly. The virus can be demonstrated in the living animal at the start of the disease by taking swabs (nose, throat).
However, a bacteriological examination is more important than the demonstration of the virus. This is done by taking swabs from the living animal, and by examining the organs of dead animals. If one or more pathogens regularly recur in several bacteriological examinations, it is appropriate to have a resistance test carried out.
The demonstration of the virus and the bacteriological examination are less suitable for the treatment of an individual animal, but are important in determining the further action to be taken in the prevention and treatment of the disease in the entire stock.

**Similar symptoms**

In contrast to infectious bronchopneumonia, a pneumococcal infection (cf. page 134) takes such a rapid course that a discharge from the eyes and the nose is not normally seen. Calves contract a pneumococcal infection mainly at the age of 3 weeks.

**Treatment**

The success of treatment greatly depends on the stage in which the disease is recognised and how quickly treatment is initiated.

By careful observation of the animals, checking the feed intake and measuring the body temperature, treatment can be started as early as the time of the virus infection. Antibiotics have no effect on viruses, but kill bacteria (secondary infection) or inhibit their multiplication.

In treatment, a distinction should be made between severely affected animals and those showing only minor symptoms, and the remaining livestock.

**Severely affected animals:** For antibacterial treatment, the injection of antibiotics or sulphonamides is recommended. The following antibiotics may be used: Tetracycline, Chloramphenicol, Penicillin, Streptomycin, Ampicillin or Spectinomycin. Sulphonamides often have a very favourable effect in diseases of the respiratory tract.

Fig. 176

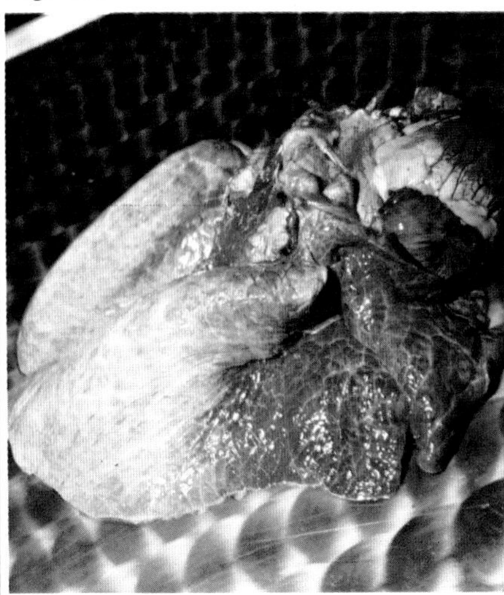

Fig. 177

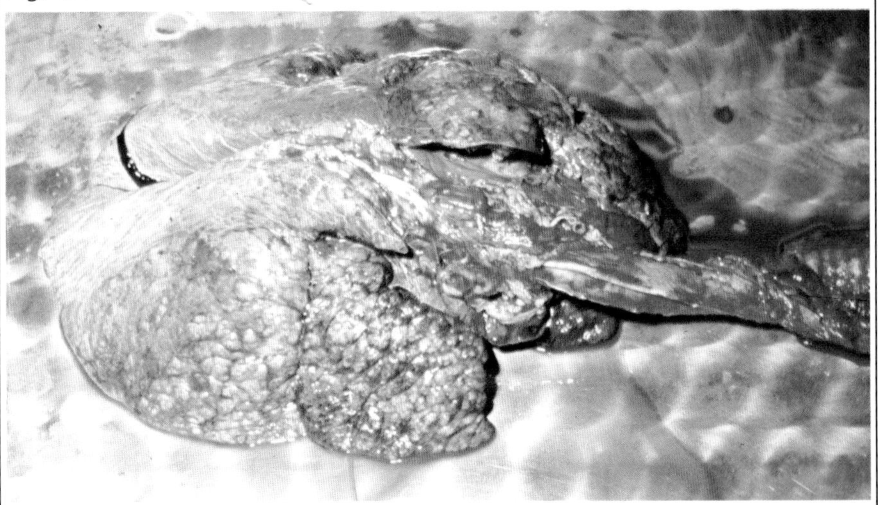

Treatment

The dosage and the period after which the treatment should be repeated, must be strictly observed. For instance, a chloramphenicol injection should be repeated after 12 hours, whereas sulphonamides are only repeated after 24 to 36 hours. In addition, we normally administer products which promote mucolysis and support the circulation.

Depending on the severity of the condition, treatment should be continued for at least 3 to 7 days, even if a single injection has brought about a considerable improvement within a short time (relapses). It takes a certain period of time for the antibiotic to achieve an effective tissue level. It would therefore be wrong to terminate treatment too early and to use some other product (see part 4; guidelines for treatment).

**Treatment of the entire stock:** If medicated feed is given in time, this will prevent the secondary bacterial infection from spreading to those animals that are not yet affected and still show normal fodder intake. Medicated feed will thus reduce the number of cases or, if the disease does occur, it will be less severe.
In our experience, a mixture of chlortetracycline, sulfadimidine, Vitamin A and Vitamin B, is suitable for this purpose. Here it should be noted that calves predominantly fed on milk can properly absorb the active ingredients only in water-soluble form (CHEVICALF). Calves with a developed compartmental stomach system can utilise the active substances better in a less prepared form (CHEVIBULL).

*Fig. 175: Frequent finding on slaughter: Liver-like appearance of a lobe of the lungs, following recovery from infectious bronchopneumonia.*

*Fig. 176: Severe pneumonia with involvement of the pulmonary pleura. As a result of the inflammation, the normally translucent pulmonary pleura has assumed a milky turbid appearance.*

*Fig. 177: Terminal stage of infectious bronchopneumonia in calves, if treatment is not carried out in time: Purulent abscess-forming pneumonia with adhesions.*

Fig. 178

| | | |
|---|---|---|
| Injection | **Severely affected calves:** FORACOL 1.5 ml/10 kg body-weight, repeat after 12 hours. BISOLVON 10 ml/calf; VITIN 20 ml/calf; CATOSAL 10 ml/calf. | 1st day |
| Injection | **Severely affected calves:** FORACOL 1.5 ml/10 kg body-weight, repeat after 12 hours. BISOLVON 10 ml/calf; PRED-NISOLONE 5 ml/calf. | 2nd day |
| Injection | **Severely affected calves:** FORACOL 1.5 ml/10 kg body-weight, repeat after 12 hours. BISOLVON 10 ml/calf. | 3rd day |
| Feed | Affected calves and **all animals** at susceptible age **being fed on milk:** 20 g CHEVICALF/calf per day for 7 days, then 10 g CHEVICALF/calf per day for 14 days. **Calves with developed rumen:** 10 g CHEVIBULL/calf per day, for 3 weeks. | 1st to 21st day |
| Injection | Continue injection treatment, if necessary. FORACOL may be replaced by KELFIZIN, VETOPRIM, SPECTAM, PENBROCK, FORAPEN and similar injectable products. | |

*Fig. 178: Treatment schedule for infectious bronchopneumonia in calves.*

**Treatment**

**Prevention**

Farms purchasing calves should operate the "in-out" method using a reception shed that is separate from the fattening house. It is only in this way that the risk of infection can be contained.

The reception shed is heated (20° C), cleaned and disinfected before the newly purchased calves are housed in it. Here the animals are exposed to those infections which they have brought with them from their respective farms of origin. Preventive treatment is indispensable and should be adapted to the time of year and the duration of transport (cf. chapter on prevention at time of re-housing, page 262).

Fig. 179

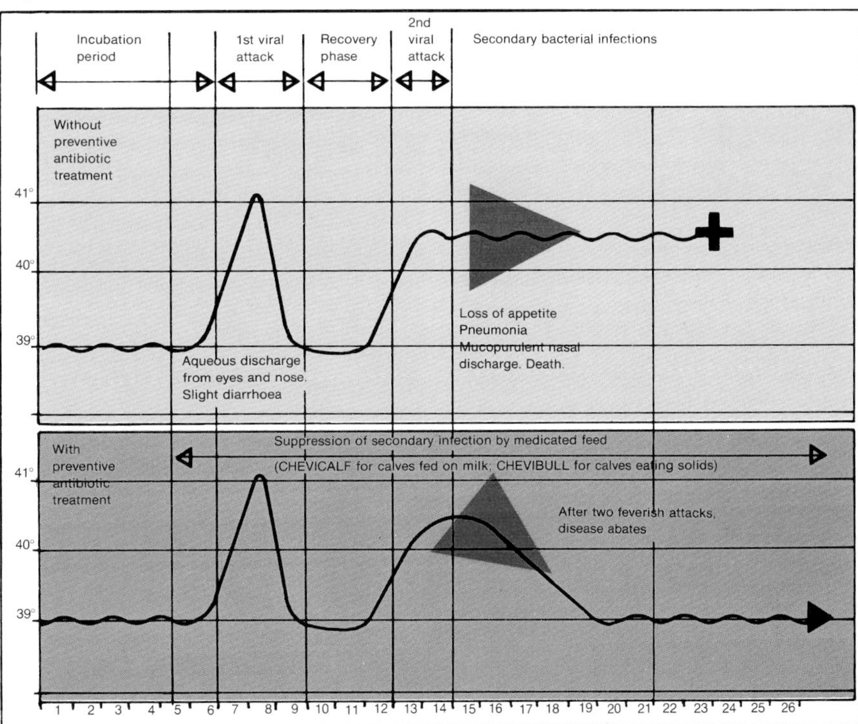


*Fig. 179: After the incubation period, the initially purely viral infection leads to the first attack of fever. This stage is usually overlooked by the animal attendant. After a brief recovery phase in which the temperature returns to normal, the second virus-induced increase in temperature occurs which is then maintained by secondary infections. These secondary infections are usually responsible for the death of the animals.*
*When the first signs of disease (fever, aqueous discharge from eyes and nose, loss of appetite) are observed in the stock, the visibly affected animals should immediately be given injection treatment. In addition, the administration of medicated feed to the entire stock is necessary, in order to prevent secondary bacterial infections. Although the animals will still suffer two attacks of fever, the severity of the condition is reduced, their appetite is maintained and losses are avoided.*

**Prevention**

Preventive vaccination against infectious bronchopneumonia in calves does not provide reliable protection, because the virus infection only constitutes one of the factors which together precipitate the disease.

If parainfluenza III viruses are predominantly involved, vaccination with parainfluenza III vaccine will bring about a substantial improvement in the condition. Vaccination is only a supportive measure. It cannot make up for an inadequate controlled environment or unhygienic housing conditions, nor can it dispense with the need for a reception shed. Vaccination does not replace preventive treatment with antibiotics, since this treatment is aimed at bacterial infections and unavoidable stress factors which occur on re-housing.

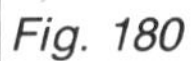

## Tympany in calves

*Fig. 180*

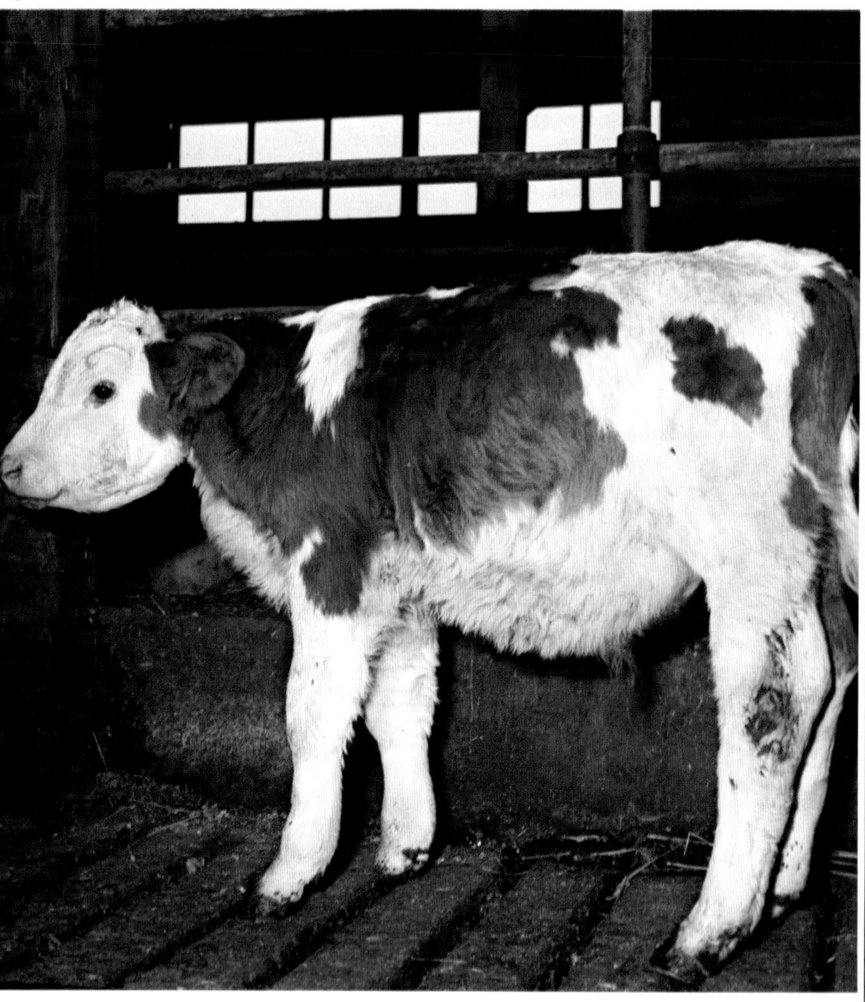

**Term**

Tympany (bloat) is the rapid, excessive distension of the rumen, the dorsal sac or the abomasum. In this condition, for a variety of reasons fermentation gases can no longer escape via the oesophagus and gullet.

We know three different types of bloat which differ in origin, progress and treatment.

- Suddenly occurring (acute) tympany of the first three stomach compartments.
- Chronic recurrent tympany of the first three stomach compartments.
- Tympany of the abomasum.

Fig. 181

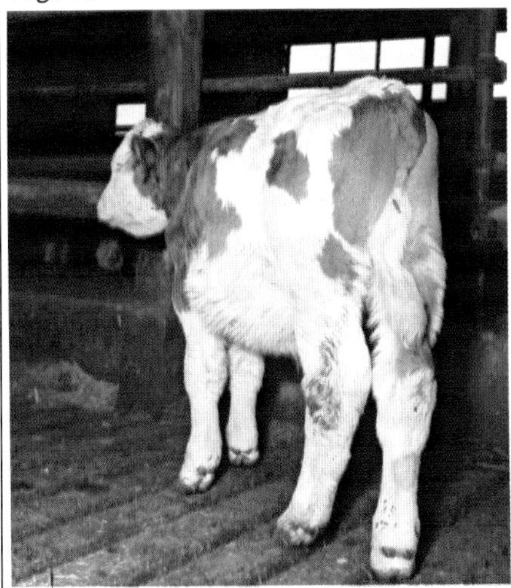

Fig. 182

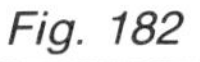

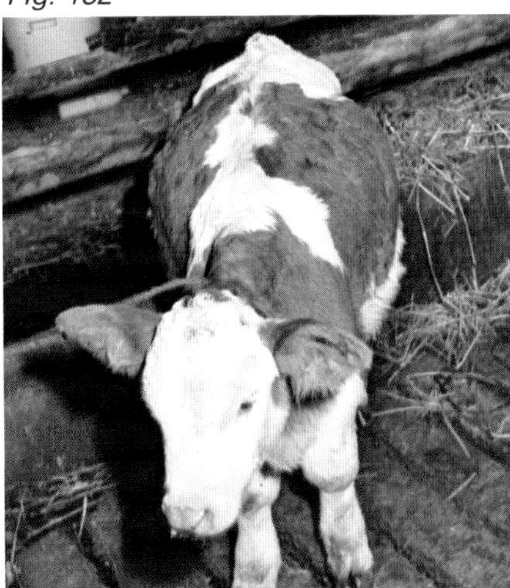

Fig. 183

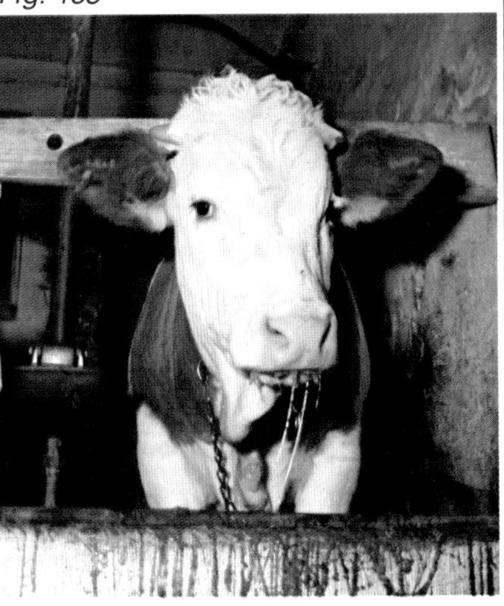

●●

## Suddenly occurring (acute) tympany of the first three stomach compartments

**Cause**

The sudden distension occurs as a result of an obstruction of the gullet by large lumps of fodder (pieces of corn-cob, apples, potatoes or pieces of turnip).
Swelling fodder, like sugar-beet chips, may cause congestion of the gullet.

**Symptoms**

When a lump of fodder becomes lodged in the oesophagus, this results in spasms of the gullet muscles, leading to the foreign body being wedged in even more tightly. Since the fermentation gases which are formed, can no longer be released by regular eructation, they accumulate in the rumen. In this way a gas bubble is formed which increases in size very rapidly and visibly expands the left side of the body between the last rib and the hip bone. On palpation in the region of the rumen, a clear sonorous sound can be heard. Having swallowed the lump of fodder, the animal refuses to feed any more and begins to salivate profusely. A frightened look and bowed head are further signs of an obstruction of the gullet.

**Treatment**

Rapid action is imperative. An injection of spasmolytic drugs (NOVALGIN, BUSCOPAN) will facilitate the removal of the foreign body. An attempt should be made either to pull the lump out carefully or to push it down into the dorsal sac (e. g. using the THYGESENEX TRACTOR). If the distension is excessive, the gas is released by introducing a trocar and cannula through the abdominal wall into the rumen.

*Figs. 180 to 182: Chronic recurrent tympany. Drum-like distension of the abdomen. Pronounced bilateral protrusion of the abdominal wall, particularly on the left.*

*Fig. 183: Obstruction of the gullet: frightened look, profuse salivation.*

## Chronic recurrent tympany of the first three stomach compartments

While the animals are being weaned from milk and after the change-over to roughage, they are very susceptible to chronic recurrent bloat. With this condition, a distinction must be made between tympany where free gas forms a gas bubble, and foamy fermentation which is rarely observed.

**Causes**

**Tympany with the formation of a gas bubble** may be due to one of the following causes:

- Flora of the rumen not functioning
  For some calves, the change-over from milk to roughage is carried out too quickly. The time when milk feeding is terminated, depends not only on age but also on the development of the stomach compartments. For the development of the stomach compartments an adequate intake of calf starter feed and roughage (calf hay) is required. Roughage and calf starter feed affect the degree of acidity in the rumen in such a way that bacteria and rumen infusoria are able to multiply. The right proportion of acetic acid to propionic acid and butyric acid (50–60 to 20–30 : 5–10) promotes the growth of villi in the rumen. Mechanical stimulation by roughage also promotes the development of the muscles of the first three stomach compartments, which are responsible for the myokinetics of the movements of these stomach compartments.
  It is only when a daily intake of 1.5 kg calf starter feed and 0.5 to 1 kg of hay has been reached that milk feeding can be terminated.
- Chronic gastrointestinal catarrh:
  An inflammation of the mucosa of the first three stomach compartments and of the abomasum is caused by drinking fluid that is too cold or too hot, by irregular feeding times and by varying quantities of feed. This disturbs the rhythm of rumination; the movements of the first three stomach compartments slow down or stop completely (atony of the rumen).
- Nerve damage (nervus vagus) as a late sequel of infectious bronchopneumonia
  Swelling and inflammation of the lymph nodes, as they occur in infectious bronchopneumonia, may produce nerve damage. Paralysis of nerves responsible for the digestive movements leads to impaired motoricity of the first three stomach compartments.
- Hair balls
  Fattening calves often sweat as a result of the high energy content of their drinking fluid.

*Fig. 184*

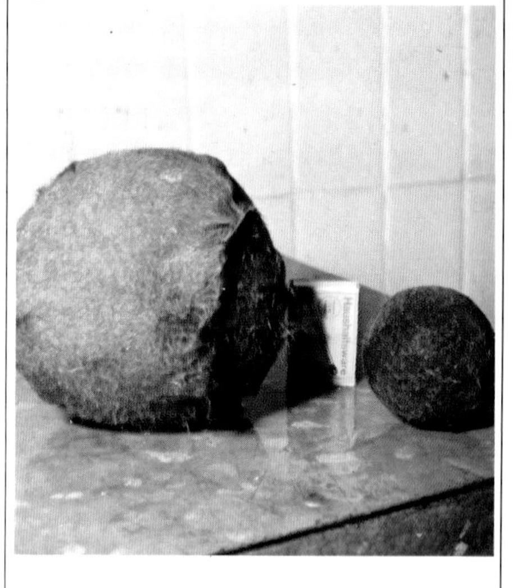

*Fig. 185*

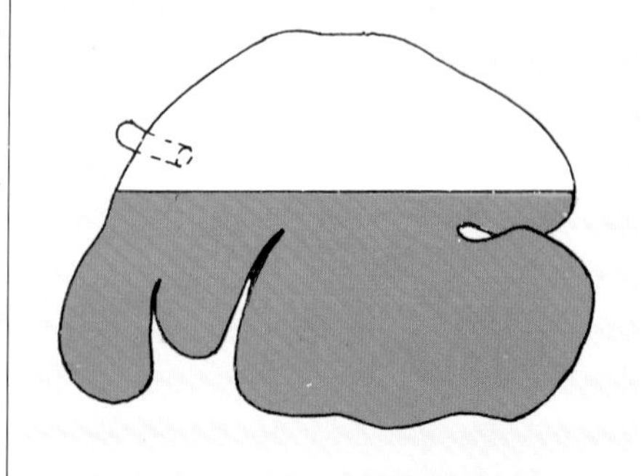

*Fig. 184: Hair balls of calves. These hair balls are often the cause of digestive disorders and bloat.*

*Fig. 185: Diagram of tympany with dorsal gas bubble.*

*Fig. 186: Diagram of tympany with foamy permeation of rumen contents.*

*Fig. 187: Ulcers in the mucosa, the dorsal sac and the oesophageal groove (arrows): These ulcers impair the function of the oesophageal groove.*

*Fig. 188: Dried-out contents in the omasum due to lack of water cause colic-like digestive disorders with tympany.*

*Fig. 187*

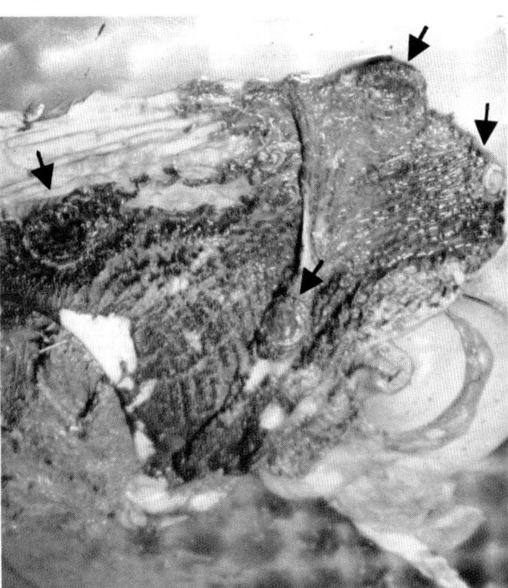

*Fig. 188*

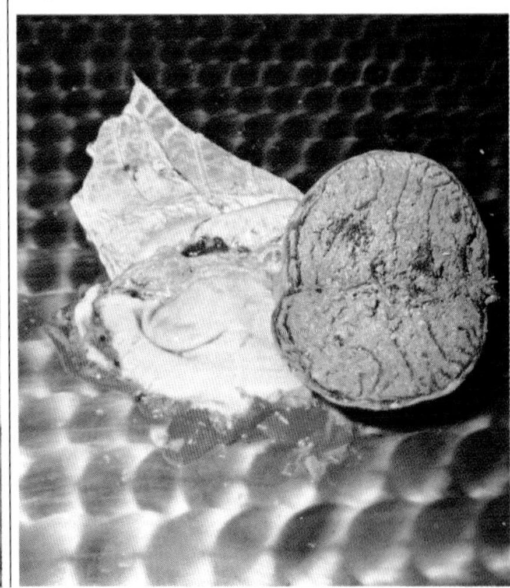

*Fig. 186*

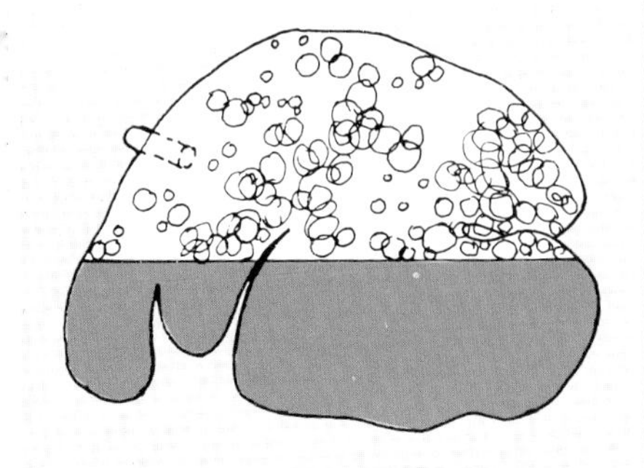

**Causes**

Sweating makes the animals feel uncomfortable, and they try to lick themselves dry. In doing so, they constantly swallow hairs which may become matted and form hair balls in the abomasum or the rumen. This licking is often wrongly interpreted as compulsive licking (vitamin and mineral deficiency). In calf rearing, mutual licking is seen particularly after drinking (cf. page 264).

- Inappropriate feedstuffs

  This includes the feeding of green forage while the calves still receive milk. At this age, swill and brewer's grains also cause fermentation.

Tympany caused by **foamy fermentation** may be due to the following causes:

- Young green forage which is deficient in crude fibre and rich in protein, is swallowed without any significant formation of saliva. The saliva contains mucins which suppress the formation of foam. If salivation is inadequate, the fine gas bubbles being formed are not dissolved. The fine bubbles permeate the contents of the rumen and lead to tympany (foamy fermentation). The fact that young fresh grass contains foam-stabilising substances (saponins) further aggravates the condition.
- If the crude fibre content is low, bacteria form enzymes (mucinases) which render the foam-suppressing substances of the saliva (mucins) ineffective.

In tympany caused by the formation of a bubble of free gas, a tube is introduced through the oesophagus to release the excessive gas volume. In bloat due to foamy fermentation, the numerous small bubbles which are intermingled with the rumen contents, must be dissolved by surface-active agents, so that a large gas bubble is formed which can then be released via the tube. For this purpose TYMPANOL or SICADEN is introduced through the oesophagus. In urgent cases, these agents are injected direct into the rumen.

**Treatment**

Repeated introduction of the tube causes irritation and inflammation of the oesophageal mucosa. This may result in spasms of the oesphageal muscles leading to a recurrence of bloat. In such cases the best solution is the introduction of an indwelling trocar and cannula according to BUFF (cf. Figs. 189 to 198).

*Fig. 189*

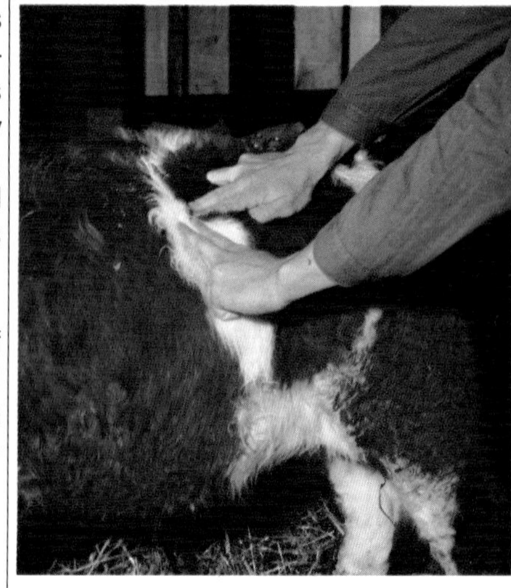

*Fig. 189: Site of introduction of the trocar in the calf: Two finger-breadths below the transverse processes of the lumbar vertebrae, two finger-breadths behind the costal arch.*

*Fig. 193: Screwing in the trocar under steady pressure: When the resistance to turning decreases, the thread of the trocar projects completely into the rumen.*

*Fig. 193*

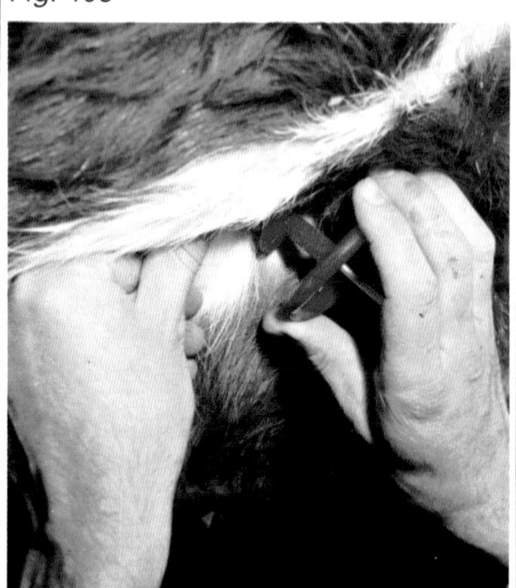

*Fig. 194: Fixation of the indwelling trocar: The space between the skin and the trocar disc is filled by tight bandaging with gauze dressing. In this way the wall of the rumen is firmly pressed against the inside of the abdominal wall.*

*Fig. 194*

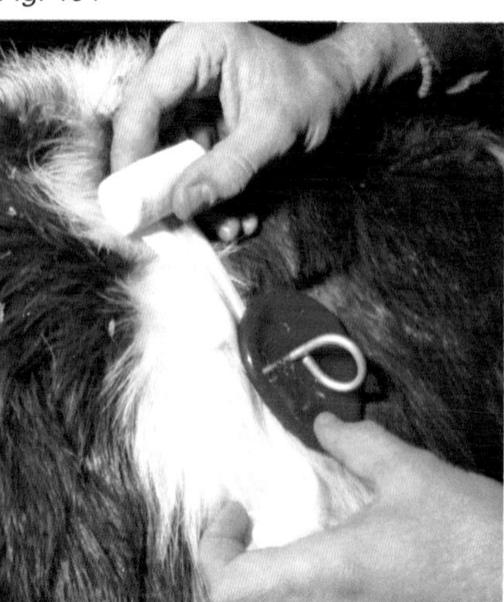

*Fig. 195: Correct position of indwelling trocar.*

*Fig. 195*

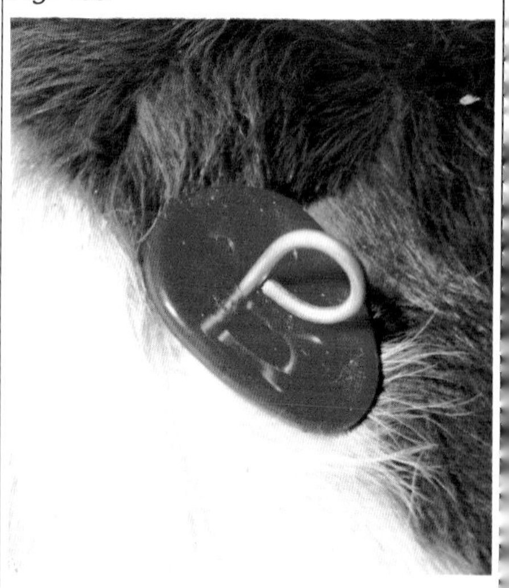

*Fig. 190*

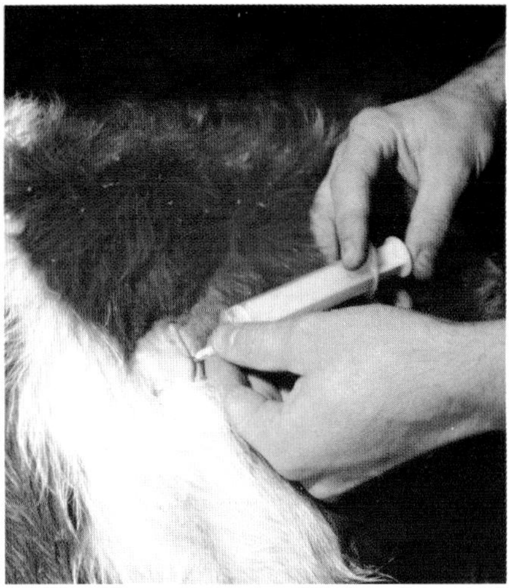

*Fig. 190: Local anaesthesia for the incision into the skin by injecting a local anaesthetic (e. g. HOSTACAINE, PROCAINE).*

*Fig. 191*

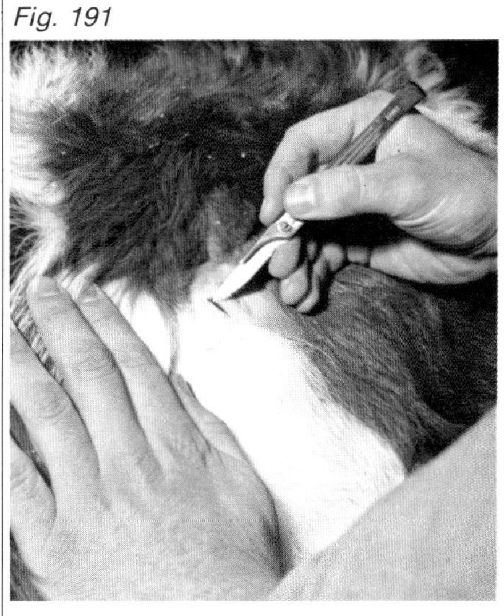

*Fig. 191: An incision into the skin approx. 1 cm in length facilitates the introduction of the trocar.*

*Fig. 192*

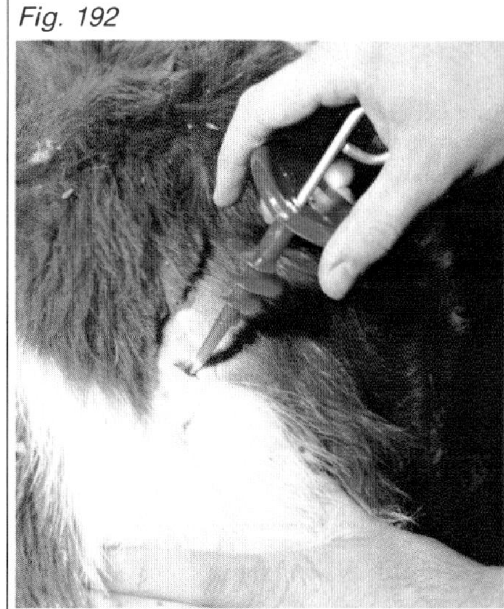

*Fig. 192: Positioning and introducing the trocar: The puncture is made in the direction of the elbow joint of the right foreleg.*

*Fig. 196: To keep the trocar clean and to prevent any obstruction, a metal rod (mandrin) is introduced. When the mandrin is withdrawn, excessive gas escapes.*

*Fig. 196*

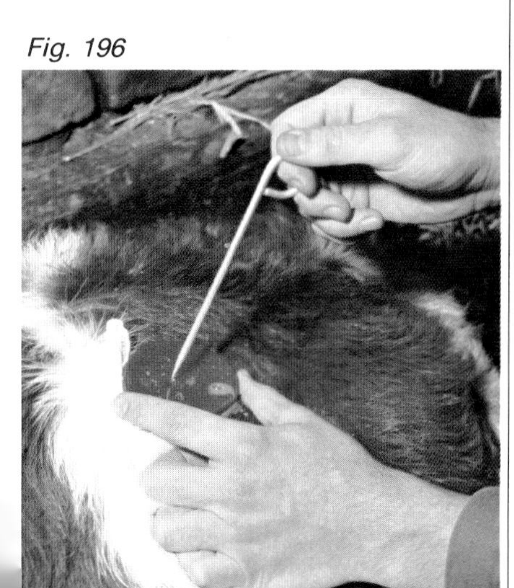

*Fig. 197: The gas is released several times a day by withdrawing the mandrin. After 2 or 3 weeks the trocar can usually be removed.*

*Fig. 197*

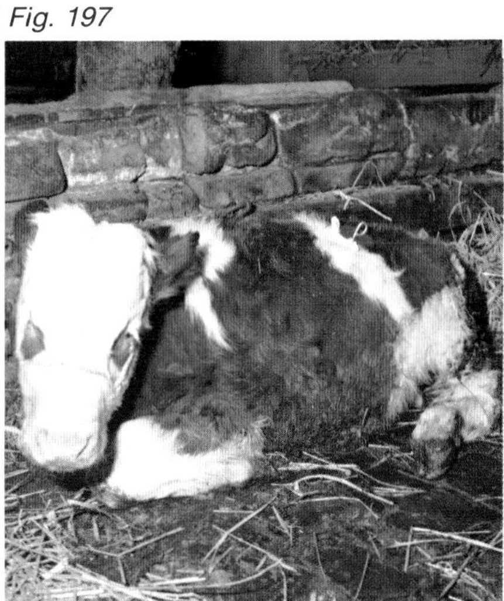

*Fig. 198: The wound closes spontaneously. Spraying with LOGWOOD TINCTURE promotes healing and prevents irritation by flies.*

*Fig. 198*

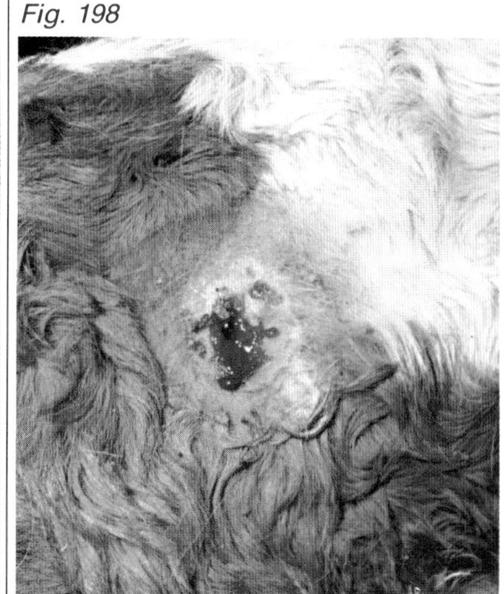

Prevention of recurrent tympany may be attempted as follows:

- Let calves fast for one day, but water must be freely available.
- Be careful with maize silage.
- Continue feeding the calves with milk in the early stages of weaning.
- Give 2 tablespoonsful of TYMPANOL three times daily.
- Transfer fresh rumen juice, warmed to body temperature.
- In persistent cases, start weaning all over again.

## Tympany of the abomasum

**Incidence**

In sucking and fattening calves tympany of the abomasum is observed in isolated cases. With tympany of the abomasum, as distinct from bloat of the first three stomach compartments, protrusion of the abdominal wall occurs on the right-hand side in the lower part of the costal arch.

**Causes**

During the first few weeks of life, the abomasum cannot hold more than 4 litres per feed. Bloat is caused in particular by the ingestion of large volumes of milk.

*Fig. 199*

| Age | Rumen | | Abomasum |
|---|---|---|---|
| 1st to 4th week | 1 | : | 2 |
| 4th to 8th week | 3 | : | 2 |
| 8th to 12th week | 4 | : | 2 |
| Adult cattle | 9 | : | 1 |

Further possible causes of tympany of the abomasum:

- Ulcers and inflammations of the abomasum occur if the drinking fluïd taken up by the animal is too hot or too cold. Nervous disorders caused by re-housing, transport, overcrowding and a change of attending personnel, produce ulcers and inflammations which disturb acid production in the abomasum. The chyme is no longer sufficiently acidified, so that putrefactive and gas-forming bacteria predominate and induce tympany.
- Hair balls may obstruct the pylorus. The contents of the abomasum can then only partly pass into the intestine, or not at all. The abomasum becomes congested and tympany results.
- With hasty eating, a great deal of air is swallowed at the same time, resulting in impairment of enzyme action on the chyme and multiplication of bacteria.

Fig. 200

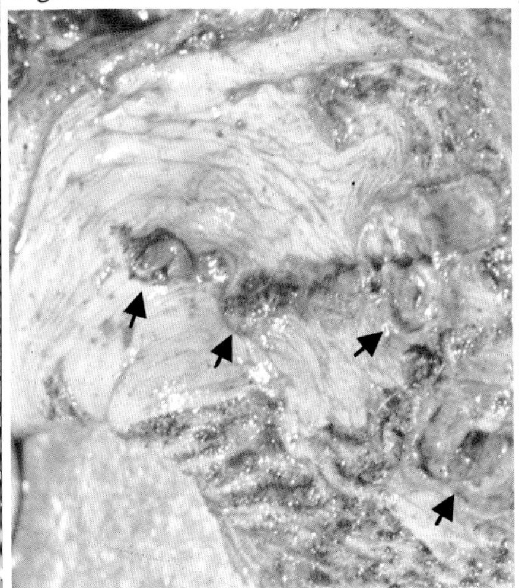

Fig. 201

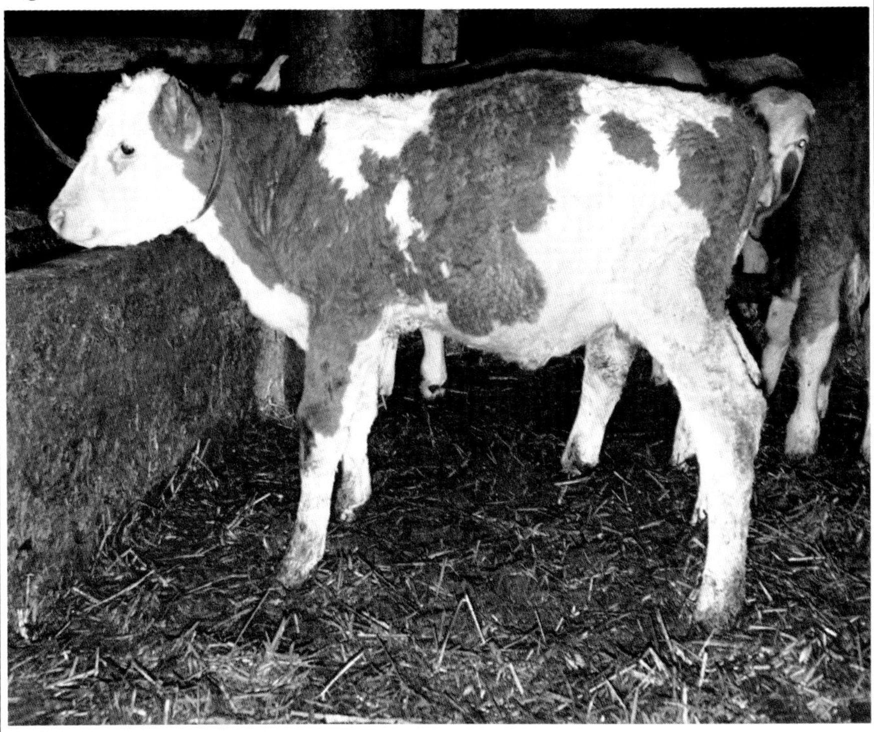

**Symptoms**

The calves show signs of severe colic. Arched back and kicking out with the legs are observed. Initially, faeces and urine are passed frequently and in small quantities.

**Diagnosis**

On palpation of the abdominal wall in the region of the costal arch a clear, sonorous sound is heard. This type of tympany cannot be remedied by the introduction of a tube through the oesophagus.

**Treatment**

By injection of NOVALGIN or BUSCOPAN the smooth muscle spasms are relieved within a short period, enabling the gas to be released by eructation.
In persistent cases puncture of the abomasum is necessary.

*Fig. 199: Size ratio of rumen to abomasum in the different periods of life.*

*Fig. 200: Abomasum ulcers (arrows) in a calf: The mucosa has been destroyed. A bulging mucosal margin forms around the ulcer.*

*Fig. 201: Bloat and pain in the abdominal region may have various causes. A protrusion on the left-hand side is not always due to bloat of the rumen. In this calf the abomasum was displaced towards the left. This results in tympany which cannot be remedied by the introduction of a tube.*

# Nutrition-induced loss of hair

Fig. 202

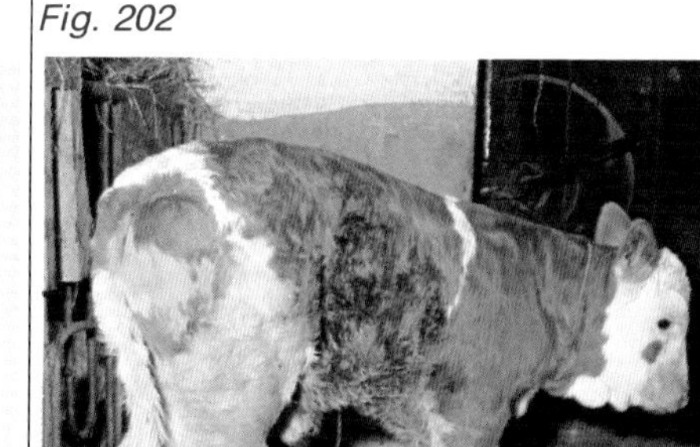

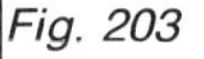

Fig. 203

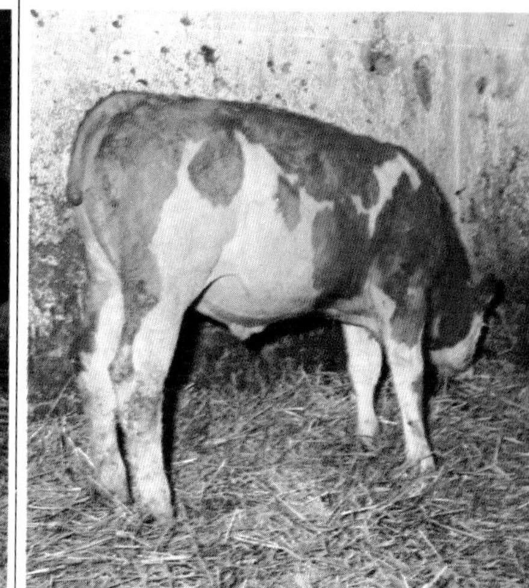

**Term**

The condition of the calf's coat is a reflection of its state of health. A smooth, shining coat with a good colour is a sign of good housing and feeding. Inadequate feeding, particularly of incompatible fats, may cause changes in the coat and loss of hair (alopecia).

**Incidence**

Nutrition-induced loss of hair occurs from the third week of life onwards. Calves receiving milk substitutes or skimmed milk with added fat are affected if the composition of the fats is incompatible.

As soon as the compartmental stomach system has developed, the fats are converted by the bacteria present in the rumen into a form that can be absorbed by the calf. In rearing calves, nutrition-induced alopecia is therefore rarely seen. However, it occurs more frequently in fattening calves, if these animals are fed exclusively on milk, which slows down the development of the first three stomach compartments.

**Causes**

The following non-milk fat constituents are the most common causes of nutrition-induced loss of hair:

- Proportion of cetine 2% or more.
- Oilseed fats, more than 3.5% (maize germ oil, soya bean oil, cotton seed oil, palm oil).
- Deteriorated fats as a result of incorrect storage (rancidity).
- Wrong distribution of fats due to insufficient emulsification.

Fig. 204

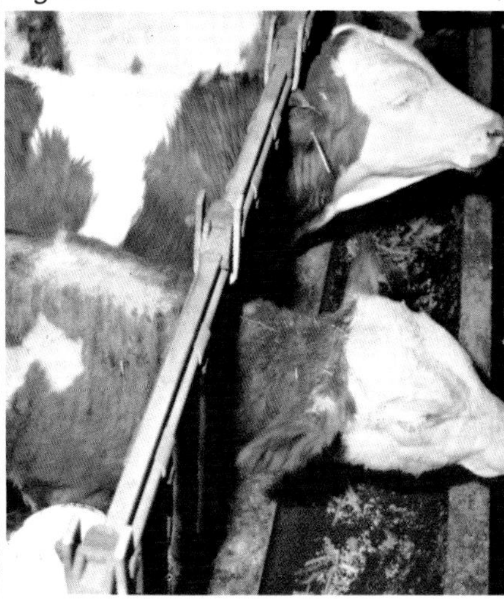

If the incompatible liquid is fed for 2 or 3 weeks, the first clinical symptoms appear. Increased greasiness of the coat, scale formation and a pronounced change in the smell of the skin are observed. A few days later, circumscribed loss of hair starts first on the head (in the region of the muzzle, the eyes and the ears), and later between the thighs and symmetrically on the extremities. The hairs can be pulled out in tufts together with the cornified outer skin layer. Completely bald patches of the skin of varying size and irregular circumscription are seen. The remaining skin is unchanged. Listlessness and diarrhoea may occur in addition to fat intolerance. Cases of death are possible.

**Symptoms**

The diagnosis must be established by excluding other skin disorders. The most important characteristics of similar conditions are as follows:

**Diagnosis**

**Similar symptoms**

- Trichophytosis (ringworm): Circular bald patches with asbestos-like desquamations.
- Mange: Strong itching, thickening of the skin; demonstration of mange mites in skin scrapings.
- Lice: Itching; broken-off hairs; demonstration of lice and nits.
- Congenital baldness: Present at birth.
- Poisoning with heavy metals: Loss of hair on the entire body surface. Haemorrhages in the subcutis. Central nervous disorders.

*Fig. 202: Loss of hair due to fat intolerance in a sucking calf: Bald patches of irregular circumscription have formed on the head and the thighs.*

*Fig. 203: Skin changes of a rearing calf following the application of an incompatible disinfectant in high concentration.*

*Fig. 204: Calf of Fig. 203 (in the foreground), compared with a calf of the same group which was not sprayed with the disinfectant.*

An immediate change of feed will arrest the loss of hair. For further feeding a milk substitute of low fat content and suitable fat composition should be used. This is then followed by a gradual change to a milk substitute with the high fat content required for fattening.
Treatment may be supported by injections of PERLACAR (10 ml per calf subcutaneously, two injections at an interval of one week).

**Treatment**

## Cerebrocortical necrosis

Fig. 205

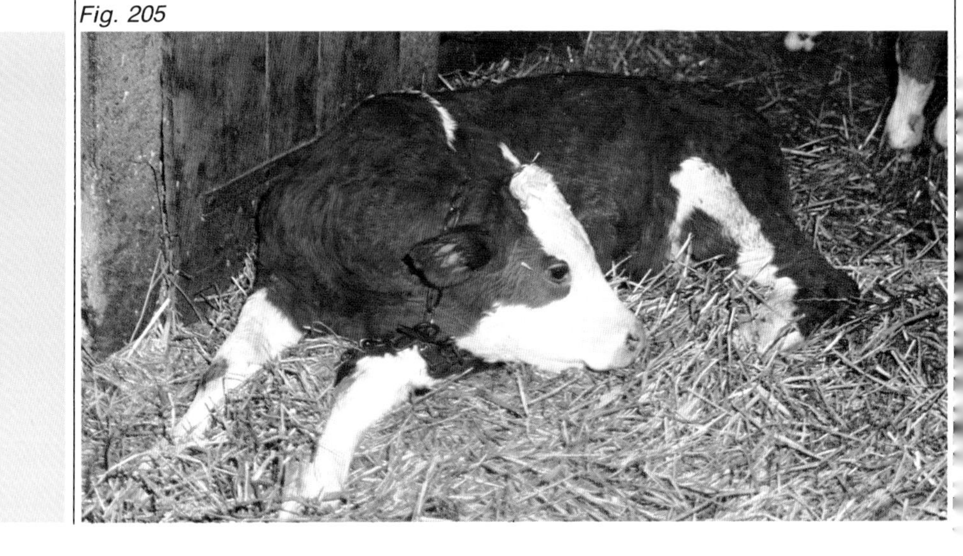

**Term**

Cerebrocortical necrosis is a non-infectious metabolic disorder. Changes in the cerebral cortex which are caused by vitamin $B_1$ deficiency lead to disorders of the central nervous system.

**Incidence**

The view, held in the past, that cattle obtain all the vitamin $B_1$ they need from the flora of the rumen, is no longer tenable, given today's requirements and modern feeding methods. Easily digestible high-energy rations and unduly rapid change-over from milk digestion to roughage digestion, as is the practice in early weaning, favour vitamin $B_1$ deficiency. The feeding of good calf hay is important for the development of a healthy rumen flora.
Vitamin $B_1$ deficiency occurs as early as the 4th week of life, but is more frequently observed after the change-over to roughage.

**Cause**

Up to the age of 10 weeks (100 kg body-weight) calves need 5 mg vitamin $B_1$ daily. In older animals this requirement rises to 5–10 mg per 100 kg body-weight.
Vitamin $B_1$ is an essential biological substance in carbohydrate metabolism. It also has an important function in conduction in the nervous system. The central nervous system can function only if sufficient glucose – and vitamin $B_1$ as intermediary carrier (co-enzyme) – is available.

*Fig. 205: Cerebrocortical necrosis in its initial stage: Head turned to the side; stretched-out forelegs. After injection of vitamin $B_1$ the symptoms disappeared within a few hours.*

*Fig. 206: Advanced stage of cerebrocortical necrosis: Animal lying down on its side with stretched-out head and neck; fixed look. The animals tend to have bloat.*

*Fig. 206*

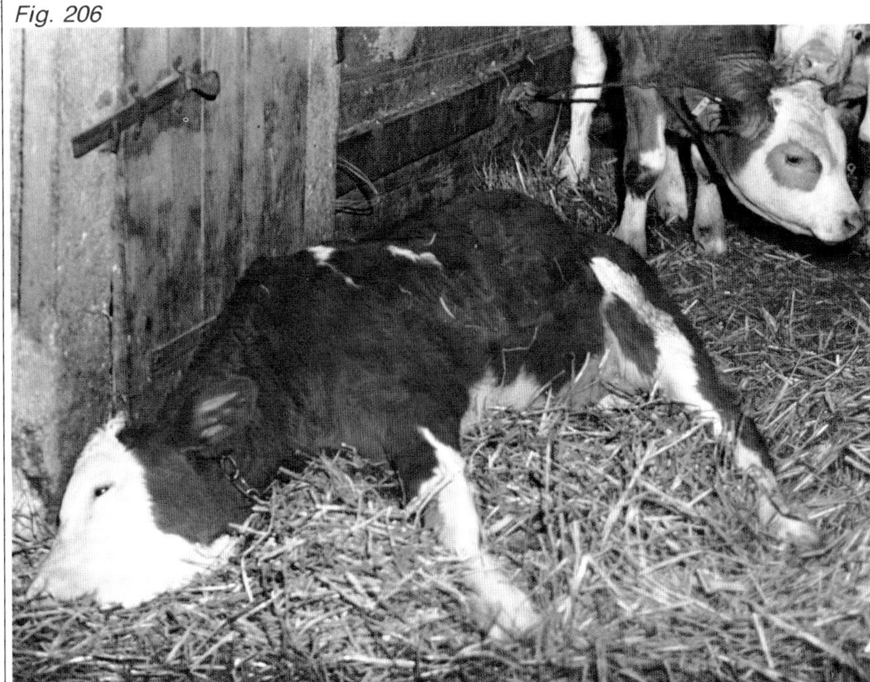

●●

**Cause**

Vitamin $B_1$ deficiency which finally leads to cerebrocortical necrosis may be due to the following causes:

- Feed does not contain sufficient vitamin $B_1$.
- Mould fungi and bacteria in the feed form enzymes (thiaminases) which destroy vitamin $B_1$.
- An abrupt change in feed disturbs the bacterial flora in the rumen, which then produces too little vitamin $B_1$.
- Sudden changes in temperature in the cattle house raise the vitamin $B_1$ requirement considerably (additional requirement of up to 20%). A change to slatted floors, for instance, may induce vitamin $B_1$ deficiency.

**Symptoms**

A disturbance of carbohydrate metabolism, caused by vitamin $B_1$ deficiency, produces a swelling of the cerebral cortex. This increases the pressure in the cranial cavity. Nerve cells in the brain die as a result (pressure necrosis) causing deficiency symptoms.

Initially the calves adopt a saw buck-like posture. They are dazed and easily frightened and stand apart from the group. Muscular tremor, at times associated with spasms, impaired vision and knocking against obstacles are observed. Occasionally attacks of acute mania are seen whereby the head is stretched upwards and backwards. The animals have a staggering gait.

In the terminal stage, the calves lie down on the side with their legs stretched out and performing "rowing" movements. If treatment is not carried out in time, the animals die within 2 or 3 days.

**Diagnosis**

If calves and young cattle show central nervous disorders, vitamin $B_1$ deficiency and cerebrocortical necrosis should be suspected.

As an immediate measure, vitamin $B_1$ should always be injected in high dosage. This treatment also has "diagnostic" value because any improvement seen after the injection of vitamin $B_1$ will indicate the presence of vitamin $B_1$ deficiency.

In the living animal the diagnosis is confirmed by determining the blood levels of pyruvic acid, lactic acid and glucose (cf. Fig. 207).

The autopsy of animals that have died of the disease, reveals yellow patchy changes in the cerebral cortex as well as an accumulation of blood in the meninx. Under the microscope, liquefaction of nerve cells (necroses) may be seen.

**Similar symptoms**

Diseases associated with central nervous disorders should be differentiated from cerebrocortical necrosis. Such diseases include rabies, listeriosis, furazolidone poisoning and ISTME. The most important distinguishing characteristics of these diseases are as follows:

- Rabies: Profuse salivation, bloat, sudden collapse.
- Listeriosis: Raised body temperature and difficulty in breathing.
- Vitamin E/selenium deficiency: Pale appearance of mucosae, muscular weakness, haematuria.
- ISTME (hypersomnia): Raised body temperature, no response to vitamin $B_1$ injection.

*Fig. 207*

| Blood levels |
|---|
| Lactic acid |
| Pyruvic acid |
| Glucose |

## Treatment

Treatment is likely to be successful only in the early stage. 0.5 to 1 g of vitamin $B_1$ should be injected. On the following two days, half the initial dose should be given.

As complementary treatment, roughage and medicated feed with a high vitamin $B_1$ content has proved of value.

If the cerebral changes are advanced, disorders of the central nervous system will remain.

*Fig. 208*

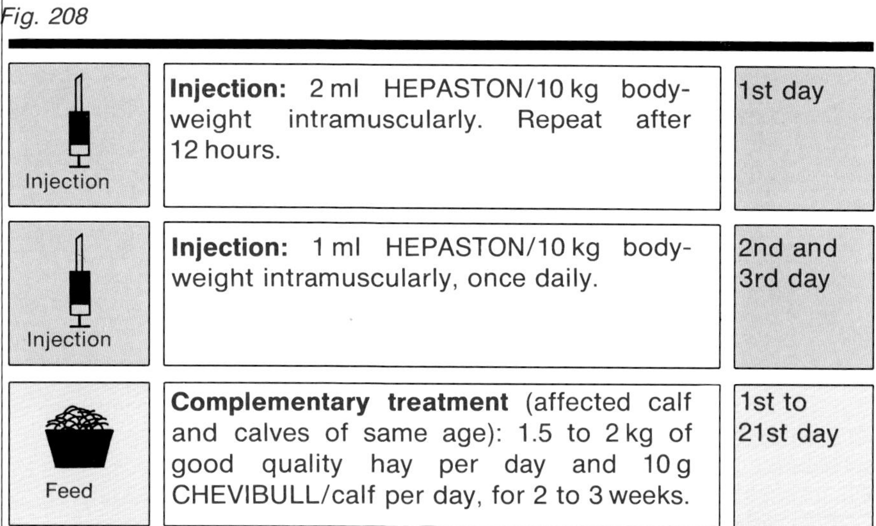

| | | |
|---|---|---|
| Injection | **Injection:** 2 ml HEPASTON/10 kg bodyweight intramuscularly. Repeat after 12 hours. | 1st day |
| Injection | **Injection:** 1 ml HEPASTON/10 kg bodyweight intramuscularly, once daily. | 2nd and 3rd day |
| Feed | **Complementary treatment** (affected calf and calves of same age): 1.5 to 2 kg of good quality hay per day and 10 g CHEVIBULL/calf per day, for 2 to 3 weeks. | 1st to 21st day |

*Fig. 208: Treatment schedule for cerebrocortical necrosis.*

| Healthy animal | Cerebrocortical necrosis |
|---|---|
| 12 mg/100 ml | 240 mg/100 ml |
| 0.6-1 mg/100 ml | 5.5 mg/100 ml |
| 50 mg/100 ml > | 200 mg/100 ml |

*Fig. 207: Summary of blood levels which may be useful in the diagnosis of cerebrocortical necrosis.*

## Prevention

Feeding appropriate to ruminants (hay, straw), vitamin $B_1$ supplements via medicated feed and avoiding sudden changes in feed, will help to counteract the development of cerebrocortical necrosis. Medicated feed (CHEVIBULL) should be given for a period of 2 to 3 weeks at the end of the weaning phase and when the animals are re-housed on slatted floors. Fattening calves that have been purchased need to be given a medicated feed with an appropriate vitamin $B_1$ content.

# Vitamin E/Selenium Deficiency

Fig. 209

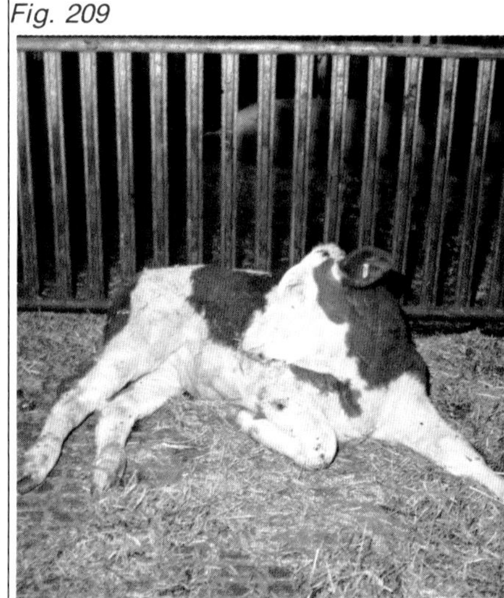

Fig. 210

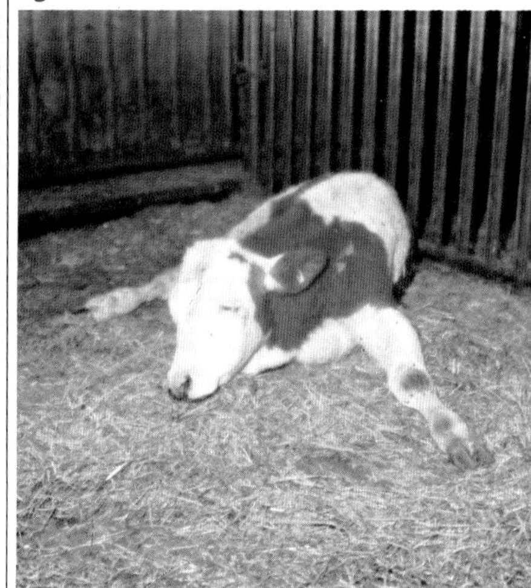

**Term**

Vitamin E has the capacity to protect feedstuffs with a high content of unsaturated fatty acids from being destroyed by oxidation. In this way the vitamin E contained in the fodder is used up and is no longer available to the animal.

There is a close correlation between vitamin E and the trace element selenium. The two substances have a mutual "saving" effect, but cannot replace each other.

Vitamin E deficiency in the feed ration can cause changes in the cardiac and skeletal muscles. These are known as white muscle disease or "white meat" disease.

**Incidence**

If deteriorated milk substitutes (inadequate or excessively long storage) are fed during calf fattening, white muscle disease is seen with increasing frequency.

If the calf is fed by its mother or another lactating cow, this condition will occur only if the vitamin E and selenium supply of the cows is grossly inadequate. In some areas, the soil is poor in selenium leading to a deficiency in the basic fodder (hay). The vitamin E content of all feedstuffs steadily decreases with storage.

**Cause**

If milk substitutes are fed which contain too many unsaturated fatty acids in large quantities, vitamin E deficiency symptoms appear. If milk substitutes are stored for too long or incorrectly, the fats decay and peroxides are formed.

Fig. 212

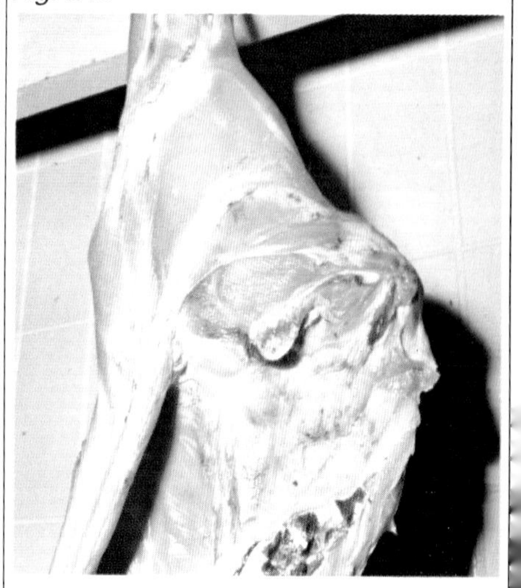

Fig. 211

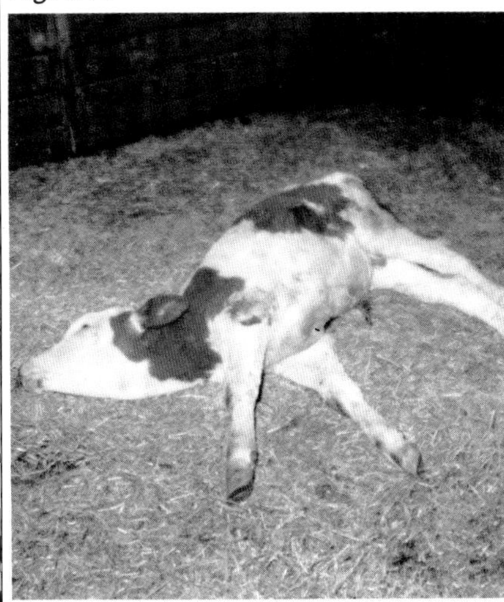

The daily requirement of the calf is 20 mg vitamin E and 0.25 mg selenium.

**Symptoms**

This deficiency manifests itself particularly in muscular weakness. Stiff gait and arched back are usually the first signs of muscular changes in this condition. The animals frequently lie down and have an unsteady gait. The extent of the disorder depends on the group of muscles affected. With severe vitamin E/selenium deficiency, the animals lie down permanently on the chest or side and show nervous disorders.

**Diagnosis**

The animals tire very quickly. They pass bright red to dark brown urine, since the cell disintegration leads to increased myohaematin levels in the blood. The serum level of vitamin E is greatly reduced:

Affected animal – 0.04 mg vitamin E/100 ml serum
Normal animal – 0.15 mg vitamin E/100 ml serum.

The muscles of animals that have died or have been slaughtered show dark red patches with greyish white foci (necrotic foci). The carcass meat of such animals has a light pale colour and is classed as low-quality meat.
If vitamin E/selenium deficiency occurs, the milk substitute used should be checked (age, storage, degree of freshness and type of fats used).

**Treatment**

For the treatment of this condition, vitamin E and selenium are given by injection and via the feed. Animals with nervous disorders should be given vitamin $B_1$ in addition.

Fig. 213

| | | |
|---|---|---|
| Injection | **Immediate treatment** of the affected animal: 5 ml VITAMIN E + SELEN per calf injected intramuscularly without delay. After 24 and 48 hours give a further 2 ml per calf. | 1st to 3rd day |
| Fodder/ Fluid | **Treatment of stock:** 10 g MULTIVITAMIN R 12/calf per day to be stirred into the drinking fluid or admixed to the fodder. | 1st to 10th day |

**Prevention**

Commercially available milk substitutes with a fat content of 20% should contain at least 20 mg vitamin E per kg of dry substance.

*Figs. 209 to 211: vitamin E/selenium deficiency: Severe leg and muscle weakness with central nervous symptoms. As distinct from the very similar symptoms of vitamin $B_1$ deficiency, pale mucosae and urine with reddish discoloration are seen here.*

*Fig. 212: White carcass meat, classed as low-quality meat.*

*Fig. 213: Treatment schedule for vitamin E/selenium deficiency.*

## Coccidiosis

Fig. 214

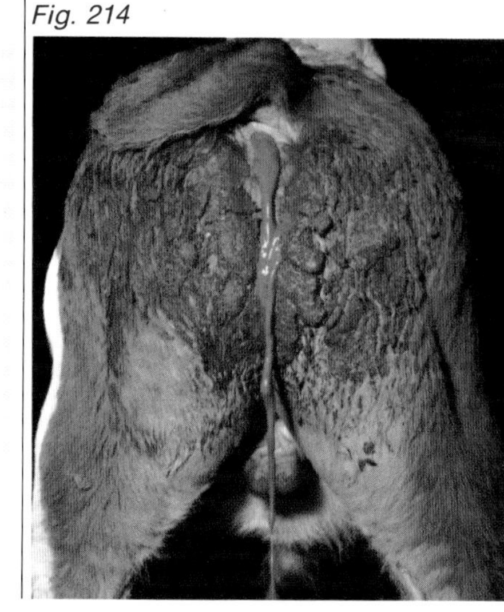

Fig. 215

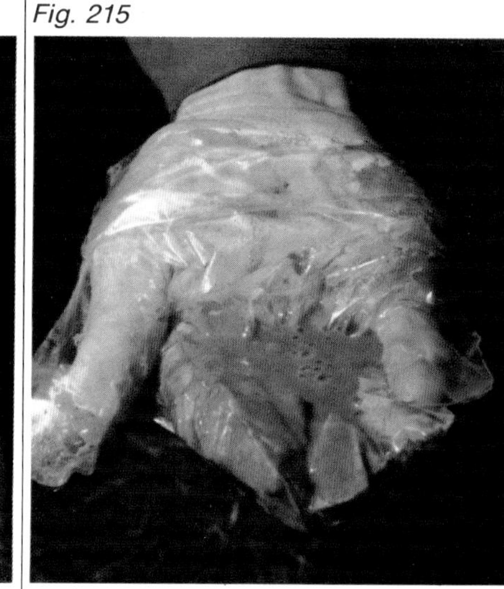

**Term**

Coccidiosis is an intestinal disease which is caused by monocellular parasites (protozoa). Severe infestation with coccidia leads to diarrhoea with bloody faeces, for which reason the disease is also known as "red dysentery".

**Incidence**

Coccidiosis occurs in all domestic animals. In cattle, it appears particularly at the age of 10 weeks to 2 years.

**Pathogen/ Cause**

The causative organisms, coccidia, are monocellular protozoa. In cattle, mainly the Eimeria species is found, particularly Eimeria bovis and Eimeria zürni.

**Importation/ Route of infection**

Infected animals pass coccidial oocysts in the faeces. These oocysts mature outside the animal organism into sporulated oocysts. In order to reach maturity outside the animal body, the oocysts require moisture, oxygen and warmth. Mature oocysts are taken up in the fodder or drinking-water and pass into the intestine. Their outer shell is dissolved and the sporozoites attack the intestinal mucosa. They multiply in the mucosal cells, at first asexually, and later sexually.

Fig. 216

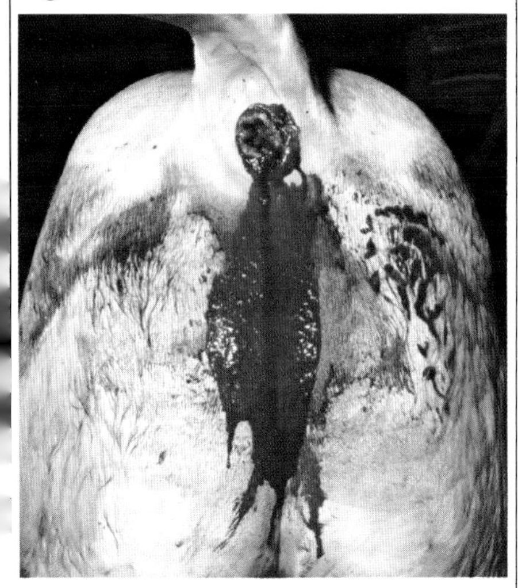

Fig. 217

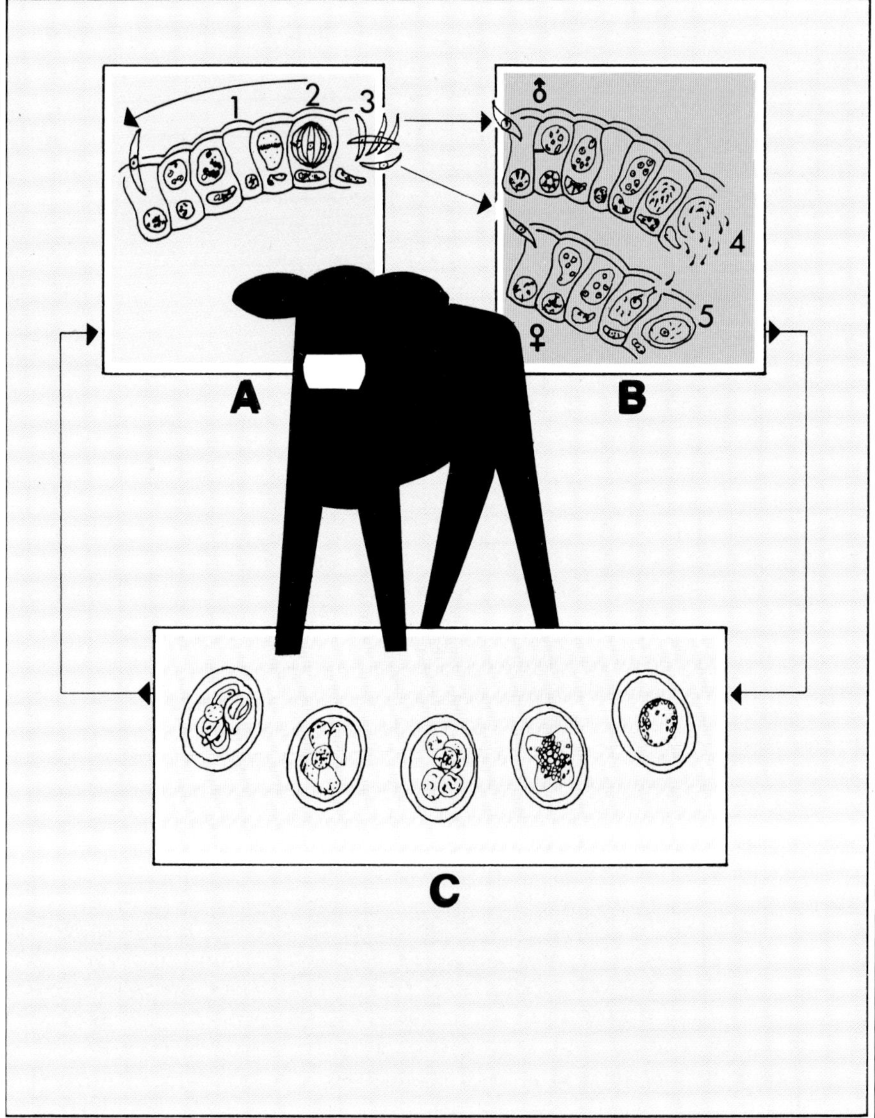


Importation / Route of infection

*Figs. 214 and 215: Coccidiosis. Thinly pappy, chocolate-coloured faeces, tending to be bubbly.*

*Fig. 216: Coccidiosis with severe bloody diarrhoea. An examination of the faeces does not reveal a corresponding number of coccidial oocysts in all cases.*

*Fig. 217: Life cycle of coccidia in cattle: A and B = endogenous development in the intestinal mucosa.*
*A = asexual reproduction (schizogony):*
*1-trophozoite*
*2-schizont*
*3-merozoite*
*B = sexual reproduction (gametogony):*
*4-microgamete*
*5-macrogamete*
*C = exogenous development in the environment: Maturation (sporulation) of the oocysts.*

Oocysts may remain infective for more than a year. Moist areas in cattle houses and on pastures offer favourable conditions for the development and survival of oocysts. Dry conditions and extremes of temperature (above + 40° C and below − 7° C) will quickly kill them off.

The course of the disease depends on the number of oocysts ingested and on the resistance of the animals. Diarrhoea occurs one or two days after ingestion of the oocysts. Initially, the faeces are thinly pappy to aqueous, then become mucoid with the admixture of some blood.

**Symptoms**

At the same time a progressive deterioration in the animals' general condition with symptoms like dullness, emaciation and drawn-in abdomen, is observed. The body temperature is not raised, but is in fact often below normal. In severe cases, the loss of blood leads to pale mucosae, and the loss water (dehydration as a result of diarrhoea) to desiccation of the body.

In the terminal stage, the animals are extremely weak (staggering gait; lying down all the time). If treatment is not instituted in time, death may ensue as early as after 3 days.

*Fig. 218*

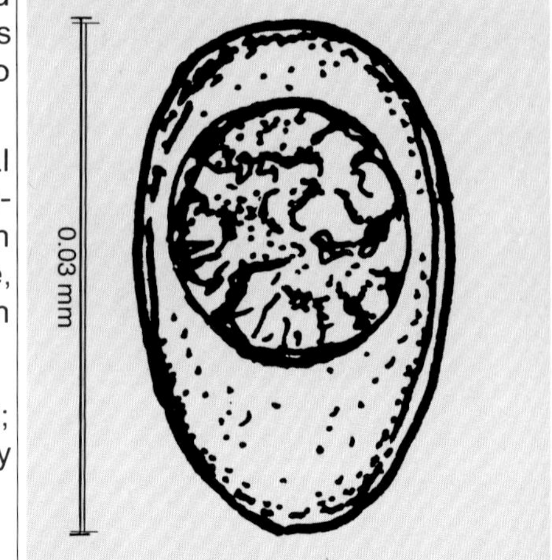


**Diagnosis**

Coccidiosis should be suspected if diarrhoea with the admixture of blood is observed in calves. A parasitological examination of the faeces will show if coccidial oocysts are present (cf. Fig. 374). However, the number of oocysts found does not necessarily give an indication of the severity of the disease, since oocysts are excreted irregularly and only in batches.

**Similar symptoms**

The diarrhoea seen in salmonellosis, poisoning, inappropriate diet and worm infestation resembles the diarrhoea observed in coccidiosis. Bacteriological and parasitological tests enable a differential diagnosis to be established (cf. pages 42 and 194).

**Treatment**

Sulphonamides are used for the treatment of coccidiosis. With persistent diarrhoea, electrolyte solutions should be given in addition. Together with sulphonamide therapy, hygienic measures are taken, e. g. moving animals to another grazing ground, keeping feeding and watering points dry and changing them repeatedly, dry litter and keeping water troughs clean.

Fig. 218: *Freshly excreted coccidial oocyst of cattle.*

*Fig. 219: Treatment schedule for coccidiosis.*

*Fig. 220: Measures for the prevention of coccidiosis.*

**Treatment**

*Fig. 219*

| | | |
|---|---|---|
| Given by mouth | **All animals of the stock:** 1 bolus BOVIBOL/150 kg body-weight per calf, to be given once. (Not to be administered to animals fed on milk) | Imme-diately |
| Given by mouth | **Calves with persistent diarrhoea:** 2 litres of electrolyte solution with 90 g ELRISAL, to be given 2 or 3 times daily. | 1st and 2nd day |
| Fodder | **Follow-up treatment:** 10 g RP. CHEVIBULL/calf per day, for 3 weeks. | 1st to 21st day |

With low-grade coccidial infestation without symptoms, hygienic measures will be sufficient to interrupt the development cycle of the infection and to prevent the outbreak of the disease.

**Prevention and disinfection**

The basis of all prevention is an improvement of hygienic conditions in the cattle house or on the pasture. Fig. 220 summarises the most important preventive measures in coccidiosis.

*Fig. 220*

| Cattle house | Pasture |
|---|---|
| ■ Keep drinking troughs free from faeces and clean regularly.<br>■ For deep litter house, provide dry bedding; avoid moist places. | ■ Reinforce and immobilise drinking troughs; avoid moist feeding and watering points.<br>■ Clean water troughs regularly, remove faeces.<br>■ Change position of movable drinking troughs daily. |

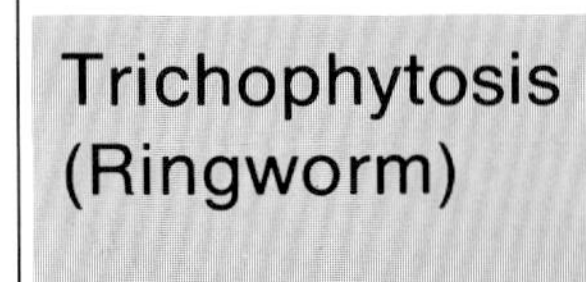

# Trichophytosis (Ringworm)

*Fig. 221*

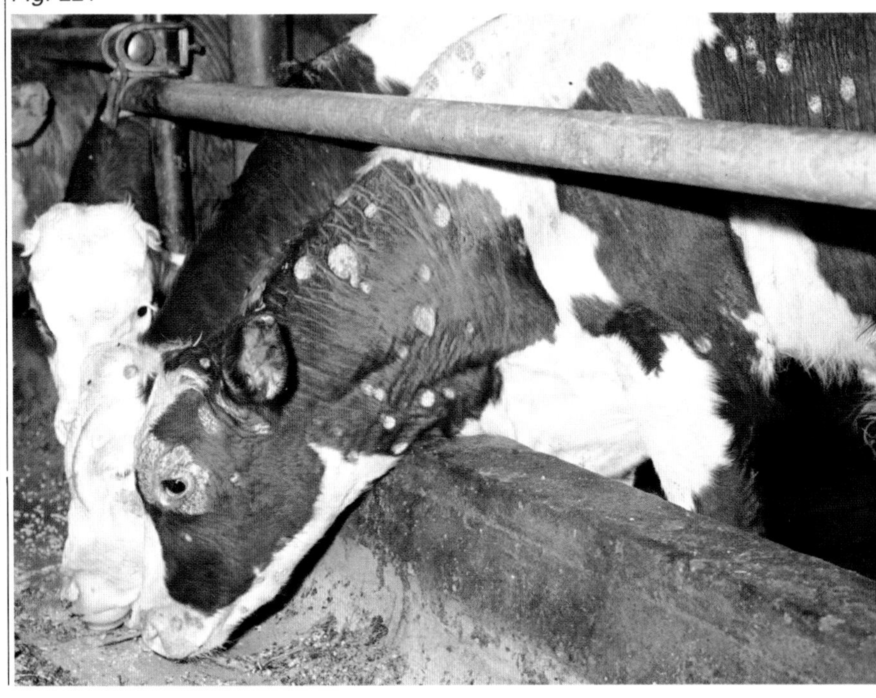

**Incidence**

Being the most common skin disease in calves and young cattle, trichophytosis is often seen on rearing farms. Adult cattle are rarely affected.

Due to the higher degree of air humidity, ringworm occurs more frequently in winter when the animals are kept in the cattle house. When they are put out to graze, the condition usually heals without treatment. However, on fattening or rearing farms the disease may be observed throughout the year.

**Term**

Trichophytosis is an infectious disease of the outer skin layers producing typical skin changes. It is caused by fungi and is also known as ringworm.

Ringworm may be transmitted to man, particularly children.

**Pathogen / Cause**

Ringworm is caused by thread fungi (Trichophyton verrucosum) which penetrate into the outer skin layers where they multiply. The fungi develop highly resistant permanent stages (spores) which remain infective for years in dry places (wood; places against which the animals rub themselves).

*Fig. 221: Trichophytosis distributed over the entire body (advanced stage): Circular bald, dry patches with asbestos-like crusts.*

*Fig. 222: Incipient trichophytosis on the head: Round bald patches with reddening of the skin.*

*Fig. 223: Growth of trichophyton fungi on a special culture medium.*

*Fig. 222*

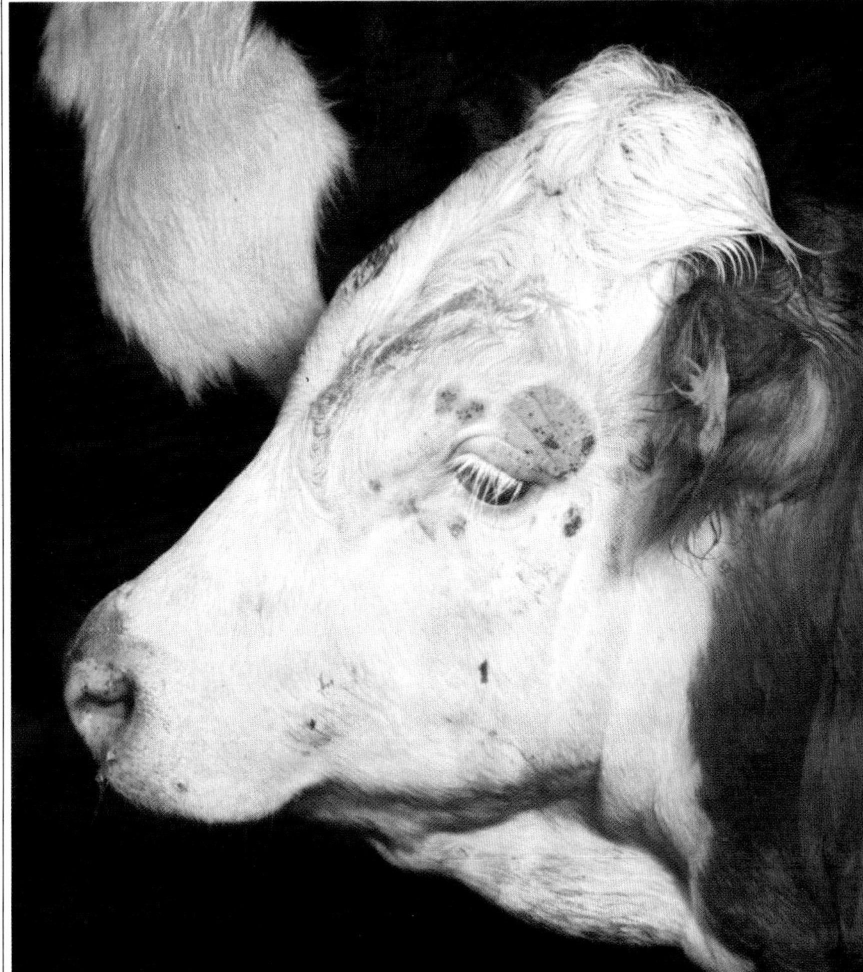

*Fig. 223*

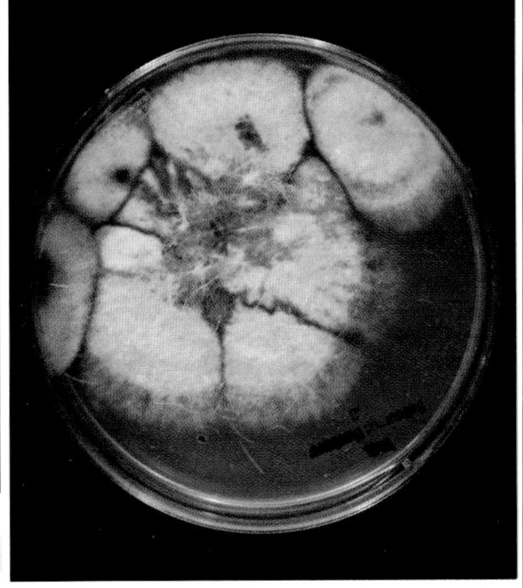

**Importation / Route of infection**

The disease is mainly transmitted by contact between the animals. Indirect transmission (walls of cattle house, implements) is possible. Furthermore, lice, flies or biting lice may be regarded as vectors of the spores. They spread the infection particularly on animals already affected. Trichophytosis spreads through transmission by these parasites to other animal species (change of host). Man may also act as a carrier (cf. Fig. 224).

*Fig. 224*

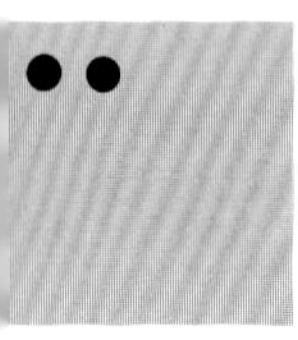

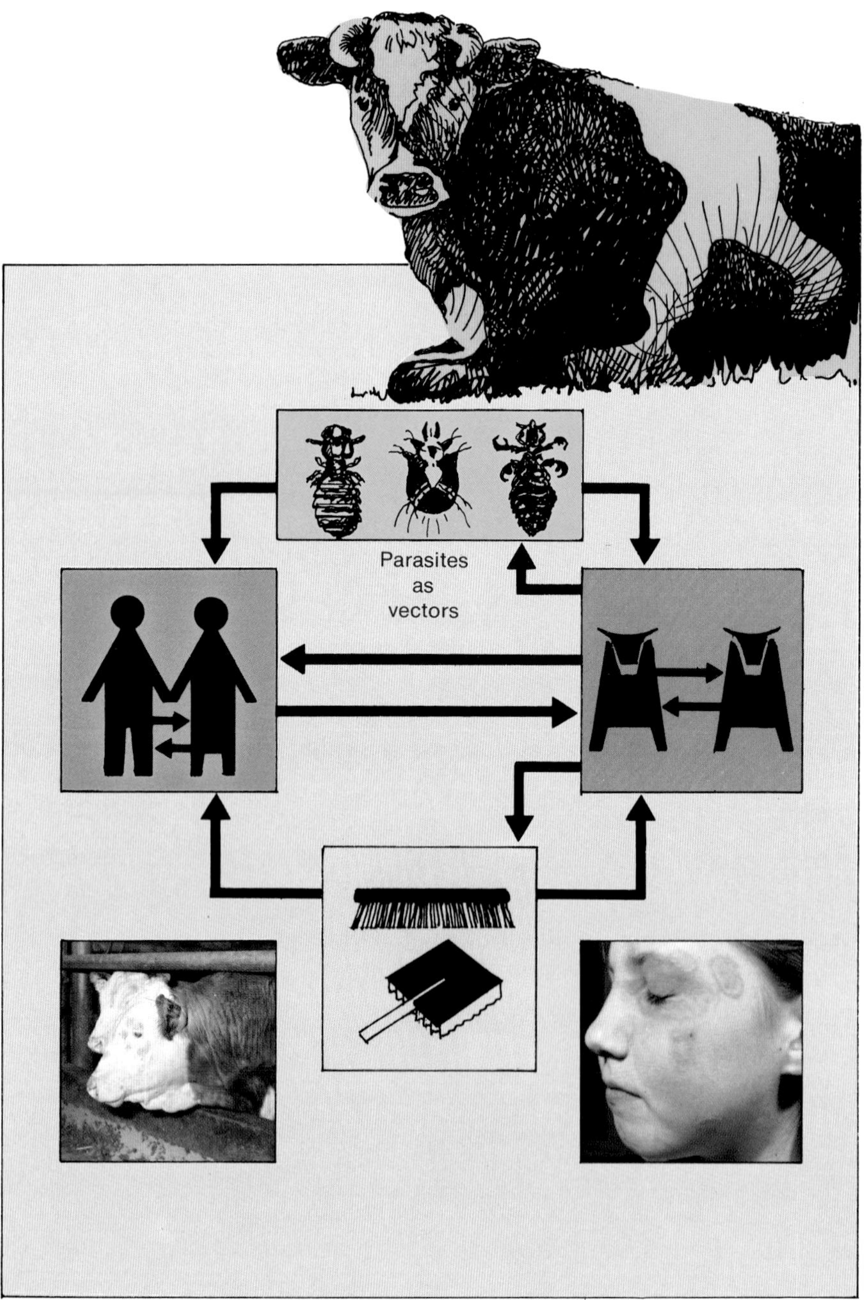


*Fig. 224: Possibilities of the transmission of trichophytosis: Direct transmission from animal to animal and from animal to man.*

*Indirect transmission by biting lice, mites and lice and by cleaning utensils, cattle house implements and equipment is possible.*

*Figs. 225 to 227: Trichophytosis on the bridge of the nose, the back of the head and the corner of the mouth.*

Fig. 225

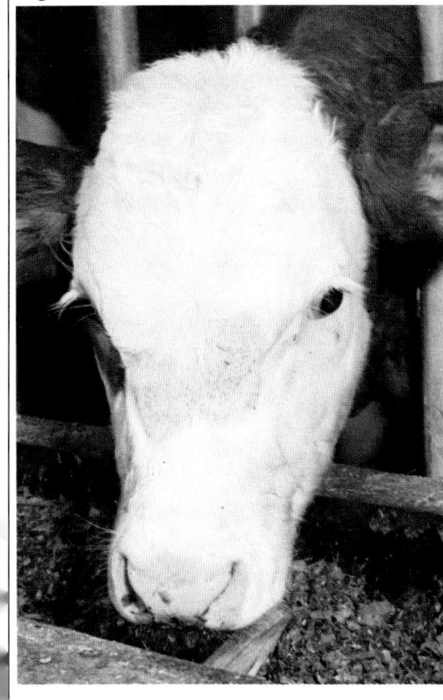

Fig. 226

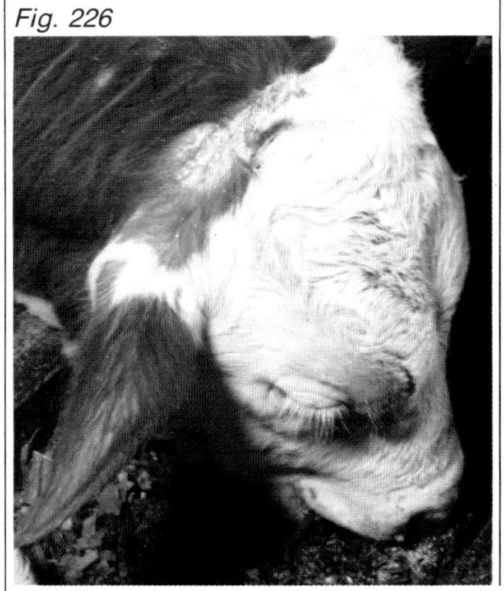

Fig. 227

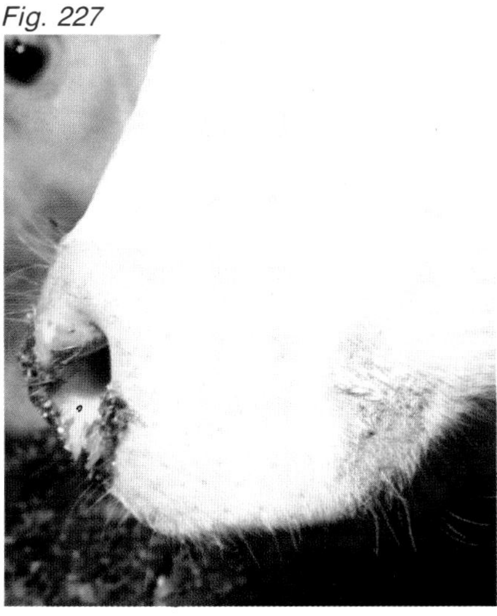

**Importation / Route of infection**

The spores germinate on the skin and the resulting mycelium penetrates into the hair follicles. The hairs break off and fall out. The mycelium continues to grow in the skin forming circular lesions.

In our experience, the nutritional state of the animal has no bearing on the incidence of the infection. Lice infestation and mange favour the spread of trichophytosis.

**Symptoms**

Initially the head, particularly the orbital margin, and the neck are affected. Ringworm may then spread over the entire body surface, but rarely involves the lower extremities or the abdomen.

Approx. 4 weeks after the infection, nodules, initially of lentil size, are formed on the skin where the hairs stand on end. At these sites the hair follicles are inflamed. The hairs break off leaving round bald patches. At first these patches show some redness. Eventually a dry asbestos-like crust remains on the skin. The circular spread of the infection whereby the lesions heal evenly with hair growing again in the centre, results in annular changes. Given favourable climatic conditions, the disease may heal spontaneously after 3 to 5 months, even if no treatment is carried out. During the infection the animal develops lasting immunity. This is why the disease is rarely seen in older animals.

With fresh infections and where no other pathogens are involved, there is no itching. In the healing phase or with concomitant parasite infestation (lice, mange mites), restlessness due to itching is observed.

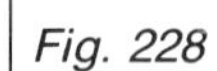

**Diagnosis**

The disease can clearly be recognised from the typical skin changes. In the laboratory, the diagnosis can be confirmed by protracted culturing of the pathogen and by microscopic examination.

**Similar symptoms**

The condition may possibly be confused with squamous eczema, skin allergies and mange. Differentiation from mange and infestation with lice is possible by demonstration of the parasite (cf. pages 205 and 211).

*Fig. 228*

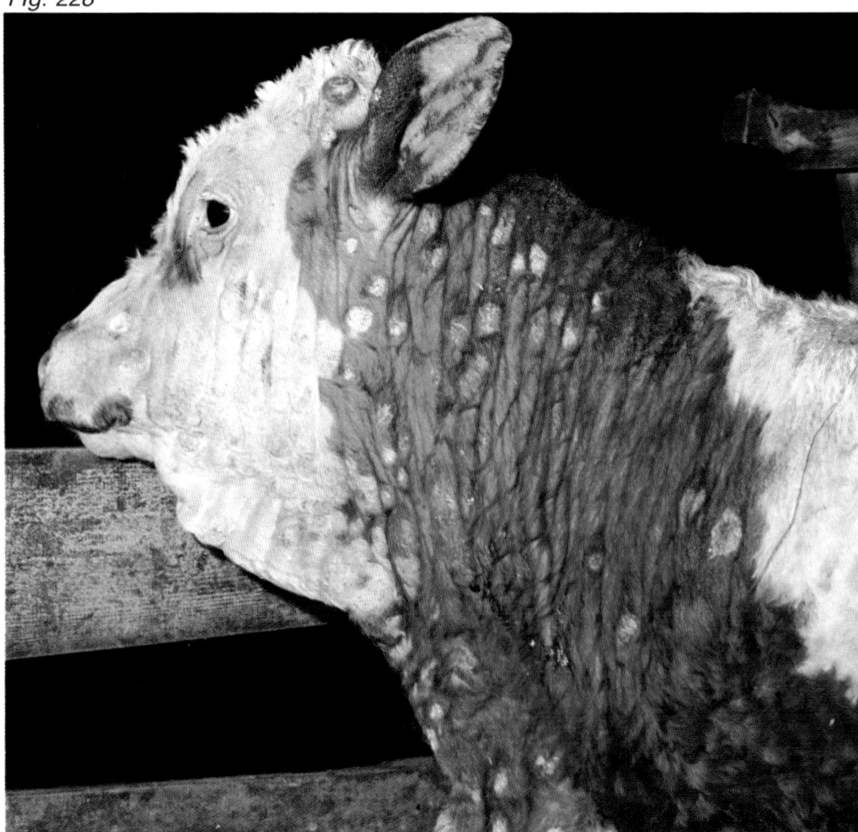

*Fig. 229*

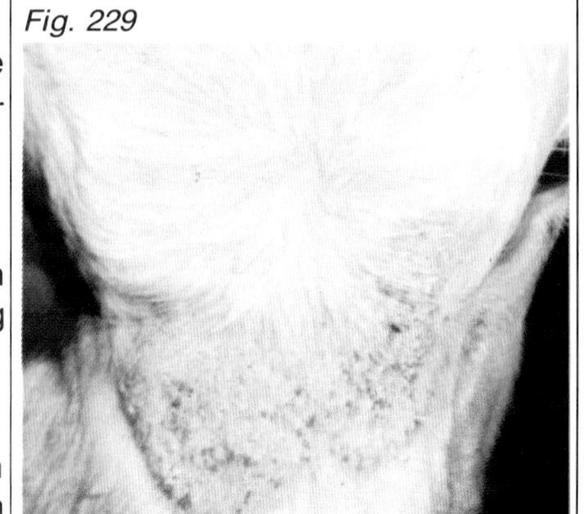

Fig. 230

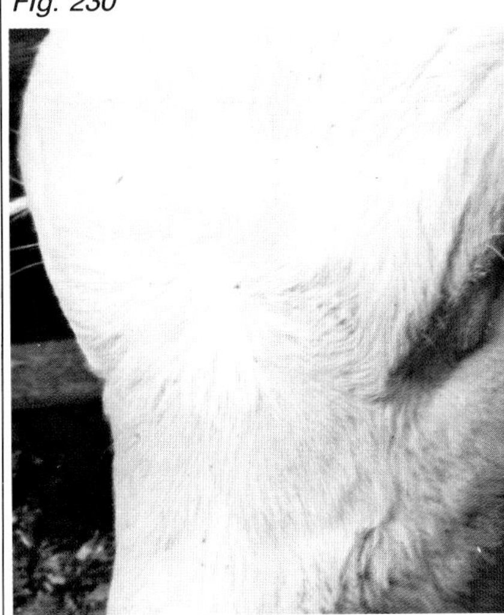

Treatment is carried out by partial or total ablution with special fungicidal products (DEFUNGIT, DERMA-TRICHEX). It should be repeated after 3 to 5 days.

The animals may be sprayed with suitable spraying equipment, but experience has shown that brushing-in enhances the effect of the fungicidal product. At the same time the cattle house and implements should be disinfected after cleaning, using disinfectants (CHEVI 45) or the medicinal solution employed for ablution.

If larger groups of animals are affected, treatment with GRISEOFULVIN, given in the fodder, is indicated. We also prefer this treatment in unfavourable weather conditions and in poor controlled environment.

The products mentioned are only effective against fungi. In the event of mixed infections (lice, mange mites) appropriate additional treatment must be carried out (cf. treatment of mange).

**Treatment**

Fig. 231

| | | |
|---|---|---|
| 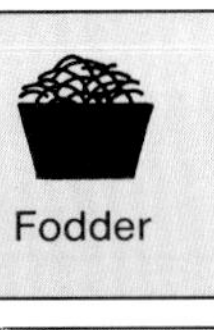 Fodder | **Treatment of animal groups,** particularly in case of unfavourable controlled environment: 10 g GRISEOFULVIN/100 kg bodyweight, to be given for 7 days in the fodder. | 1st to 7th day |
| 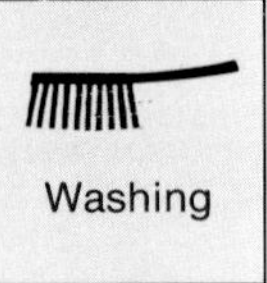 Washing | **Affected calves – treatment of individual animals:** Brush in 0.5% DEFUNGIT solution or 5% DERMA-TRICHEX. Repeat after 5 days. | 1st and 5th day |
| 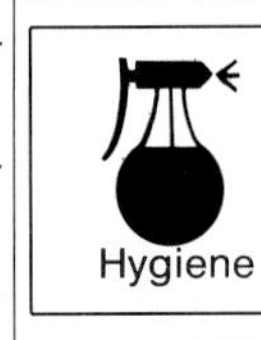 Hygiene | **Disinfection:** Cleaning and disinfection of cattle house (walls of pens) and implements with 2% CHEVI 45 solution. | 1st day |

*Fig. 228: Mixed infestation with lice and trichophytosis. The lice contribute to the distribution of the fungal spores over the entire body surface.*

*Figs. 229 and 230: Extensive trichophytosis on the bridge of the nose before and after treatment (approx. 3 weeks).*

*Fig. 230 still shows a faint redness. The hair is growing again.*

*Fig. 231: Treatment schedule for trichophytosis.*

Fig. 232

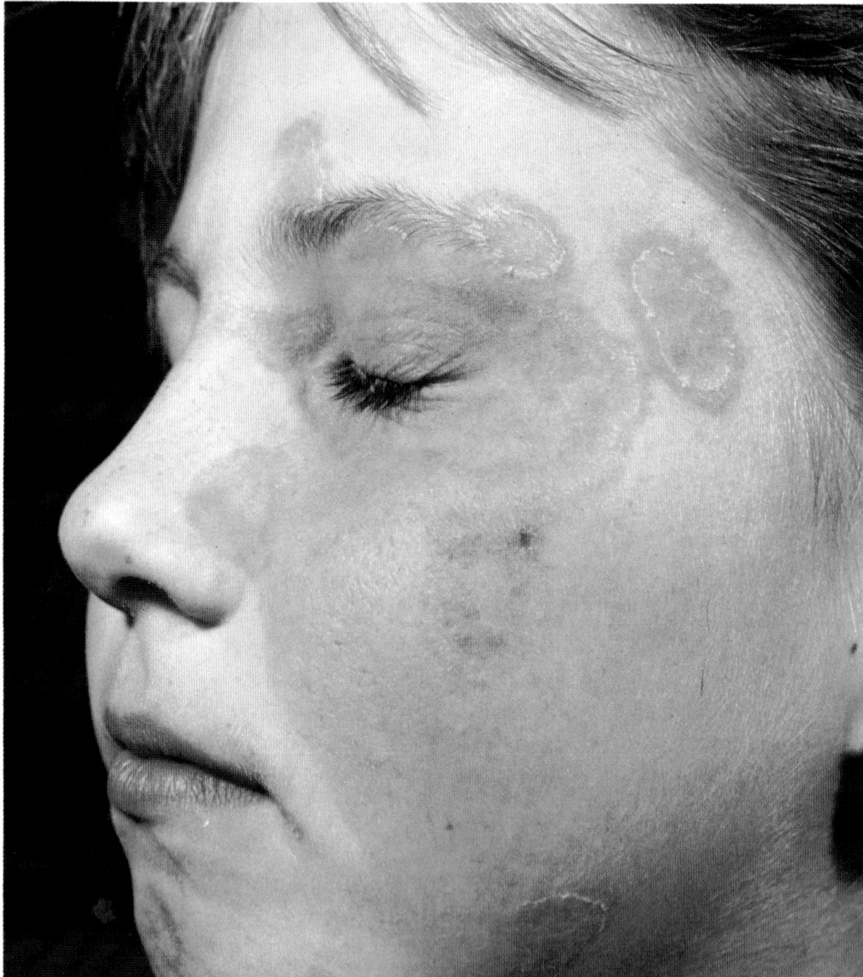

Fig. 233

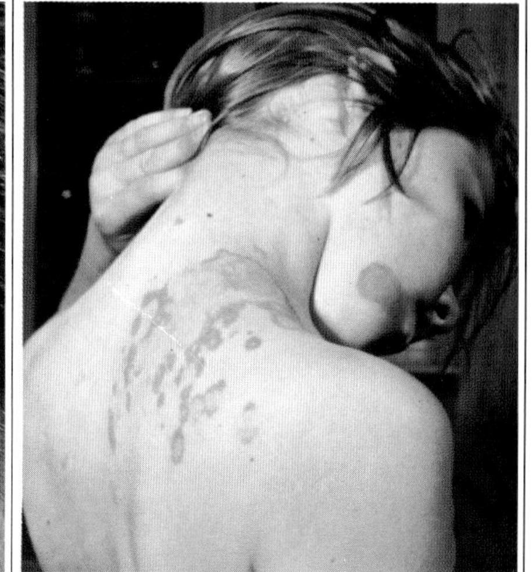

Fig. 234

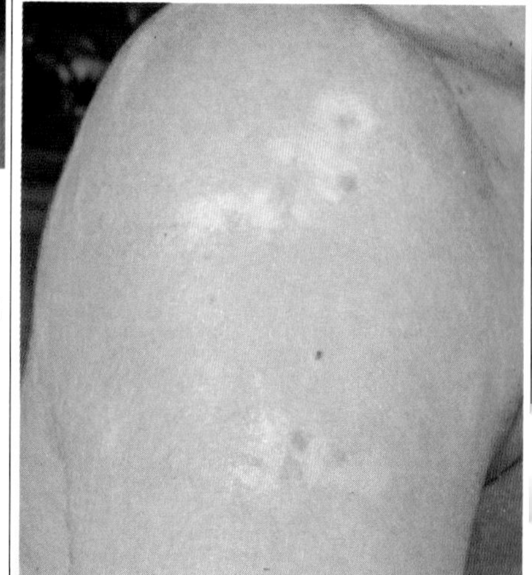

**Danger to animals and livestock farmers**

Trichophytosis is often transmitted from cattle to other domesticated animals (horses, dogs, cats) and to man. Children are particularly at risk. Medical treatment is required in the event of infestation.

*Figs. 232 and 233: Trichophytosis in man. The annular distribution of the mycelia, which gave rise to the name ringworm, is clearly visible.*

*Fig. 234: Trichophytosis on the arm, in the process of healing.*

*Fig. 235: Jaundice: Pronounced yellow discoloration of the conjunctiva and sclera in copper poisoning.*

*Fig. 236: Trace element copper: Copper requirements and quantities causing poisoning.*

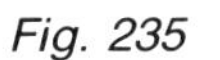

*Fig. 235*

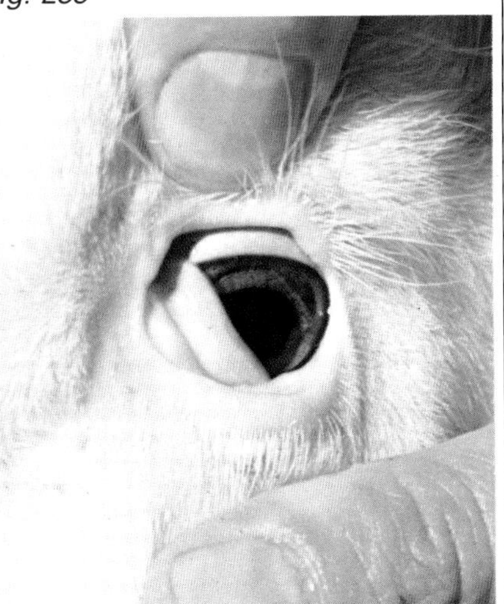

# Copper Poisoning

**Term**

The trace element copper plays a part in the formation of red blood cells. The pigmentation of the hair, the function of the central nervous system and the formation of bones are also influenced by copper.
If feedstuffs with excessively high copper content are fed or if copper-containing feedstuffs are given in unduly large quantities, symptoms of intoxication appear.

**Incidence**

Copper poisoning is usually observed when calves have received excessive quantities of copper in their feed over a prolonged period. Cattle with a fully developed compartmental stomach system require a higher copper content in the fodder than sucking calves being fed on milk. Calves are therefore more sensitive to excessive copper intake.

Copper requirements and quantities causing intoxication are shown in Fig. 236.

*Fig. 236*

| Age of the animals | Copper requirement | Copper intake leading to poisoning |
|---|---|---|
| Up to 12th week of life | 7 to 10 mg/day | more than 70 mg/day |
| Cattle with compartmental stomach system | 10 to 20 mg/kg dry substance | more than 250 mg/kg dry substance |

Fig. 237

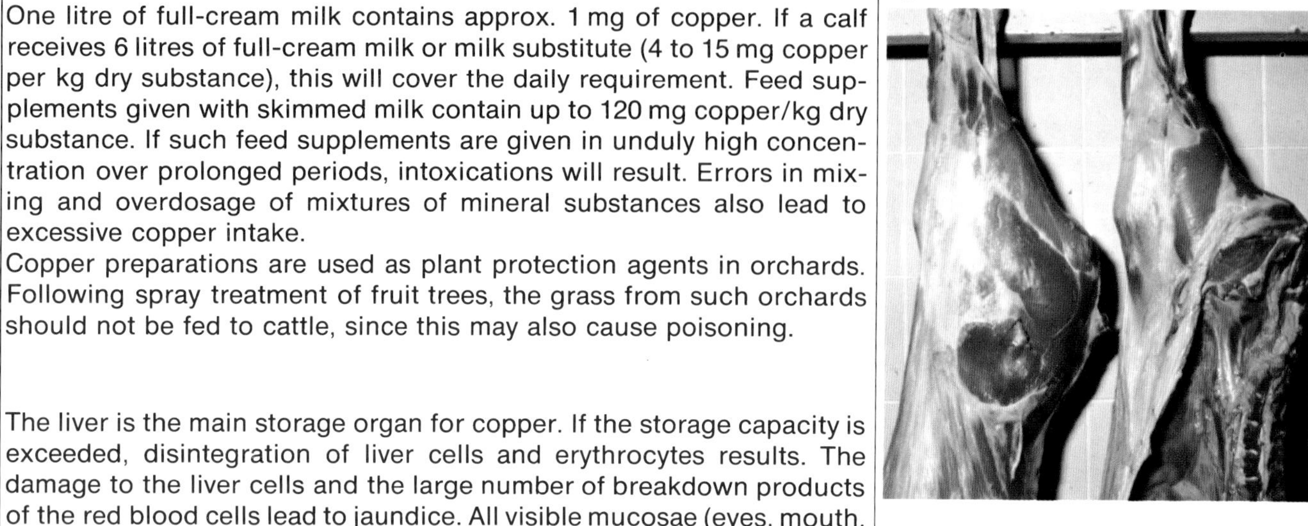

**Cause**

One litre of full-cream milk contains approx. 1 mg of copper. If a calf receives 6 litres of full-cream milk or milk substitute (4 to 15 mg copper per kg dry substance), this will cover the daily requirement. Feed supplements given with skimmed milk contain up to 120 mg copper/kg dry substance. If such feed supplements are given in unduly high concentration over prolonged periods, intoxications will result. Errors in mixing and overdosage of mixtures of mineral substances also lead to excessive copper intake.
Copper preparations are used as plant protection agents in orchards. Following spray treatment of fruit trees, the grass from such orchards should not be fed to cattle, since this may also cause poisoning.

**Symptoms**

The liver is the main storage organ for copper. If the storage capacity is exceeded, disintegration of liver cells and erythrocytes results. The damage to the liver cells and the large number of breakdown products of the red blood cells lead to jaundice. All visible mucosae (eyes, mouth, vagina) show a distinctly yellow discoloration (jaundice, icterus). The calves become dull and feed reluctantly. Their body-temperature rises; their urine shows a reddish colour. Timidity and convulsions often accompany the condition. A large number of affected animals die.

**Diagnosis**

If jaundice is observed in calves, the total copper quantity per animal and per day should be calculated and checked.
In dead animals, the diseased liver shows a copper content of more than 150 mg/kg fresh weight.

Fig. 238

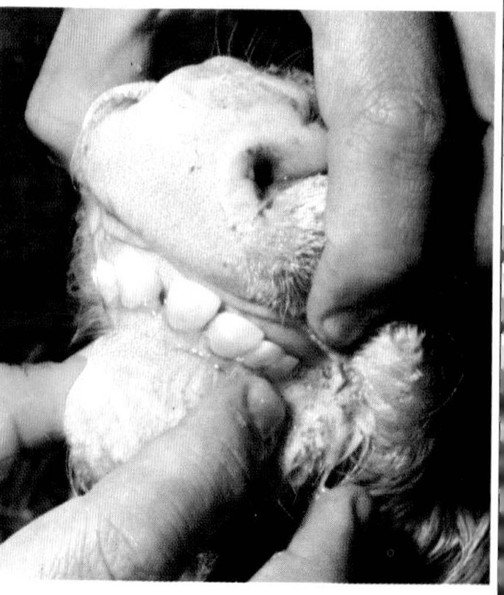

**Similar symptoms**

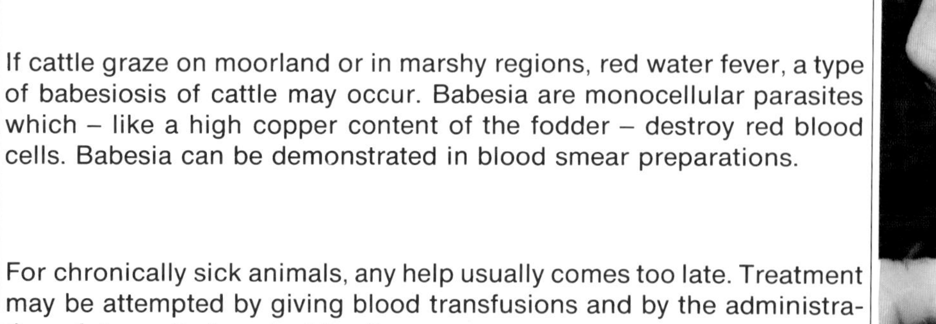

If cattle graze on moorland or in marshy regions, red water fever, a type of babesiosis of cattle may occur. Babesia are monocellular parasites which – like a high copper content of the fodder – destroy red blood cells. Babesia can be demonstrated in blood smear preparations.

**Treatment**

For chronically sick animals, any help usually comes too late. Treatment may be attempted by giving blood transfusions and by the administration of drugs that protect the liver.

In order to avoid any further cases of the disease, the correct copper concentration in the feedstuffs used is absolutely vital.

Fig. 239

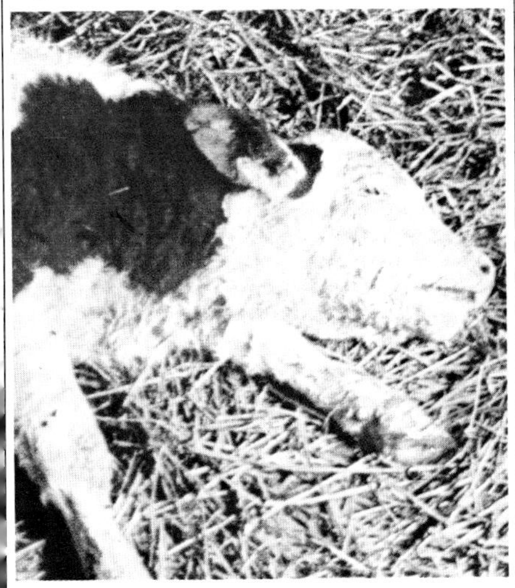

Fig. 240

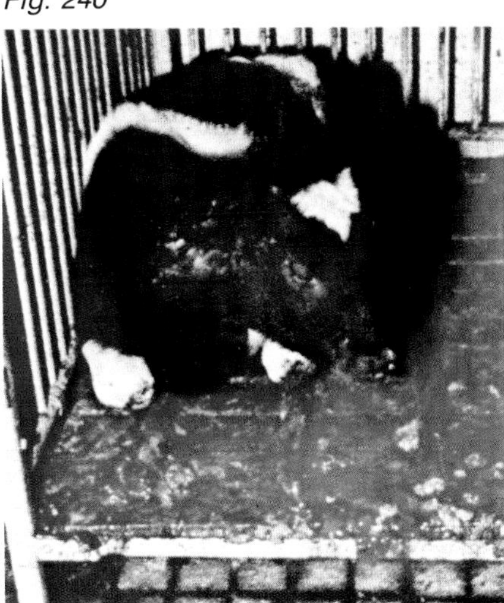

# Furazolidone poisoning

**Term**

Furazolidone used to be a permitted feed additive in many countries. In some countries this still applies today. Because of its efficacy in the intestine and its favourable price, Furazolidone is used in the treatment of diarrhoea (salmonellosis and E. coli infection). The drawback with this antibiotic is that it causes intoxication in the calf, even if it is only slightly overdosed or if it is given for too long a period. This is why inappropriate treatment of diarrhoea in calves with furazolidone-containing drugs gives rise to intoxication on quite a number of occasions.

**Cause**

If given for prolonged periods, relatively small quantities of furazolidone cause chronic poisoning. Acute intoxication is observed if very high doses are given for a few days.

Fig. 241

| Dosage | Duration | Manifestations | |
|---|---|---|---|
| 4–8 mg/ kg body-weight | for several weeks | Nervous deficiency symptoms. Punctiform or more extensive haemorrhages. Death possible; little weight gain. | chronic poisoning |
| 20–30 mg/ kg body-weight | 3–6 days | Convulsions, paralysis, muscular tremor, bleeding from body cavities, death. | acute poisoning |

*Figs. 237 and 238: Yellow discoloration of the subcutaneous tissue, the muzzle and the buccal mucosa.*

*Fig. 239: Calf lying on its side; stretched-out posture of head and neck with spasmodic spreading of forelegs: Severe central nervous disorder in furazolidone poisoning.*

*Fig. 240: Bleeding from the nostrils; fresh blood admixtures in the faeces.*

*Fig. 241: Summary of dosage, period of administration and symptoms with furazolidone use.*

●●

In veterinary medicine, furazolidone is always given in the fodder or drinking-water. The product exerts its action mainly in the intestine where it inhibits the propagation of bacteria. It is used for the treatment of salmonellosis and E. coli infection.

Fig. 242

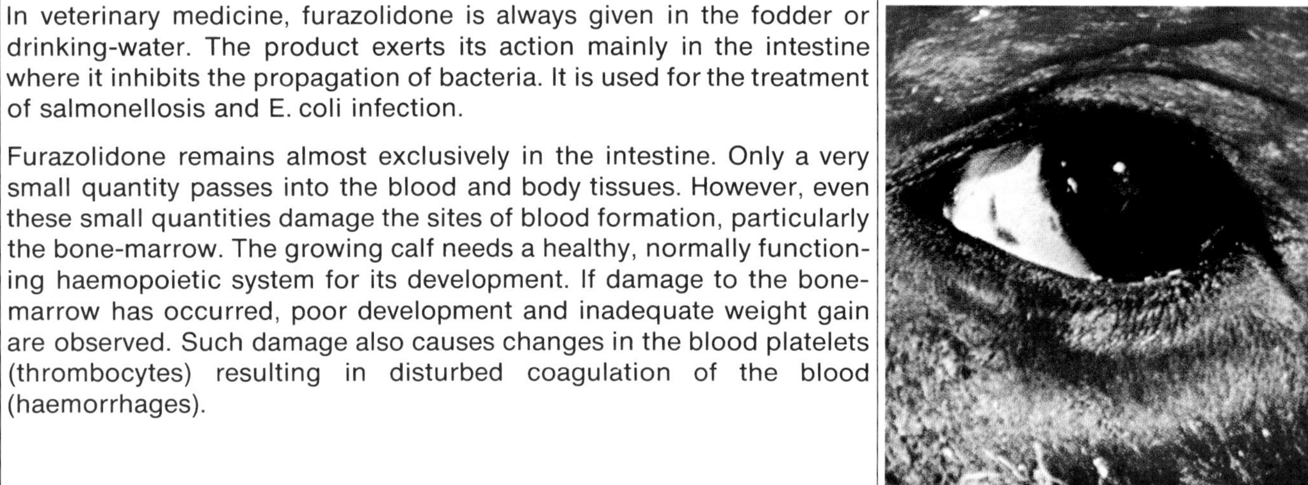

**Cause**

Furazolidone remains almost exclusively in the intestine. Only a very small quantity passes into the blood and body tissues. However, even these small quantities damage the sites of blood formation, particularly the bone-marrow. The growing calf needs a healthy, normally functioning haemopoietic system for its development. If damage to the bone-marrow has occurred, poor development and inadequate weight gain are observed. Such damage also causes changes in the blood platelets (thrombocytes) resulting in disturbed coagulation of the blood (haemorrhages).

**Symptoms**

At first, irregular drinking, heightened excitability, muscle twitching and an increase in body temperature are observed. The increased tendency to bleeding is seen from the fact that even very minor injuries bleed for a long time. Punctiform haemorrhages on the visible musosae (lips, tongue, third eyelid) and bleeding from the anus and nostrils may occur.

Convulsions and extreme debility lead to death within a few days.

**Diagnosis**

If furazolidone poisoning is suspected, feedstuffs and medicated feeds should be checked for their furazolidone content. An examination of the feedstuffs used may clarify any errors in mixing.

Furazolidone-like substances, e. g. nifurprazine or furadaltone, which are regarded as furane derivatives, should also be taken into consideration here.

In many cases intoxication occurs because, in addition to the quantities given daily in the fodder, furazolidone-containing drugs are administered.

**Similar symptoms**

All diseases with admixtures of blood in the faeces and nervous disorders show similar symptoms.
The most important distinguishing characteristics of other diseases are as follows:

Fig. 243

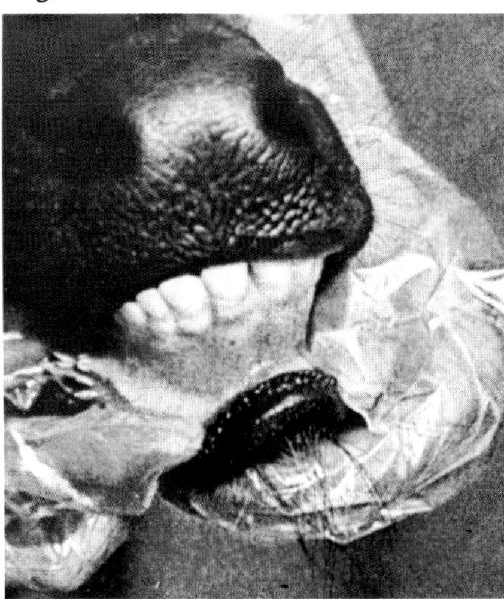

**Similar symptoms**

- Salmonellosis: Mucoid fluid faeces with whitish flakes. Demonstration of salmonellae by bacteriological examination of the faeces.
- Coccidiosis: Fluid, greyish brown and bubbly faeces. Demonstration of coccidia by parasitological examination of the faeces.
- Coumarin poisoning: Occurs if mouldy clover hay is fed. No central nervous disorder.
- Vitamin $B_1$ deficiency: No haemorrhages discernible. Typical posture with head bent backwards and upwards ("stargazing"). Rapid improvement following administration of vitamin $B_1$.

**Treatment**

If signs of intoxication are observed, any treatment of visibly affected animals has little prospect of success. All calves that have received the same furazolidone dose, but do not yet show any symptoms, should be treated with multivitamin products for several days.

Fig. 244

| | | |
|---|---|---|
| 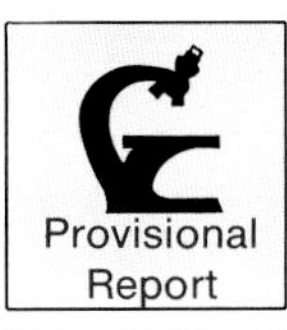 Provisional Report | Check fodder and any medicated products given for furazolidone and similar substances. Check feedstuffs for furazolidone content (errors in mixing). | Immediately |
| 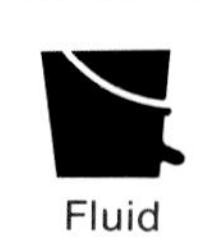 Fluid | **Stop** giving feedstuffs and drugs containing furazolidone or similar substances (e. g. nifurprazine, furadaltone). | Immediately |
| 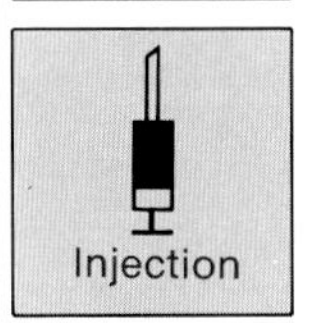 Injection | All animals having received the same fodder or treatment are given an injection of 2 ml VITIN/10 kg body-weight. | Immediately |
| 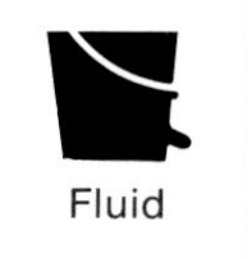 Fluid | Use milk substitute with high skimmed-milk content and low fat content. In addition, give 2 g MULTIVITAMIN R 12/10 kg body-weight daily in the milk, for 10 days. | 1st to 10th day |

*Fig. 242: Haemorrhage in the sclera.*

*Fig. 243: Punctiform haemorrhages in the buccal mucosa.*

*Fig. 244: Measures to be taken in furazolidone poisoning.*

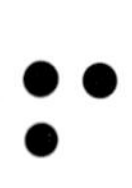

# Important characteristics of healthy cattle

## from the 13th week of life

### General behaviour

Size and development corresponding to age; lively, alert behaviour; upright posture, lively facial expression, alert eye and ear movements; shining short coat. The cattle readily approach visitors and are alert to what is happening around them.

### Body temperature

38.3 to 38.8° C

### Pulse

Rate 60 to 68, strong and regular.

### Breathing

Calm, regular, even.
Respiratory rate: 10 to 30 per minute.

### Elasticity of the skin

Raised skin folds immediately level out again.

### Urine

Thin clear amber fluid.
Daily volume: 6 to 12 litres.
pH value: 6.8 to 8.0
Specific gravity: 1,010 to 1,040

### Faeces

Pappy or formed. Colour brown to olive green, depending on feed used. Daily quantity: 15 to 25 kg.

### Blood volume

Approx. 80 ml blood per kg body-weight.

### Digestive system

Digestion has changed to multi-compartment stomach system. Capacity of first three stomachs: 180 to 230 litres. Rumination commences 30 to 45 minutes after feeding and lasts for 5 to 7 hours daily with normal feeding.

*Fig. 245*

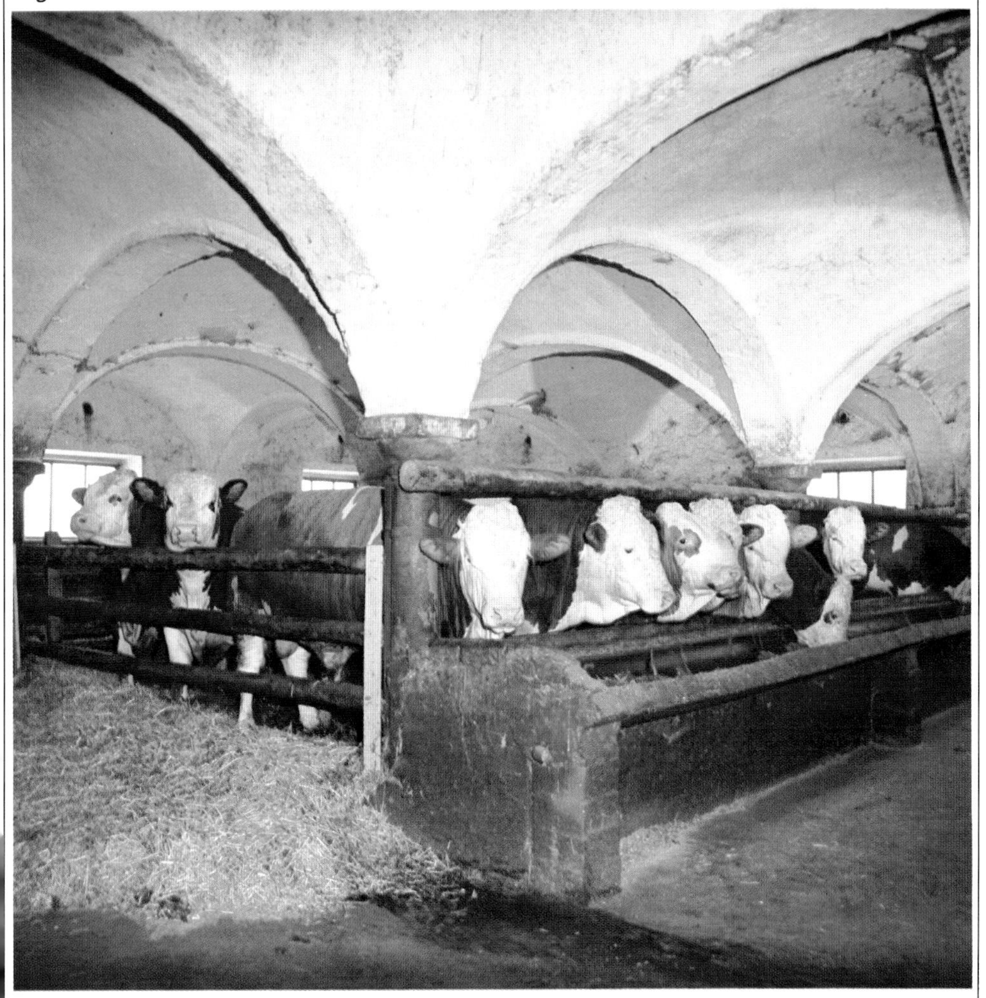

*Healthy, well-growing fattening bulls, aged 13 weeks: Balanced feeding, optimum environment and an appropriate preventive programme have resulted in evenly developed animals, despite the simple housing conditions.*

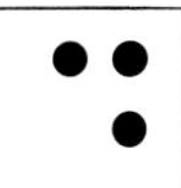

# Part 3

## The most important diseases from the 13th week of life. Rearing and fattening

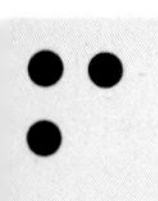

## Summary of important signs in sick cattle

## from the 13th week of life. Rearing and fattening

| | Fig. 246 | Fig. 247 |
|---|---|---|
| | 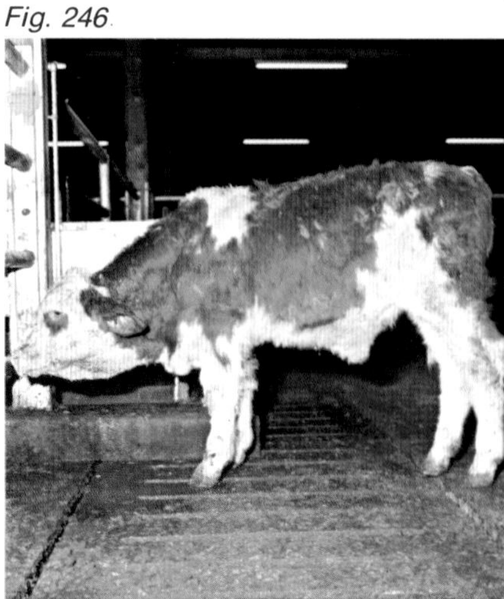 | 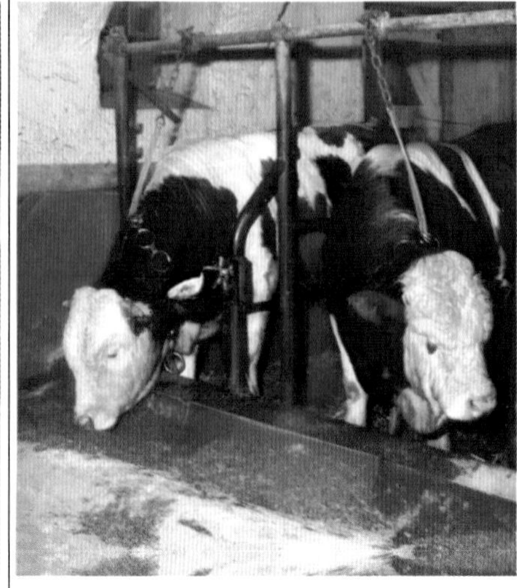 |
| Outwardly visible symptoms | Dullness, head lowered with stretched head and neck posture; drooping ears. | Eyes half closed, dull look, easily frightened; shunning light. |
| Diagnosis by examination | Standing apart from group of animals, no fodder intake. General examination. Take temperature. | Examine sclera and palpebral conjunctiva for inflammation and haemorrhage. Spinal cord puncture. Check cerebrospinal fluid. |
| Read up diseases that may be involved | Crowding disease, pages 138 and 140<br>Malignant catarrh, pages 147, 160 and 168<br>Mucosal disease, pages 138 and 162<br>IBR, pages 138 and 155 | ISTME, page 172<br>Phosphoric acid ester poisoning, page 212 |

*Fig. 248*

**Symptoms:** Animal permanently lying down on its side; stretched head and neck posture; rolling of eyes.

**Examination:** Spinal cord puncture. Check cerebrospinal fluid. Diagnostic treatment with vitamin $B_1$.

**Read up:**
ISTME, page 172
Vitamin $B_1$ deficiency, page 102
Phosphoric acid ester poisoning, page 212

*Fig. 249*

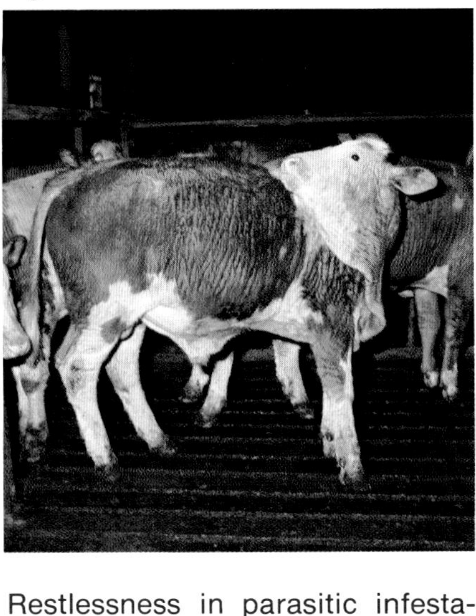

**Symptoms:** Restlessness in parasitic infestation. Rough coat due to licking and rubbing against walls and objects. Bald patches. Formation of scabs.

**Examination:** Examine skin scrapings under the microscope for mange mites. Nits and lice can be found in the hair.

**Read up:**
Mange, page 200
Lice, page 208

*Fig. 250*

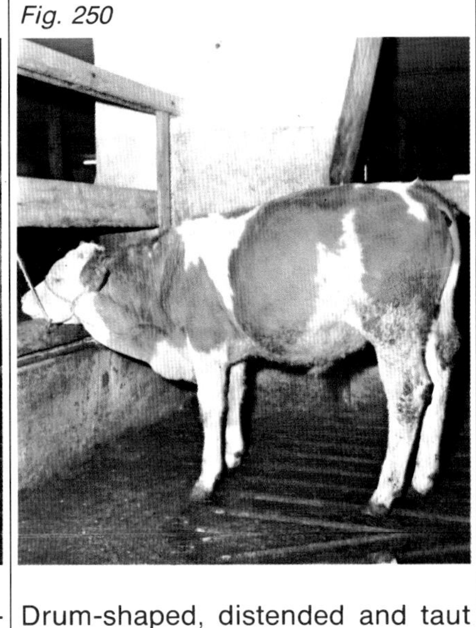

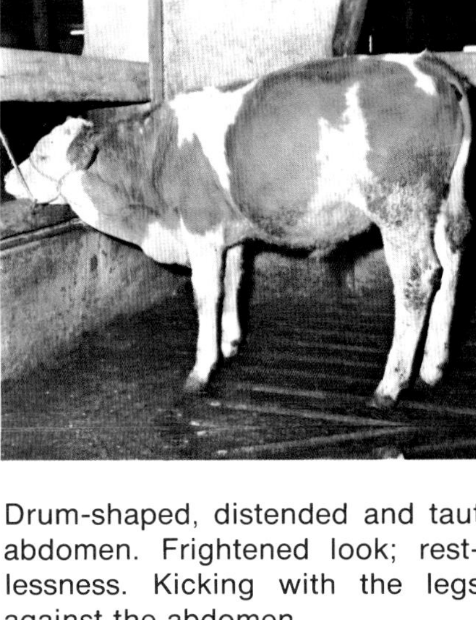

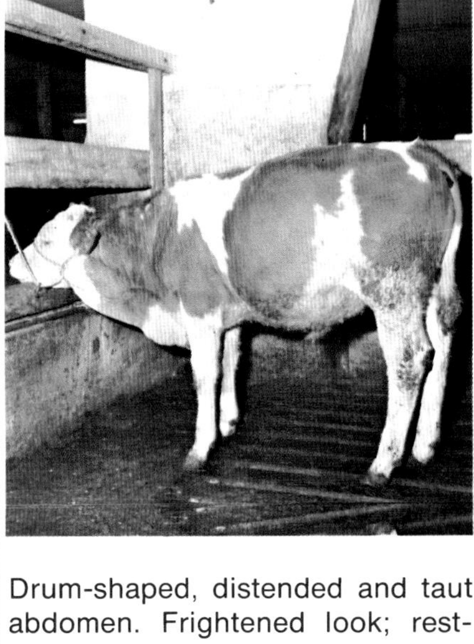

**Symptoms:** Drum-shaped, distended and taut abdomen. Frightened look; restlessness. Kicking with the legs against the abdomen.

**Examination:** Palpation of the protruded abdominal wall. Strong hollow sound. Abomasum on the right; first three stomach compartments on the left. Check urination. Examine filling of bladder rectally.

**Read up:**
Tympany, page 92
Disturbed micturition, page 178

Fig. 251

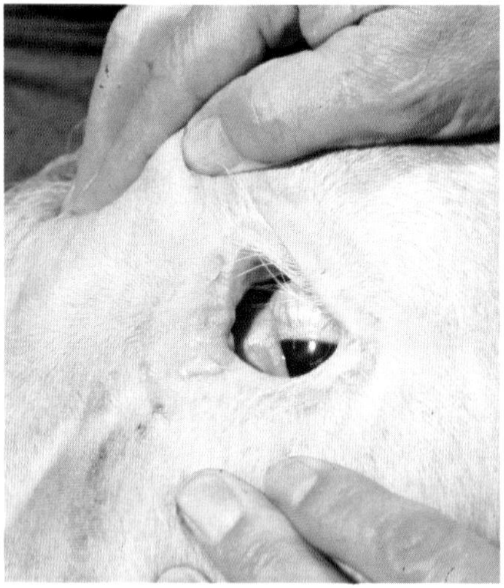

**Symptoms** Deep-set eye. Desiccation of connective tissue through loss of fluid.

**Examination** Eye lying deep in its socket, making the orbit stand out and giving the impression that the eye is getting smaller. Reduced tension of the skin. Take temperature. Diarrhoea?

**Read up** Coccidiosis, page 108
Mucosal disease, pages 138 and 162
Salmonellosis, page 36

Fig. 252

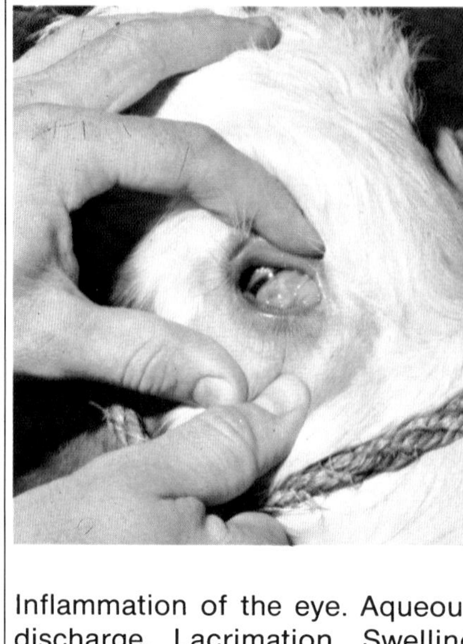

**Symptoms** Inflammation of the eye. Aqueous discharge. Lacrimation. Swelling of eyelid; later adhesion of the eye lashes. Animal shunning light, squeezing eyelids together.

**Examination** Reddening and inflammation of the palpebral conjunctiva. Protrusion of blood vessels on the sclera. Take temperature.

**Read up** Influenza-type disease complex, page 138

Fig. 253

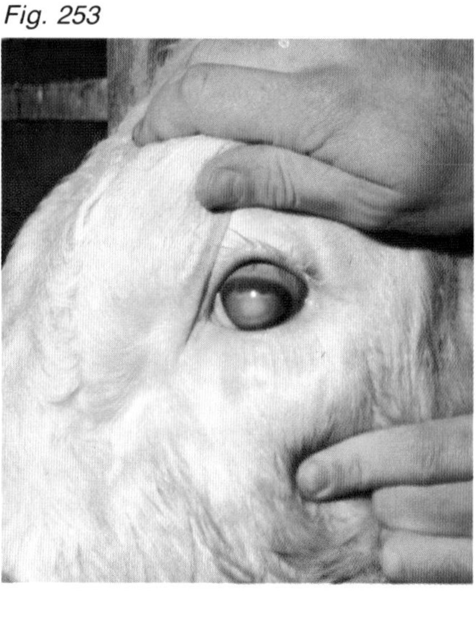

**Symptoms** Corneal turbidity. Milky grey discoloration of the cornea with vascular injection from the sclera.

**Examination** Reddening and inflammation of the palpebral conjunctiva. Look for changes of the buccal mucosa and the claw edge. Take temperature.

**Read up** Malignant catarrh, page 160
Mucosal disease, pages 138 and 162.
Injuries.

*Fig. 254*

Nostrils opened wide; stretched head and neck posture. The bull is audibly fighting for breath. Breathing through open mouth. Foaming.

Temperature raised to over 41° C. Breathing in and out with the support of the abdominal muscles (beating of flanks).

IBR, pages 138 and 155
Crowding disease, pages 138 and 140
Malignant catarrh, page 160

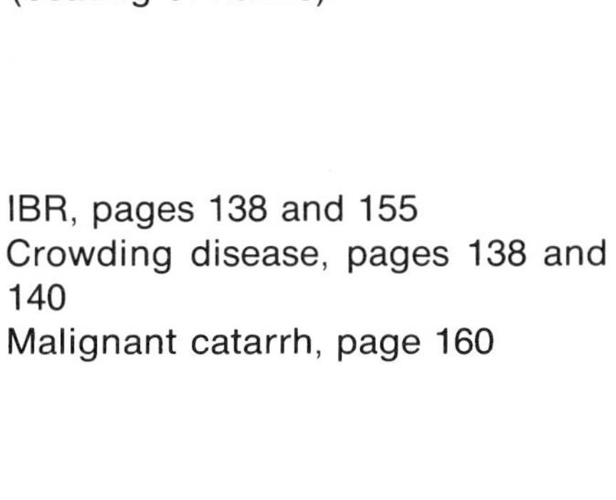

*Fig. 255*

Discharge from the nose. Viscous mucopurulent secretion.

Difficulty in breathing. Temperature varies, usually above 39.0° C. Strained facial expression. Animal ceases to feed.

Influenza-type disease complex, page 138
Malignant catarrh, pages 147, 160 and 168

*Fig. 256*

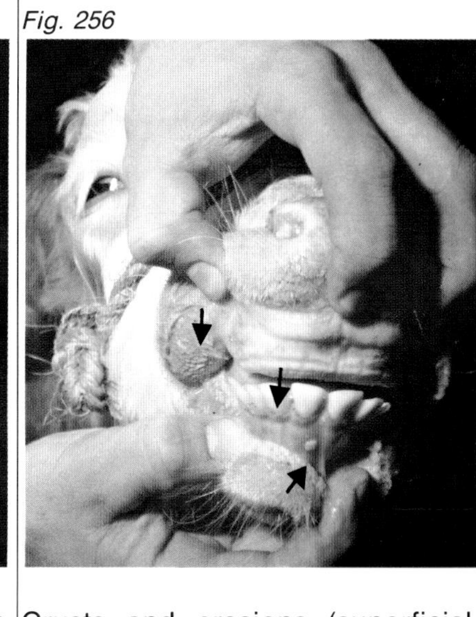

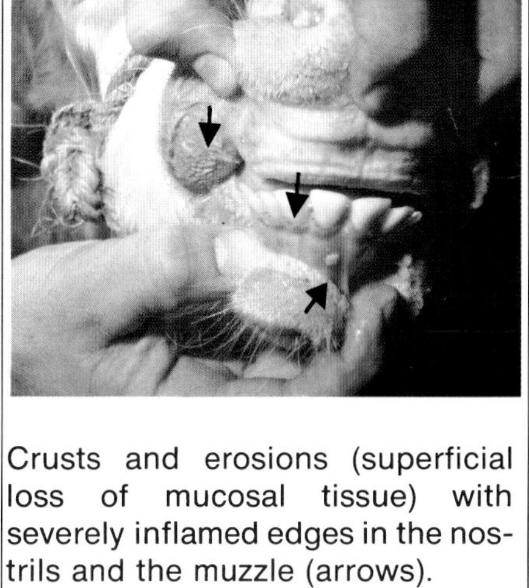

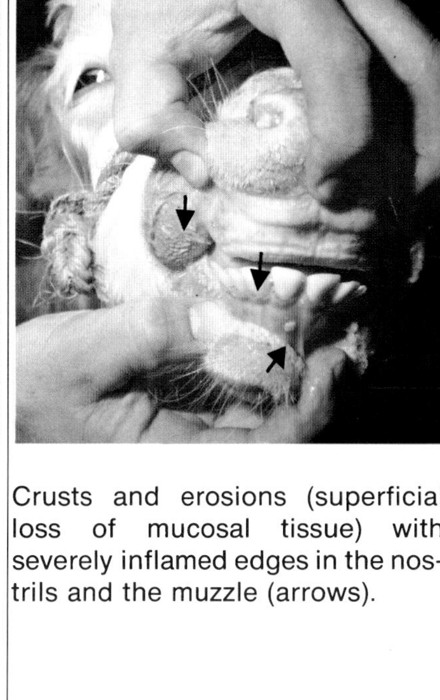

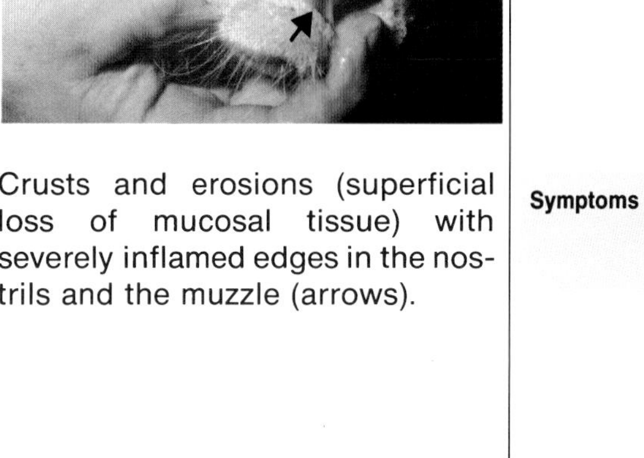

Crusts and erosions (superficial loss of mucosal tissue) with severely inflamed edges in the nostrils and the muzzle (arrows).

Temperature very high. Look for changes on the teats, the coronal edge and in the space between the claws.

Mucosal disease, pages 138 and 162.
Foot-and-mouth disease, pages 168 and 170.

Symptoms

Examination

Read up

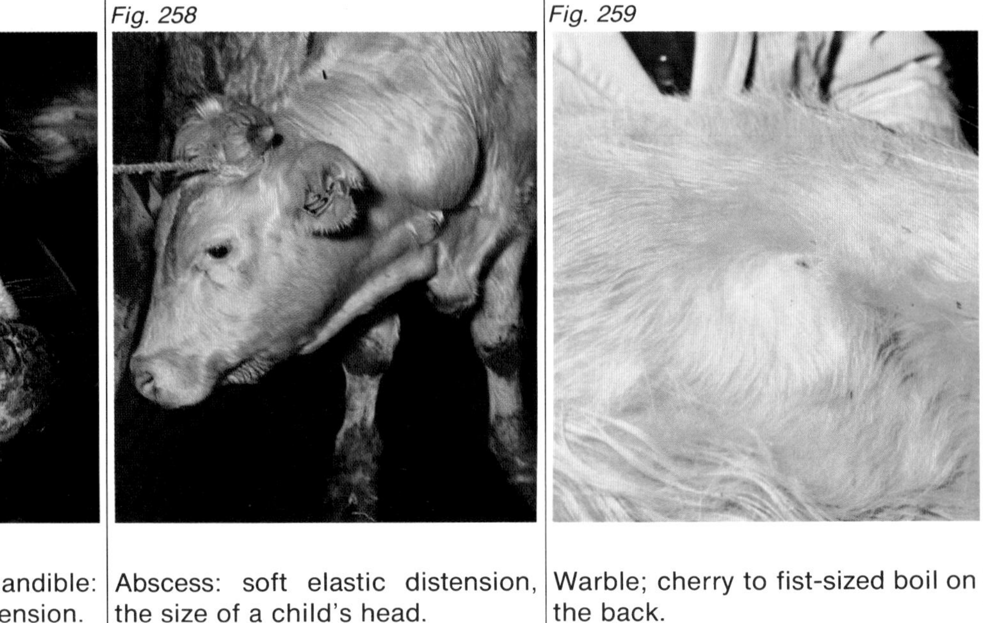

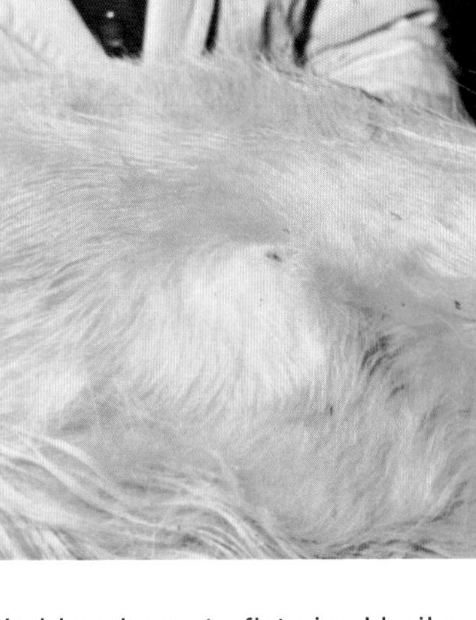

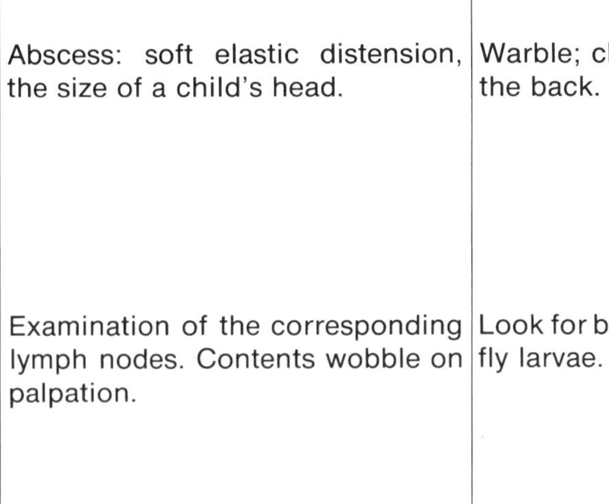

| | *Fig. 257* | *Fig. 258* | *Fig. 259* |
|---|---|---|---|
| **Symptoms** | Actinomycosis of the mandible: Fist-sized tumour-like distension. | Abscess: soft elastic distension, the size of a child's head. | Warble; cherry to fist-sized boil on the back. |
| **Examination** | Similar changes are possible in other bones and the tongue ("wooden tongue") | Examination of the corresponding lymph nodes. Contents wobble on palpation. | Look for breathing-holes of warble-fly larvae. |
| **Read up** | Actinomycosis (isolated case) | Abscess, page 222<br>Warble-fly infestation, page 196 | Warble-fly infestation, page 196 |

| | *Fig. 260* | *Fig. 261* | *Fig. 262* |
|---|---|---|---|
| **Symptoms** | Trichophytosis, ringworm: Circular bald patches, initially reddened, later asbestos-like crusts. | Infestation with lice: Bald areas in coat; broken-off hairs. | Mange: Irregular bald, raised areas with scab and crust formation. |
| **Examination** | No itching. Pathogen can be demonstrated in the laboratory. | Itching, restlessness, sucking sites of lice visible. Collect hairs for examination for lice and nits under a magnifying glass. | Itching. Examine skin scrapings under the microscope to confirm presence of mites. |
| **Read up** | Trichophytosis, ringworm, page 112 | Infestation with lice, page 208 | Mange, page 200 |

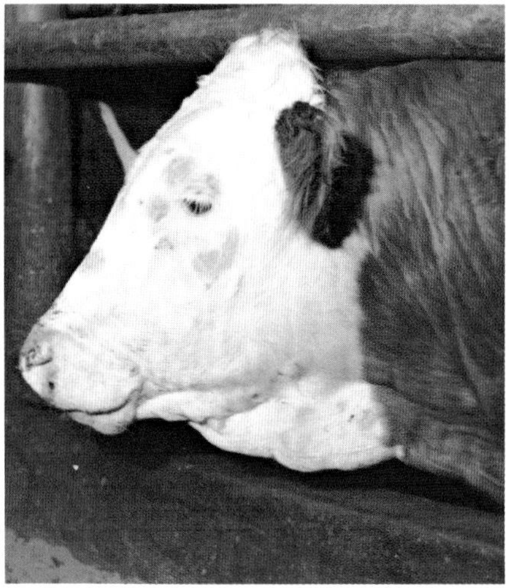

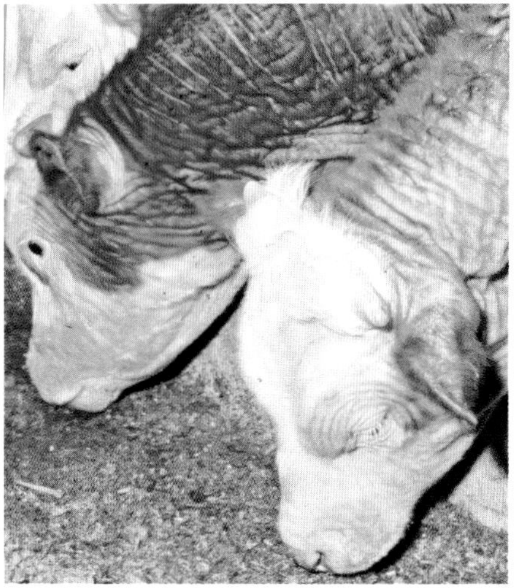

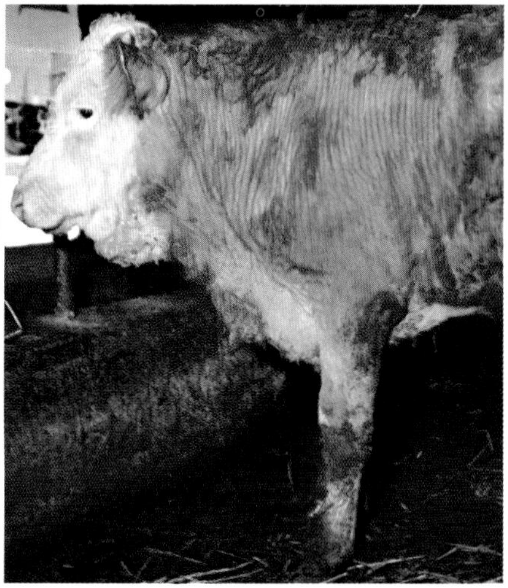

*Fig. 263*

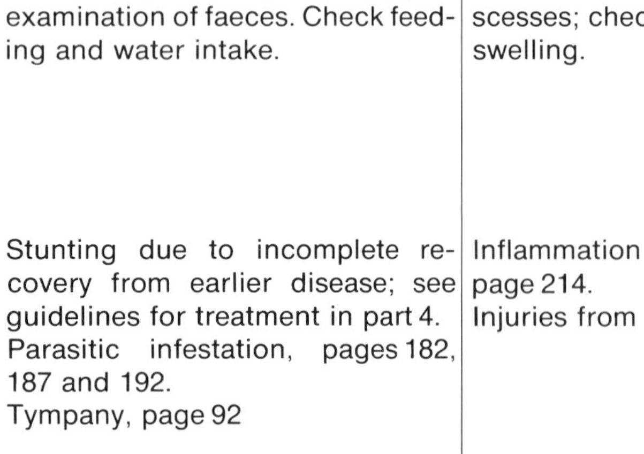

**Symptoms**: Dull, rough coat; long hair. Size and development do not correspond to the animal's age.

**Examination**: Bacteriological and parasitological examination of faeces. Check feeding and water intake.

**Read up**: Stunting due to incomplete recovery from earlier disease; see guidelines for treatment in part 4.
Parasitic infestation, pages 182, 187 and 192.
Tympany, page 92

*Fig. 264*

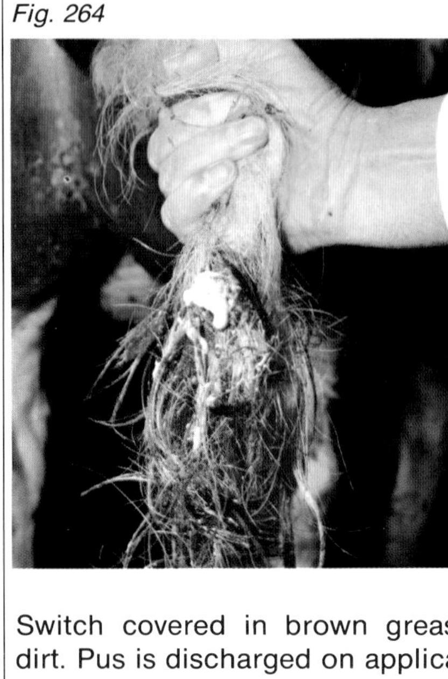

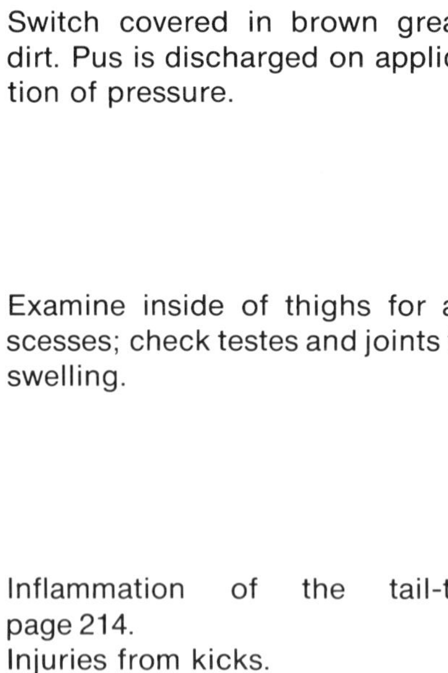

**Symptoms**: Switch covered in brown greasy dirt. Pus is discharged on application of pressure.

**Examination**: Examine inside of thighs for abscesses; check testes and joints for swelling.

**Read up**: Inflammation of the tail-tip, page 214.
Injuries from kicks.

*Fig. 265*

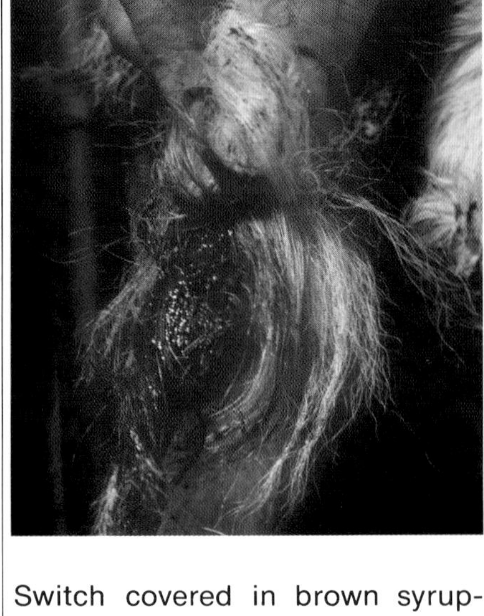

**Symptoms**: Switch covered in brown syrup-like, greasy dirt.

**Examination**: Examine inside of thighs for abscesses; check testes and joints for swelling.

**Read up**: Bite wound in cannibalism, page 218.
Inappropriate housing conditions, see part 5.
Inflammation of the tail-tip, page 214.

*Fig. 266*

Rickets-like symptoms. Carpal joints swollen; bending forwards and sideways.

Animal tied up; check measurements of feeding-trough.

Rickets, page 225
Articular inflammation, page 60

*Fig. 267*

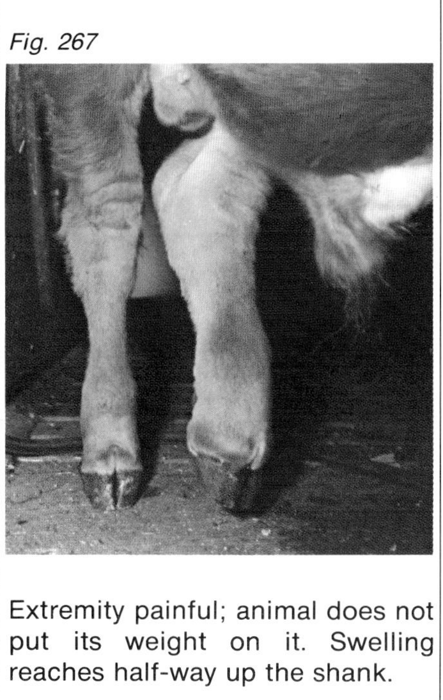

Extremity painful; animal does not put its weight on it. Swelling reaches half-way up the shank.

Check claws, interdigital space and shank.

Foul-in-the-foot, page 230
Interdigital necrosis, page 231
Bone fracture.

*Fig. 268*

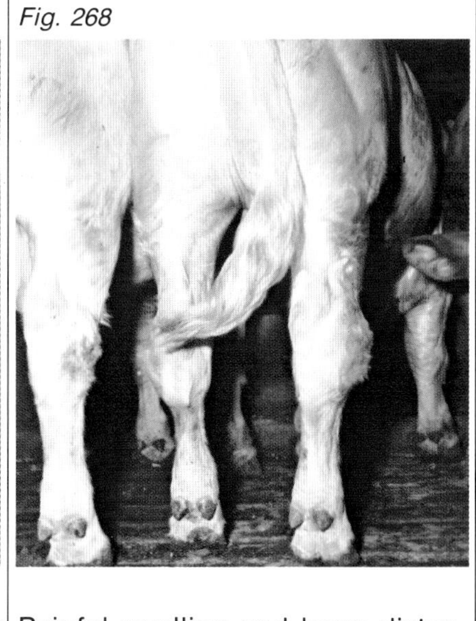

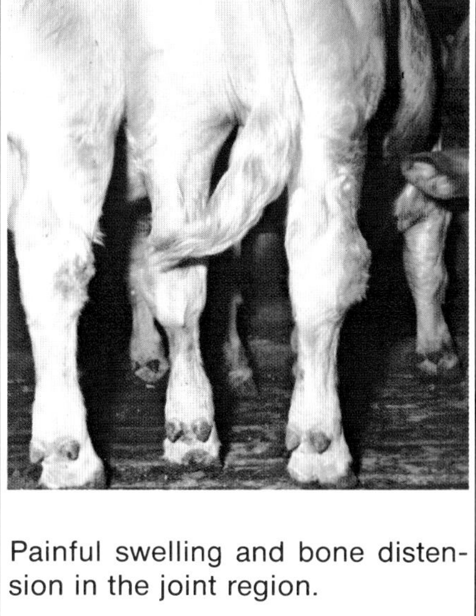

Painful swelling and bone distension in the joint region.

Check housing, slatted floor.

Rickets, page 225
Articular inflammation, page 60
Inflammation of tail-tip, page 214.

**Symptoms**

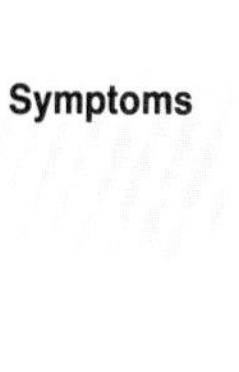

**Examination**

**Read up**

| | Fig. 269 | Fig. 270 | Fig. 271 |
|---|---|---|---|
| | 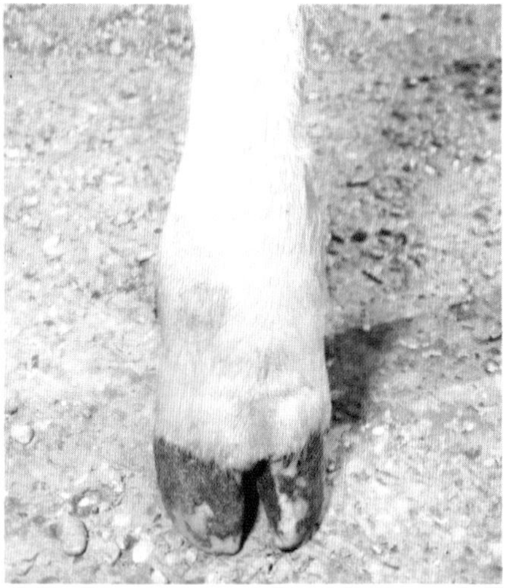 | 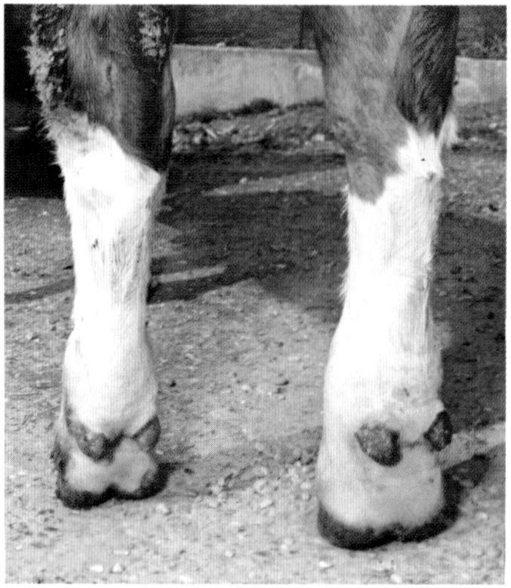 | 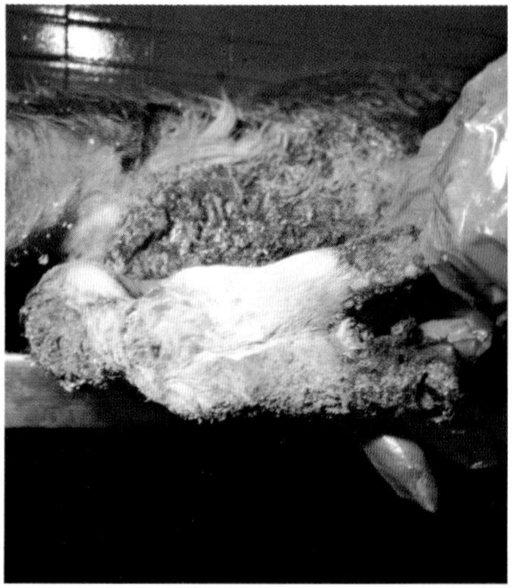 |
| **Symptoms** | Space between the claws inflamed. Swelling extending to the fetlock joint. | Skin on the ball of the foot discoloured bluish red and cracked. Swelling extending beyond fetlock joint. | Space between the claws inflamed, with furfuraceous crusts. |
| **Examination** | Clean claw carefully. Check for injuries (kicks, cuts). | Palpation of the space between the claws and of the claws. | Check remaining claws, the udder and the buccal mucosa. |
| **Read up** | Foul-in-the-foot, page 230<br>Interdigital necrosis, page 231 | Phlegmon of the ball of the foot, page 231<br>Cut, page 226 | Foot-and-mouth disease, page 170<br>Mucosal disease, page 162<br>Interdigital necrosis, page 231 |

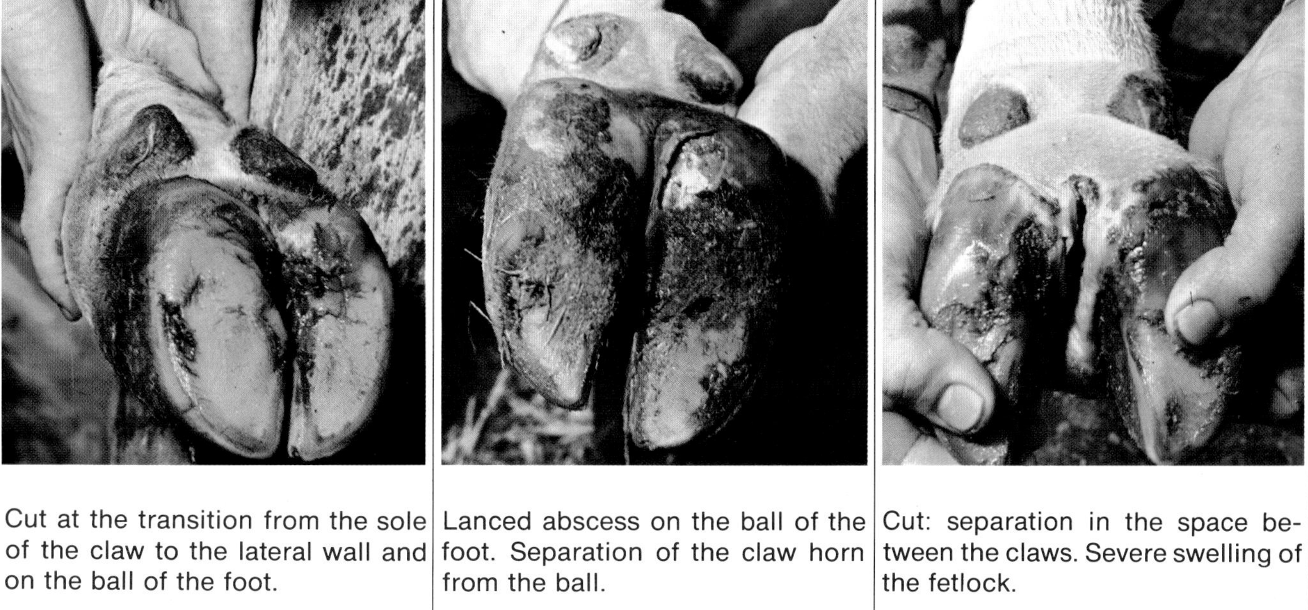

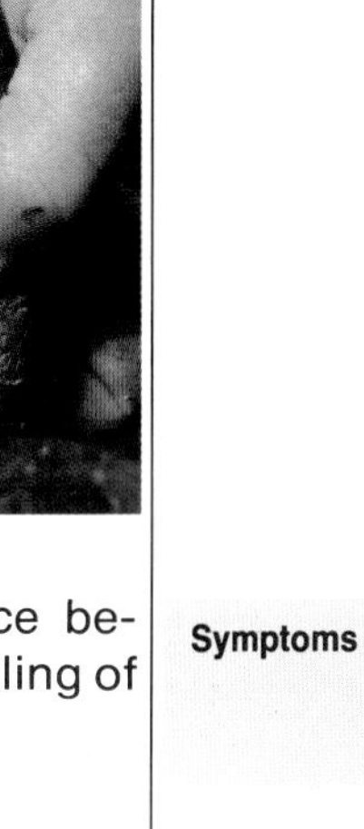

*Fig. 272*

*Fig. 273*

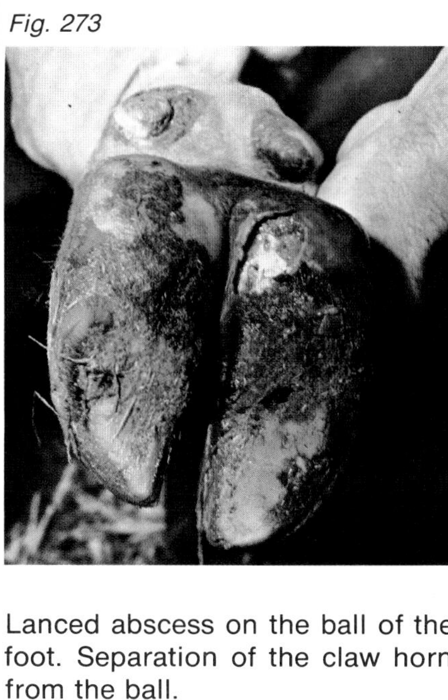

*Fig. 274*

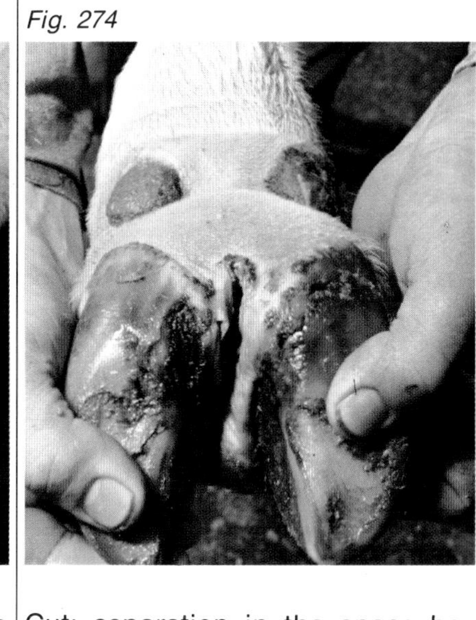

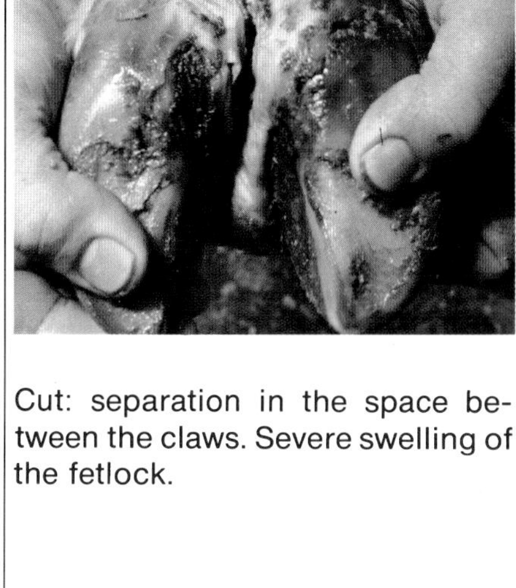

| | Fig. 272 | Fig. 273 | Fig. 274 |
|---|---|---|---|
| **Symptoms** | Cut at the transition from the sole of the claw to the lateral wall and on the ball of the foot. | Lanced abscess on the ball of the foot. Separation of the claw horn from the ball. | Cut: separation in the space between the claws. Severe swelling of the fetlock. |
| **Examination** | Examine space between the claws. Knock against wall and sole of claw to see if this is painful. | Check space between the claws; examine flexor tendons. | Examine interdigital ligaments. |
| **Read up** | Cuts, page 226<br>Ball rot, page 231 | Cut, page 226<br>Phlegmon of the ball of the foot, page 231 | Cut, page 226 |

| | *Fig. 275* | *Fig. 276* | *Fig. 277* |
|---|---|---|---|
| | | 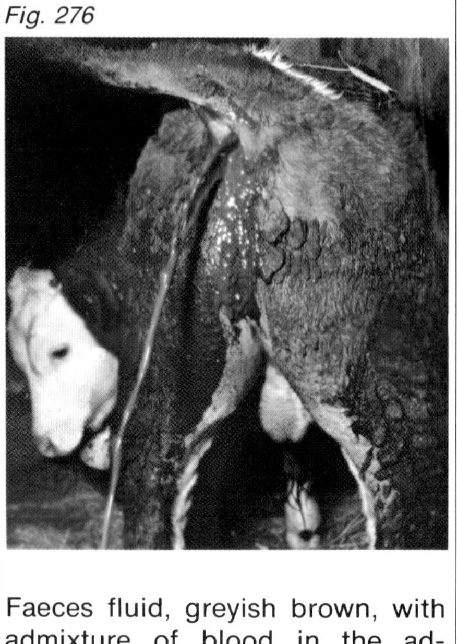 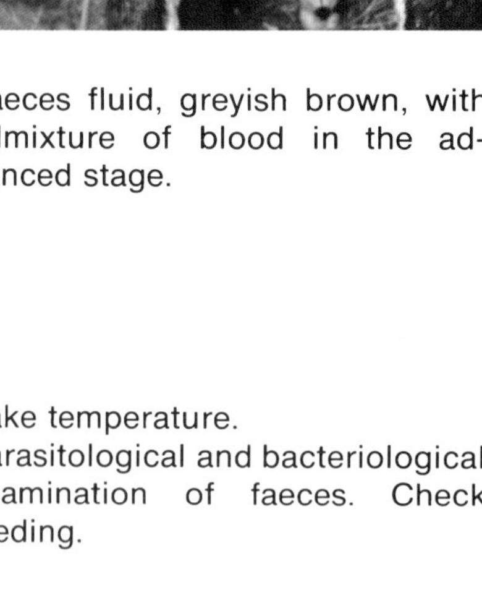 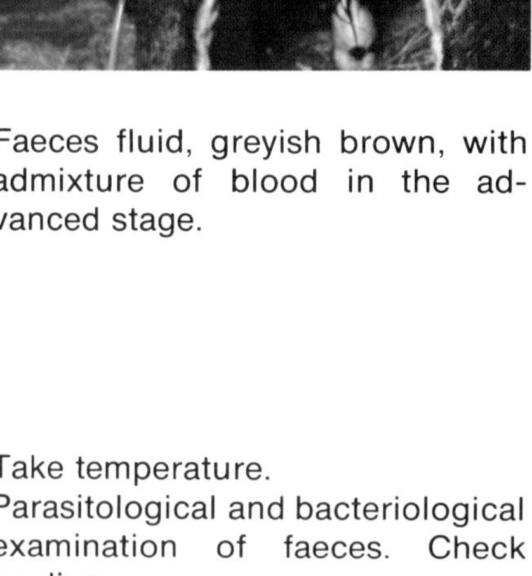 | 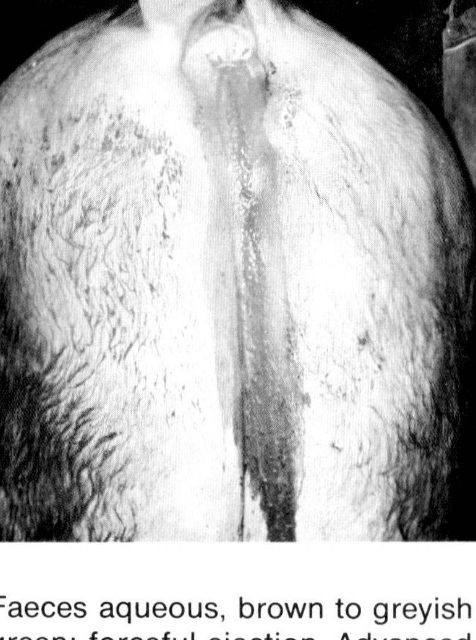 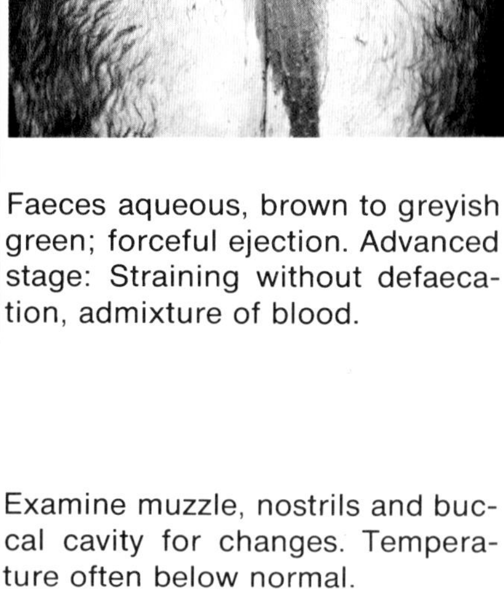 |
| **Symptoms** | "Urine drinker": Long narrow face with hair sticking together on the bridge of the nose. | Faeces fluid, greyish brown, with admixture of blood in the advanced stage. | Faeces aqueous, brown to greyish green; forceful ejection. Advanced stage: Straining without defaecation, admixture of blood. |
| **Examination** | Observe behaviour in group. | Take temperature. Parasitological and bacteriological examination of faeces. Check feeding. | Examine muzzle, nostrils and buccal cavity for changes. Temperature often below normal. |
| **Read up** | "Urine drinkers", see prevention in part 5. | Coccidiosis, page 108<br>Nutrition-induced diarrhoea, page 48<br>Salmonellosis, page 36 | Mucosal disease, page 162<br>Poisoning, pages 42 and 212. |

*Fig. 278*

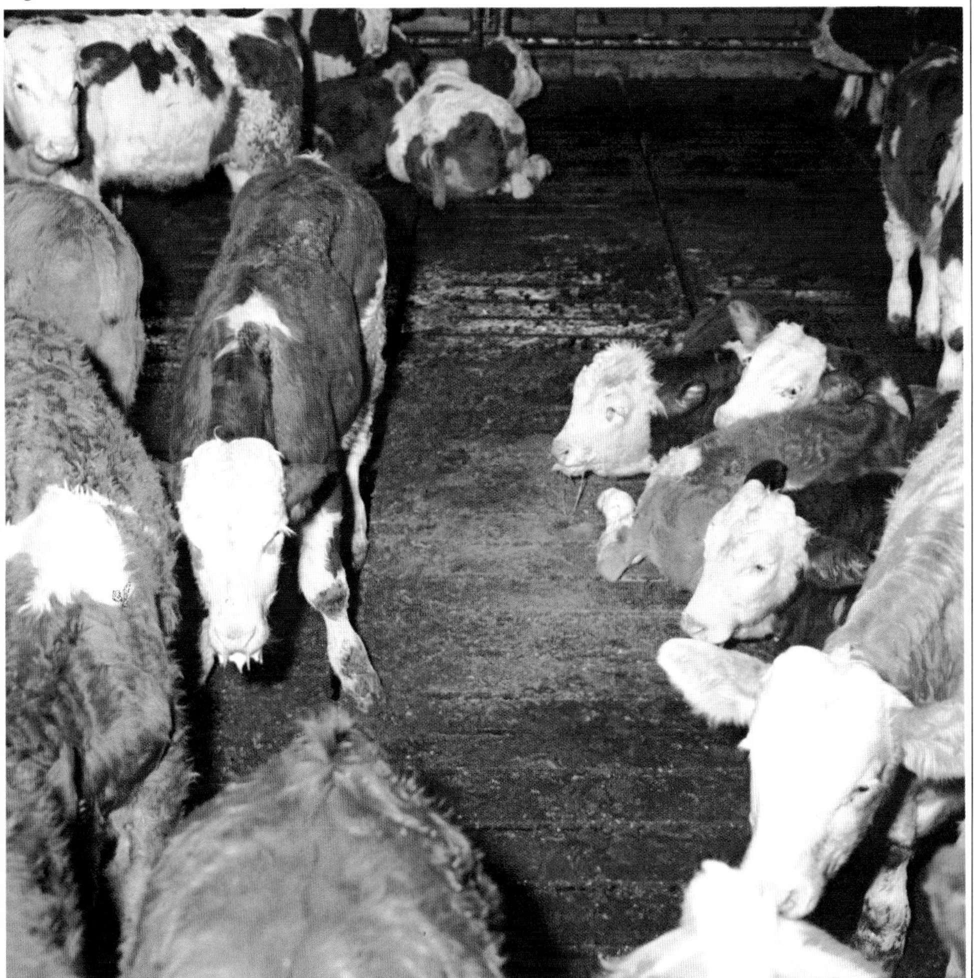

*Influenza-type disease complex in cattle: Group of affected fattening bulls. With this condition, in addition to the treatment of individual, severely affected animals, preventive treatment of all cattle at risk is necessary.*

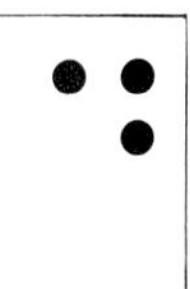

# The most important diseases from the 13th week of life. Rearing and fattening

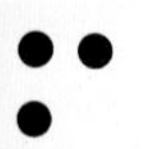

# Influenza-type disease complex in cattle

*Fig. 279*

Disease

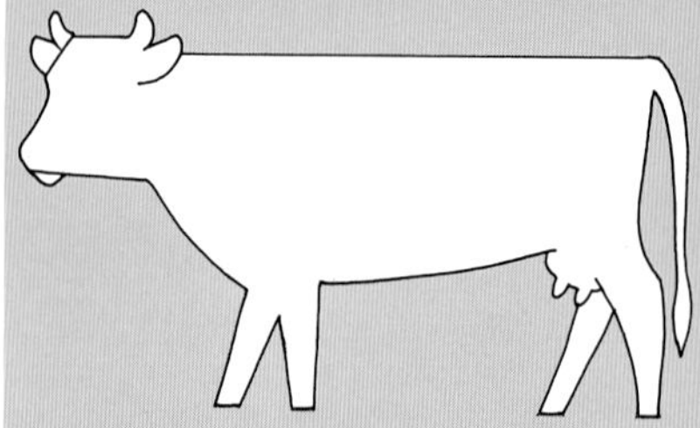

Organs affected

Pathogen(s)

Symptoms

Treatment

Prevention

The influenza-type disease complex in cattle comprises diseases affecting particularly the respiratory organs, but also the gastrointestinal tract.

In a narrower sense, "cattle influenza" is the virus influenza-type condition affecting the entire stock, or "crowding disease". The influenza-type disease complex includes two further conditions, IBR and mucosal disease, which present a similar clinical picture and may be associated with crowding disease.

Since IBR and mucosal disease – in contrast to crowding disease – are caused by known pathogens which can be well demonstrated, they are listed here as independent disease entities. Moreover, special preventive and therapeutic measures apply to these diseases.

| Crowding disease (page 140) | IBR/IPV (page 155) | Mucosal disease (page 162) |
|---|---|---|
| 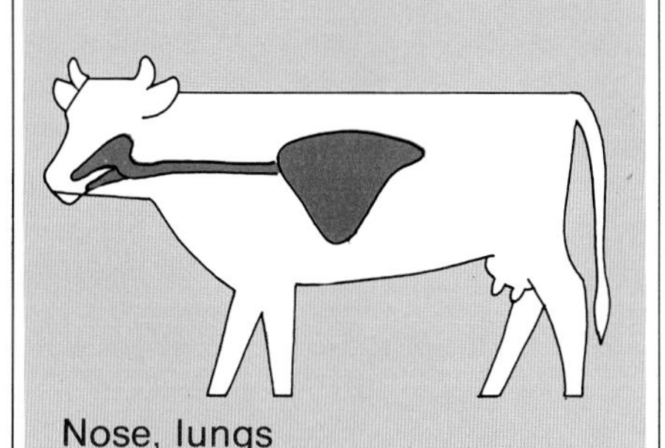 | 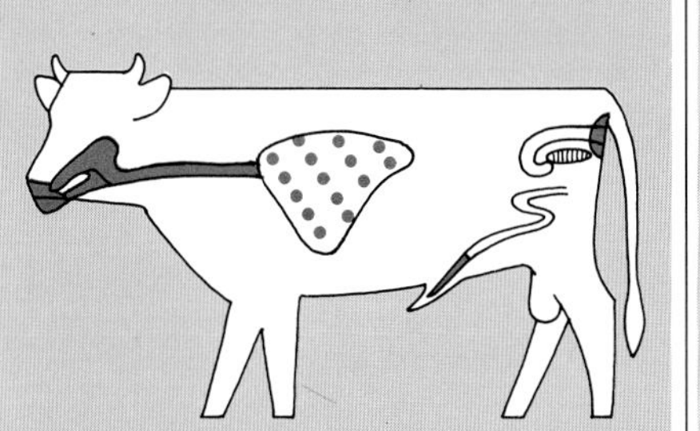 | 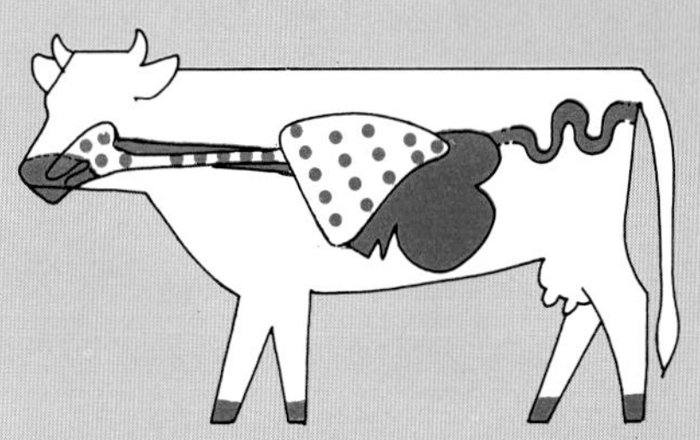 |
| Nose, lungs | IBR: Larynx, muzzle, later lungs<br>IPV: External sexual organs | Muzzle, throat, oral cavity, stomach, intestine, claws |
| Several virus types + bacteria | Herpes virus | Toga virus |
| Aqueous or mucopurulent discharge from nose and eyes, pneumonia, pulmonary emphysema. | IBR, respiratory form: "Red nose", pneumonia, respiratory distress, formation of foam at the mouth. IPV, genital form: Reddening and small pustules on the vulvae or penis. | Erosions on the muzzle and inflammation of the coronal edge on the claws. |
| Severely affected animals: Injection of antibiotics or sulphonamides; give mucolytic agents and drugs supporting the circulation. Less severely affected animals: BOVIBOL. Stock: Medicated feed. | Severely affected animals: Injection of antibiotics or sulphonamides; give mucolytic agents and drugs supporting the circulation. Less severely affected animals: BOVIBOL.<br>Stock: Medicated feed. | Severely affected animals: Treatment useless in severe diarrhoea. Stock: Emergency vaccination and medicated feed (see page 168) |
| Vaccination: BOVIGRIP or PNEUMOVAC PLUS. Only healthy animals should be vaccinated. | Vaccination: IBR/IPV VACCINE (by special permission), PNEUMOVAC PLUS. | Vaccination: BVD/MD VACCINE; PNEUMOVAC PLUS contains a BVD/MD component. |

All three infections are factor diseases. Their outbreak is induced by precipitating factors. An improvement in the conditions under which the animals are kept (controlled environment, reception house, feeding etc.) and the use of medicated feed at times of unavoidable stress, are therefore necessary. This is the most important pre-condition for avoiding influenza-type diseases. See Part 5: Housing, feeding and prophylaxis.

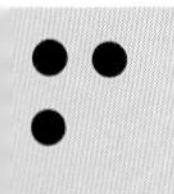

# Crowding disease

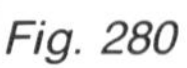

*Fig. 280*

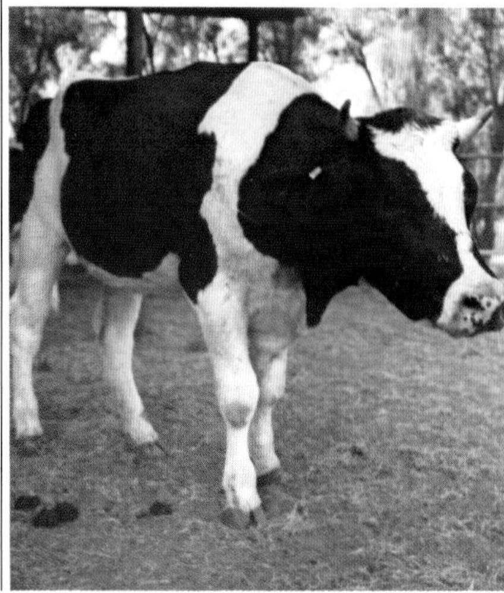

*Fig. 281*

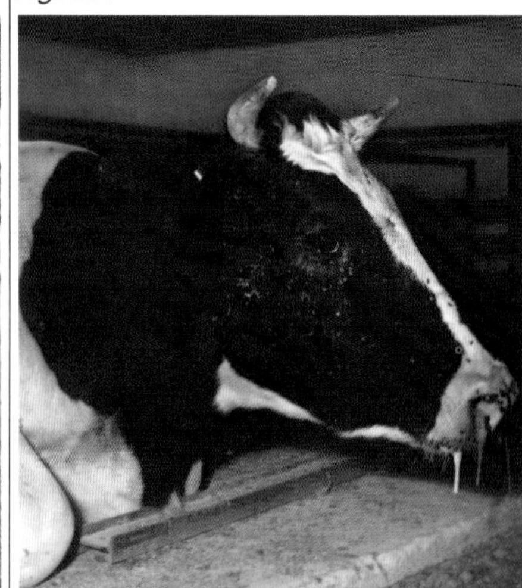

**Term**

The term "crowding disease" covers all influenza-like respiratory conditions in cattle. An unequivocal, single cause – as is the case, for instance, with FMD virus in foot-and-mouth disease – is not known for crowding disease. Here a great variety of factors, both infection-induced and housing-induced, act in concert. Housing-induced factors, e. g. inappropriate ventilation, open the door to infective organisms. Viruses take advantage of this temporary weakening of the animal's defences and multiply rapidly in the body causing a feverish condition. The viruses may be compared to an advance guard opening up a route of entry for the much slower, but more powerful bacteria. Such an additional infection is described as a secondary bacterial infection. It aggravates the initially influenza-like condition considerably and quite often causes the death of the animal (cf. Fig. 286).

**Incidence**

Crowding disease is a feverish condition of the respiratory organs occurring in entire cattle stocks. It can arise only if conditions of stress enable infective organisms to penetrate and spread in the animal body. The disease occurs in all types of stock. In stock with a large number of young animals of the same age (up to one year), crowding disease is a major problem.

**Infection- and housing-induced factors** act together in producing an outbreak of crowding disease (cf. Fig. 283). A few examples may serve to illustrate the interaction of these two groups of factors.

Figs. 280 and 281: *Heifer showing symptoms of crowding disease after transport by air from Germany to Kuwait. The restricted space in transit and the extreme change of climate produced severe pneumonia.*

*Fig. 282: The animal on the left shows typical symptoms of severe pneumonia: Head lowered, stretched head-neck posture, splayed forelegs, nostrils opened wide, drooping ears.*

*Fig. 282*

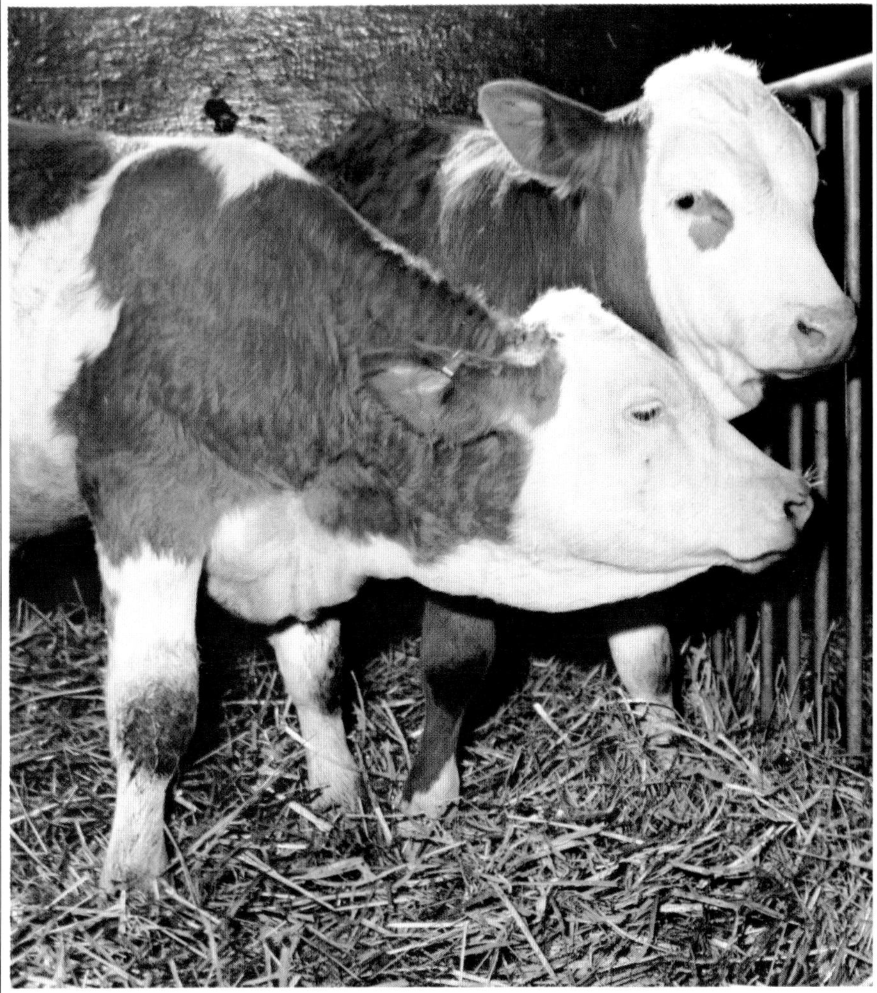

Pathogen / Cause

## ■ Poor controlled environment and inappropriate ventilation

If there is a sudden change in the weather, the ventilation is often adjusted too late to the new weather conditions. The animals which are confined to a restricted space in the house, are exposed to cold moist draughts and catch a chill. The change in the weather also leads to an increase in air humidity and to high concentrations of ammonia which irritate the airways. These stresses reduce the animals' resistance. This is why an increased incidence of the disease is observed during the months in which the external climatic conditions change rapidly, i. e. in the spring and the autumn.

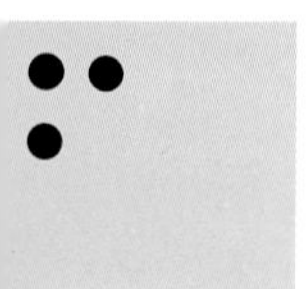

Pathogen / Cause

## Purchase

Every animal has its own intrinsic defence mechanism which is adapted to the pathogens in its environment. If this environment is changed, for instance by the purchase of young animals which are then housed with other cattle in a different location, the animals are exposed to new pathogens that may be present and have to rebuild their intrinsic defence mechanisms. Given favourable conditions, the animal overcomes this stress without ill effect. However, if there are too many pathogens present (high infective pressure) which have to be overcome in addition to the extra stress, crowding disease may result.

When animals are purchased, additional stress occurs as a result of transport, placing in dealers' cattle houses, disturbance, changes in housing, feeding and attending personnel. Diseases caused by this stress at the time of purchase, are grouped together under the term "crowding disease".

## Re-housing

Re-housing on slatted floors very often involves a change from warm straw litter to draughty, moist and cold floors. Leg discomfort and the changed environment combine to reduce the animal's appetite. This quickly leads to an inadequate intake of nutrient substances, minerals and vitamins. The coat becomes rough, the animals lose weight and are particularly susceptible to crowding disease at this stage.

In crowding disease, several virus types and subsequently various bacteria are responsible for the **infection.** The viruses involved are mainly parainfluenza III virus, reovirus, rhinovirus, adenovirus, toga virus and herpes virus. The bacteria are mainly pasteurellae, streptococci, staphylococci, micrococci, E. coli and corynebacteria. Mycoplasms and chlamydia are also involved. Many of these pathogens are present in the stock. However, the spectrum of pathogens varies from one stock to another. It is always several pathogens from this spectrum that interact to cause the outbreak of crowding disease in the presence of the stress mentioned.

*Fig. 283: Interaction of infection and environment in the outbreak of crowding disease.*

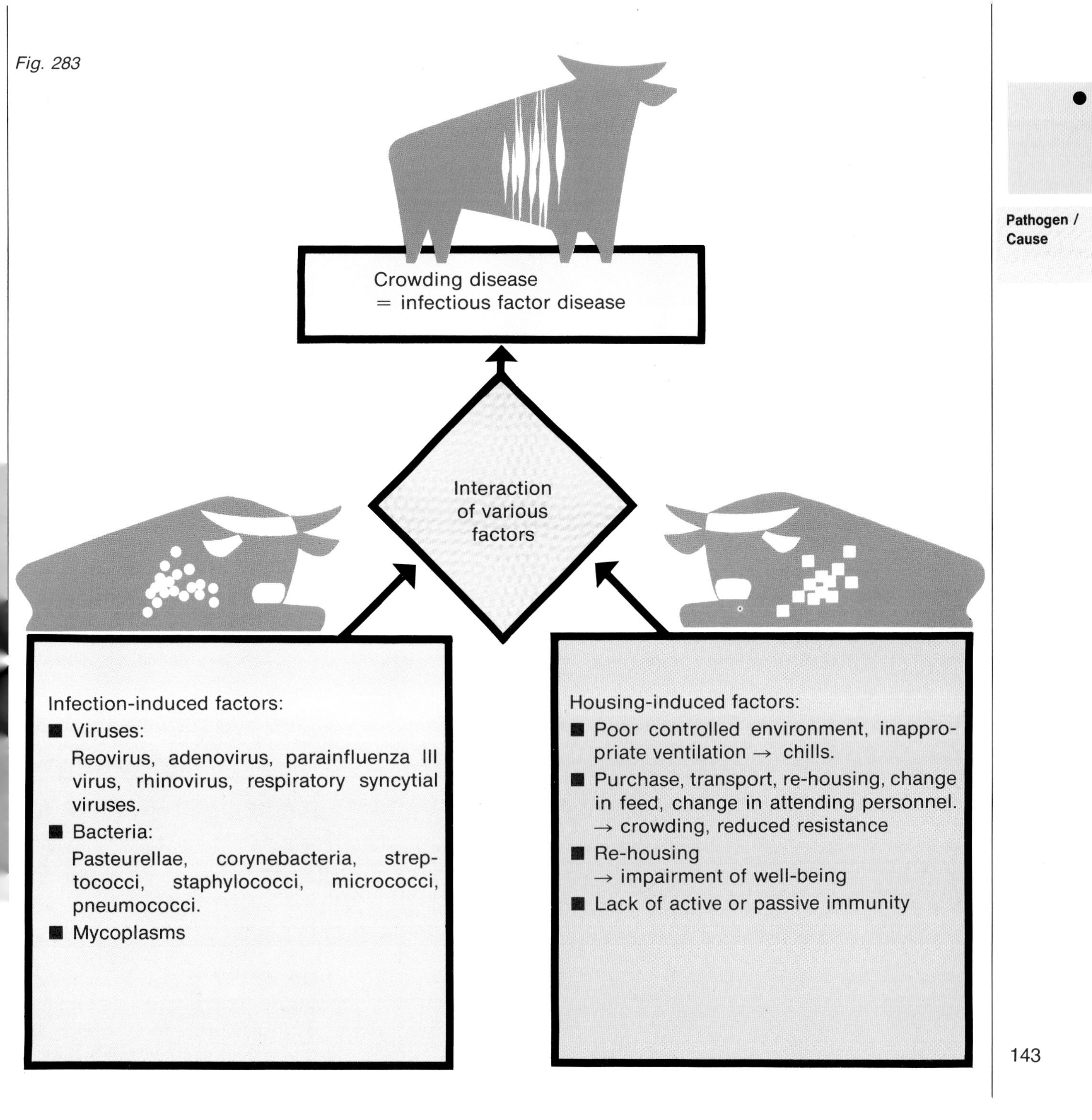
Fig. 283
Crowding disease
= infectious factor disease
Interaction
of various
factors
Infection-induced factors:
■ Viruses:
Reovirus, adenovirus, parainfluenza III virus, rhinovirus, respiratory syncytial viruses.
■ Bacteria:
Pasteurellae, corynebacteria, streptococci, staphylococci, micrococci, pneumococci.
■ Mycoplasms
Housing-induced factors:
■ Poor controlled environment, inappropriate ventilation → chills.
■ Purchase, transport, re-housing, change in feed, change in attending personnel. → crowding, reduced resistance
■ Re-housing
→ impairment of well-being
■ Lack of active or passive immunity

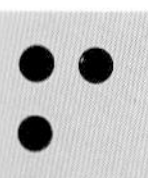

**Importation / Route of infection**

The viruses and bacteria are mainly transmitted by droplet infection. The mucus containing the pathogens is dispersed into fine particles by coughing and is inhaled by other animals, thus passing into the throat and the upper respiratory tract. Poor controlled environmental conditions and a high concentration of ammonia (acceptable levels see page 265) irritate the mucosae and reduce the activity of the cilia in the windpipe. The pathogens inhaled can therefore adhere to the mucosa.

*Fig. 284*

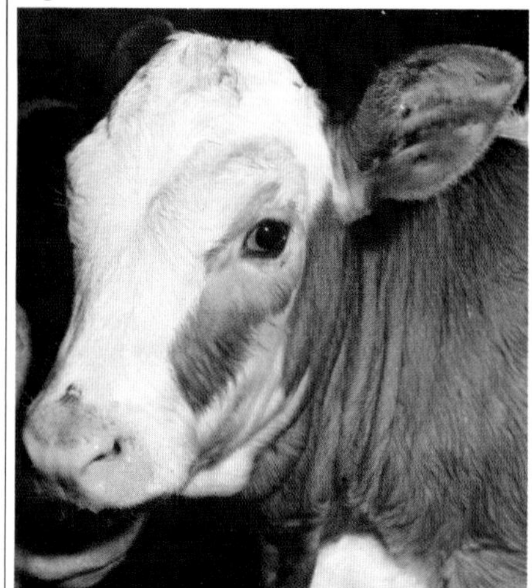

**Symptoms**

Crowding disease takes a uniform course and can be divided into two clearly defined stages:

■ **Virus-induced infection**

The spread of the initially purely viral infection, favoured by the factors mentioned above, results in an inflammation of the airways (windpipe and bronchi). The visible symptoms are not very pronounced: Sudden rise in temperature to 40–41° C, accelerated breathing, aqueous discharge from the eyes and nose and occasionally slight cough. The increased body temperature returns to normal after 1 or 2 days. In younger animals the symptoms are usually somewhat more pronounced than in older cattle. This stage of the disease is often overlooked, particularly in intensive beef bull fattening with the animals being kept in covered yards.

*Fig. 285*

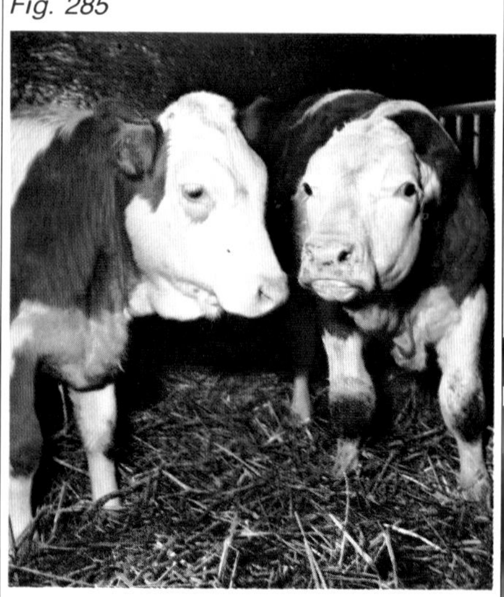

■ **Second viral attack and bacterial infection**

After a brief period in which the temperature is normal, a second viral attack occurs within a few days and the body temperature rises again to high levels. Some animals now show pronounced symptoms of disease. They refuse to feed, have difficulty in breathing, their heart rate is increased and they suffer bouts of persistent coughing. The nasal discharge becomes turbid or mucoid. Breathing has a "pumping" action. The nostrils are opened wide and the animal breathes through the mouth with formation of foam. These are symptoms of pneumonia with pulmonary emphysema. In rare cases, death through cardiac arrest may occur within one day.

It is at this stage that secondary bacterial infections with pasteurellae, staphylococci, streptococci and corynebacteria occur and aggravate the condition. The nasal discharge becomes mucopurulent, the raised body temperature shows diurnal fluctuations.

Fig. 284: Initial stage of crowding disease: Some aqueous discharge from the eyes and nose.

Fig. 285: Animal on the right: dirty muzzle, strained look, nostrils opened wide.

Fig. 286: After the incubation period, the initially purely viral infection causes the first feverish attack. This stage is usually overlooked by the animal attendant. After a brief recovery phase in which the temperature returns to normal, a second virus-induced increase in temperature occurs which is then maintained by secondary bacterial infections. These secondary infections are usually responsible for the death of the animals.

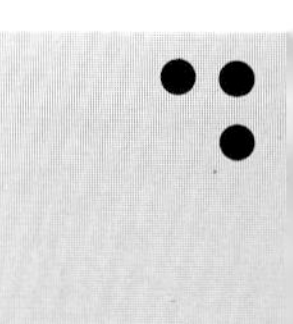

Fig. 286

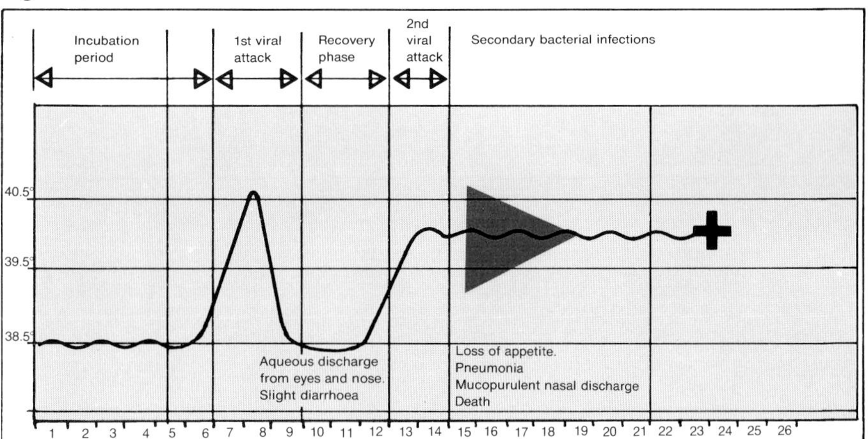


Symptoms

The animals stand listlessly with splayed forelegs and the head stretched forwards. The outer skin in the region of the lungs is painful to the touch. Apart from respiratory symptoms, some animals have diarrhoea. Unless treatment is initiated immediately at this stage, the existing bacterial pneumonia develops into chronic purulent pneumonia with alternating feverish attacks. Emaciation with concomitant severe dyspnoea and, finally, death through cardiac failure are the result.

Infection with bacteria may also occur without a preceding viral infection. Prolonged transport under extreme conditions and severe chill alone are sufficient to provoke the bacterial disease described above. This also explains why vaccination against influenza-type disease, which only provides immunity to virus infection, does not always have the desired effect.

Diagnosis

The characteristic course with two attacks of fever and the visible signs of respiratory disease point to the presence of crowding disease. The demonstration of causal viruses is necessary in stocks where crowding disease occurs regularly. In the living animal, the virus involved can be demonstrated only at the start of the disease by taking swabs (nose, throat, conjunctiva of the eye).

It is particularly important to ascertain whether IBR and mucosal disease viruses are involved, since the prevention and treatment of these diseases call for different measures to be taken.

*Fig. 287*

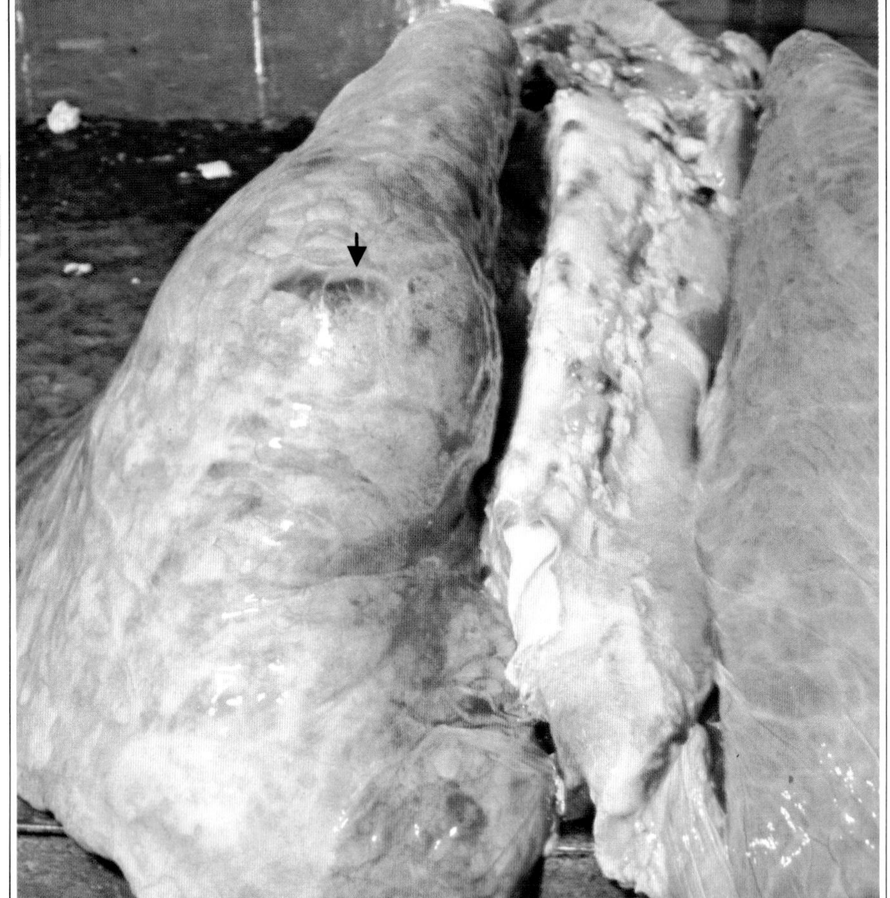

*Fig. 287: Lungs in crowding disease. Pleura shows milky turbidity. Pulmonary emphysema (arrow) by tearing of pulmonary alveoli.*

*Fig. 288: Secondary infection in crowding disease. Purulent pneumonia. Accumulation of pus in the bronchi.*

*Fig. 289: Old, incompletely healed pneumonic lesions. Adhesion of connective tissue to windpipe.*

*Fig. 290: Incision into the lungs: total pyosis of the lung tissue.*

**Similar symptoms**

In a wider sense, the influenza-type disease complex includes infectious bovine rhinotracheitis (IBR) and mucosal disease (MD). It is possible to differentiate these two conditions from crowding disease and to identify the causal pathogens involved. Further diseases with similar manifestations are listeriosis, malignant catarrh and lungworm infestation. The most important distinguishing characteristics of these diseases are as follows:

*Fig. 288*

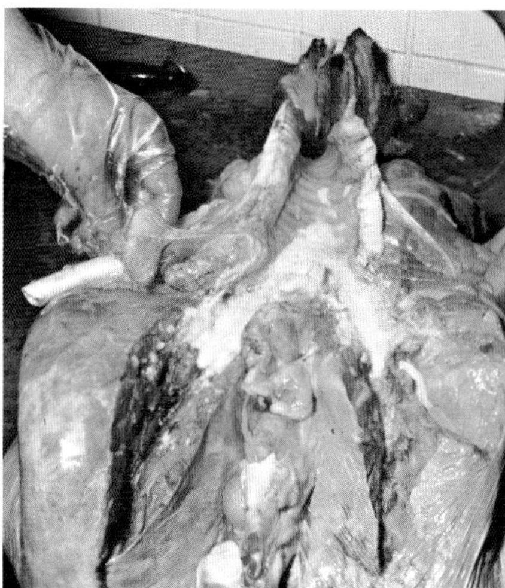

*Fig. 289*

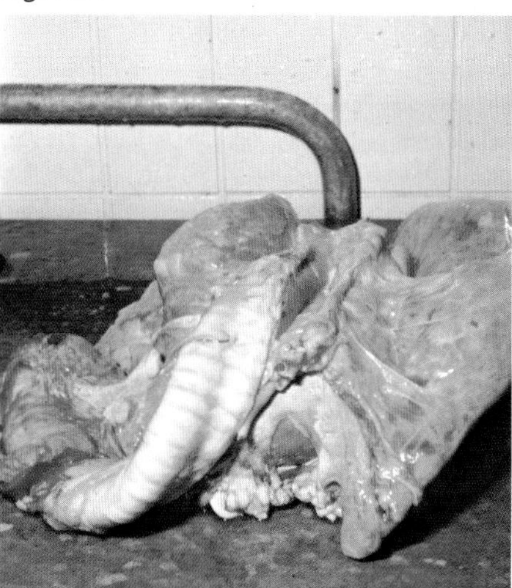

*Fig. 290*

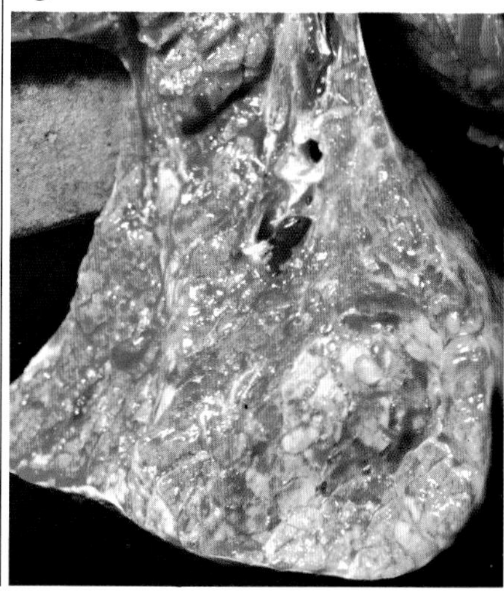

**Similar symptoms**

- IBR: Severe dyspnoea due to congestion of the upper respiratory tract with mucus. "Red nose" (reddened muzzle, particularly at the point of transition from the mucosa to the hairy skin).

- Mucosal disease: Inflammation of the gums, mucosal erosions (superficial loss of tissue), severe diarrhoea, inflammation of the coronal edge on the claws.

- Listeriosis: Central nervous disorders. The animals move in circles, always holding the head to the same side.

- Malignant catarrh: Changes in the eyes (corneal turbidity). Heavy mucoid discharge from the nose and mouth.

- Lungworm infestation: Lungworm larvae can be demonstrated in the faeces, particularly in animals grazing on infested pastures (approx. 4 weeks after being put out to graze).

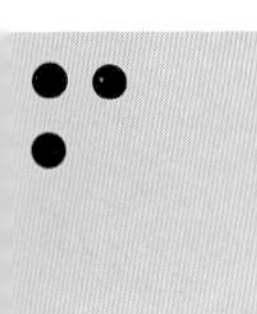

Treatment

The success of treatment depends essentially on how early the disease is recognised and how early therapeutic measures are initiated. As soon as the first signs of disease appear in some of the animals, the remaining cattle that do not yet show any symptoms should be carefully monitored. With close observation of the animals, checking their feed intake and measuring their body temperature, treatment can be started as early as the viral infection.

The administration of antibiotics prevents the appearance or the spread of secondary bacterial infections. In treatment, a distinction should be made between severely affected and slightly affected animals on the one hand, and the remaining stock on the other.

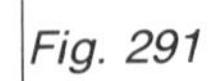

Fig. 291

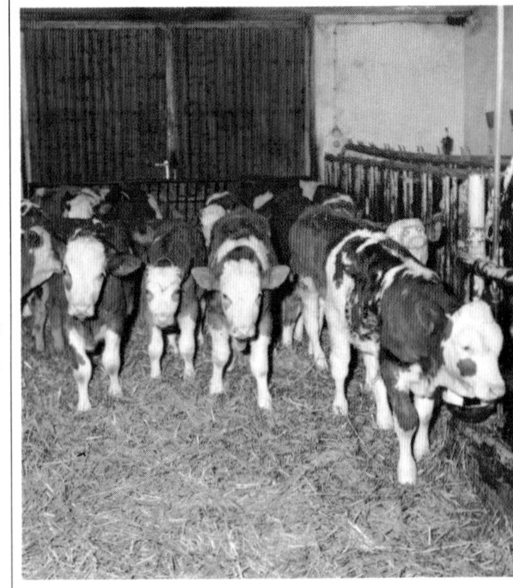

### ■ Severely affected animals

In group penning, the affected animals should be separated from the remaining stock as far as possible ("sick pen"). Injection therapy with antibiotics should be supplemented by the administration of mucolytic agents and products activating the circulation. Additional injections of vitamins and excitometabolic substances are advisable. If the fever persists, we usually administer anti-inflammatory and antipyretic products. Even if the animals' condition shows rapid improvement, injection therapy should be continued for at least 5 days.

### ■ Slightly affected animals

Treatment should be initiated by an injection of sulphonamides. At the same time, we administer a sulphonamide bolus by mouth, which remains in the dorsal sac of the rumen and maintains high blood levels over a period of 4 days (see Fig. 482). Additional administration of vitamins, particularly vitamin A, C and the B-complex, will increase resistance to infection.

### ■ Treatment of remaining stock

As soon as the first signs of disease appear in some of the animals, those not yet affected – especially animals of up to 400 kg bodyweight which are particularly at risk – are given medicated feed (CHEVIBULL) to prevent the spread of the bacterial infection. This will reduce the number of further cases of the disease as well as the severity of the condition if it does appear.

*Fig. 291: Dry, well ventilated cattle house with warming straw litter and adequate air space are the pre-conditions for avoiding crowding disease.*

*Fig. 292: After the incubation period, the initially purely viral infection leads to the first attack of fever. This stage is usually overlooked by the animal attendant. After a brief recovery phase in which the temperature returns to normal, a second virus-induced increase in temperature occurs which is then maintained by secondary infections. These secondary infections are usually responsible for the death of the animals. When the first signs of disease (fever, aqueous discharge from eyes and nose, loss of appetite) are observed in the stock, the visibly affected animals should be treated immediately. In addition, the administration of medicated feed to the entire stock is necessary, in order to prevent secondary bacterial infections. Although the animals will still suffer two attacks of fever, the severity of the condition is reduced, their appetite is maintained and losses are avoided.*

Fig. 292

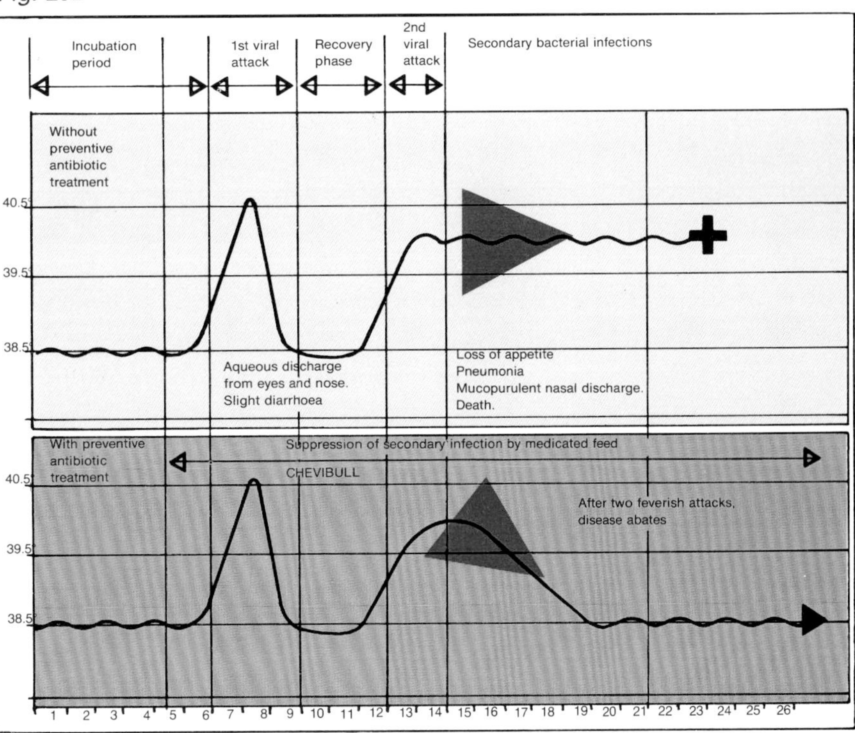


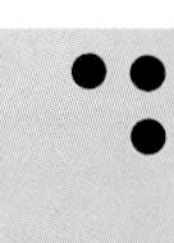

**Treatment**

This treatment should be carried out for at least three weeks. The long period of treatment and keeping within the prescribed dosage limits are necessary. Overdosage of antibiotics and sulphonamides administered via the fodder disturbs the flora of the rumen resulting in digestive disorders, loss of appetite and tympany.

Correct use of medicated feed maintains the animals' appetite. They get over the disease without showing severe symptoms and recover quickly in the follow-up period of treatment. Stunting with poor appetite and poor weight gain, often seen after crowding disease, is thus largely avoided.

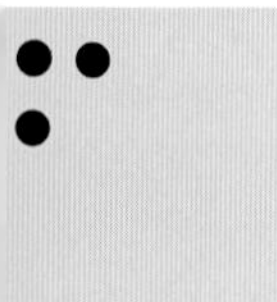

**Treatment**

*Fig. 293*

| | | |
|---|---|---|
| 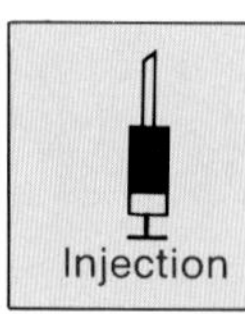 Injection | **Severely affected animals:** 1.5 ml FORACOL/10 kg. Repeat after 12 h. 1 ml BISOLVON and 0.3 ml CAFFEINE/10 kg. 10 ml VITAMIN-AD$_3$EC-100/animal. | 1st day |
| Injection | **Severely affected animals:** 1.5 ml FORACOL/10 kg body-weight. Repeat after 12 hours. 1 ml BISOLVON/10 kg body-weight. 0.2 ml VOREN/10 kg body-weight. | 2nd day |
| 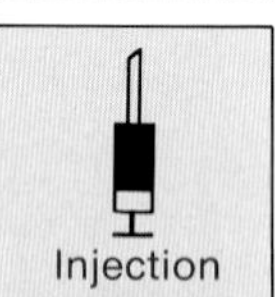 Injection | **Severely affected animals:** 1.5 ml FORACOL/10 kg body-weight. Repeat after 12 hours. 1 ml CATOSAL/10 kg body-weight. Continue injections of antibiotic. | 3rd to 5th day |
| 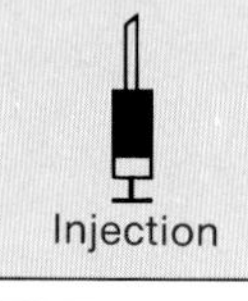 Injection | **Slightly affected animals:** Injection: 1 ml KELFIZIN/10 kg body-weight. Give 1 BOVIBOL/150 kg body-weight by mouth. | 1st day |
| Fodder | **Affected animals and all those at risk:** Give 10 g CHEVIBULL/animal per day for at least 3 weeks. If necessary, continue with half the dosage. | 1st to 21st day |
| 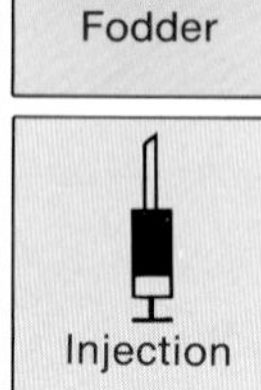 Injection | FORACOL may be replaced by KELFIZIN, VETOPRIM 24%, SPECTAM, AMPICILLIN, FORAPEN and similar products. Note directions for use in each case! | |

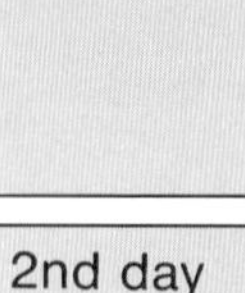

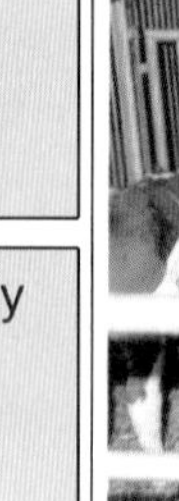

*Fig. 294*

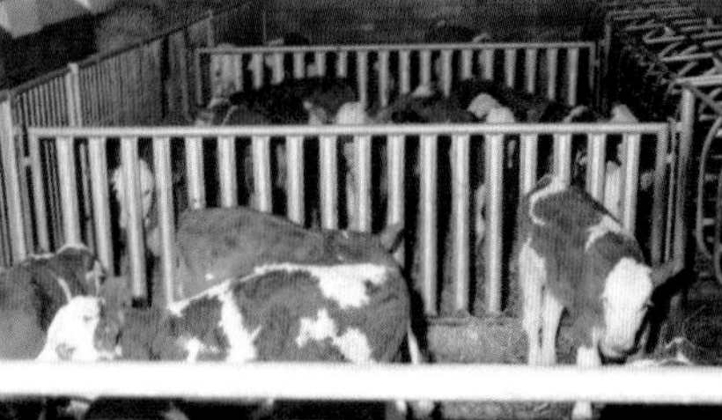

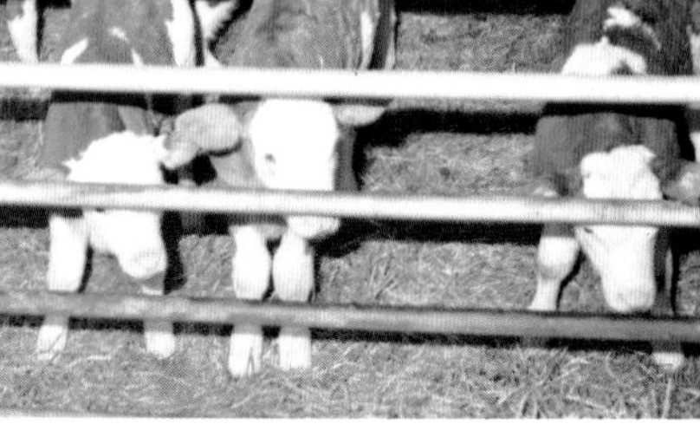

**Prevention**

Calves reared under optimal conditions in a controlled environment appropriate for cattle, are less susceptible to crowding disease. Prevention aims to create the pre-conditions necessary for good health and good performance and to counteract conditions of special unavoidable stress. In our experience, livestock farms have little trouble with crowding disease, if the points listed in Fig. 296 are observed in rearing and housing.

*Fig. 295*

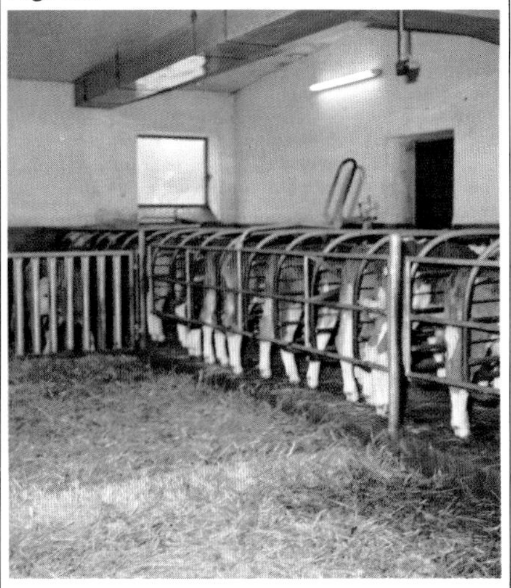

*Fig. 296*

| 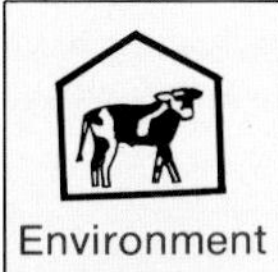 Environment | **Separate reception house:** In-out method. Cleaning and disinfection. Allow to stand empty for one week before occupation, and pre-warm; cf. page 264. | Before arrival of the calves |
|---|---|---|
| Laboratory | **Health check:** General condition, discharge from eyes and nose; navel, faeces, body-temperature; cf. pp. 70 to 80 and page 261 (check list). | On arrival of the calves |
| 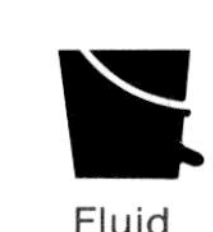 Fluid | **Prophylaxis on housing:** Depending on duration of transport, preventive treatment with CHEVICALF or BUSAL via the drinking fluid and injections; cf. page 262. | 1st to 14th day after arrival |
| 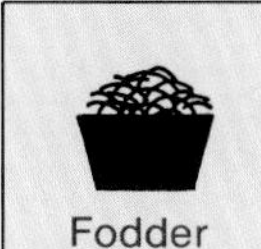 Fodder | **Correct weaning:** Milk substitute: quantity, temp. Water should always be available. Necessary to give hay. Calf starter feed ad lib. up to daily max. of 1.5 kg; cf. page 268. | 1st to 6th week |
| 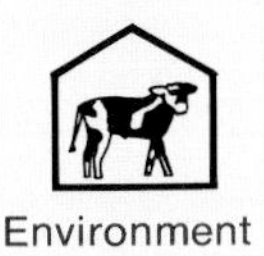 Environment | **Re-housing on slatted floor:** Heating, CHEVIBULL, from 1 week before until 2 weeks after. Observe discharge from nose and eyes, fodder intake; cf. page 272. | Rehousing |
| 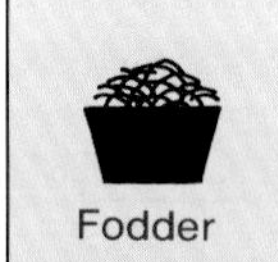 Fodder | **Purchase of fattening calves:** Observe appetite, discharge from eyes and nose, coughing. Preventive treatment on housing with BOVIBOL and CHEVIBULL. | Purchase |
| 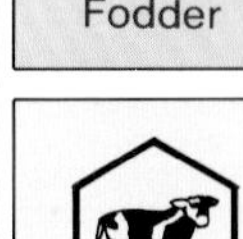 Environment | 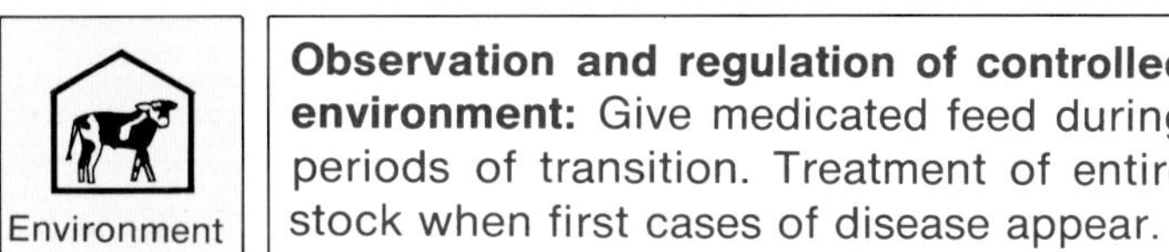 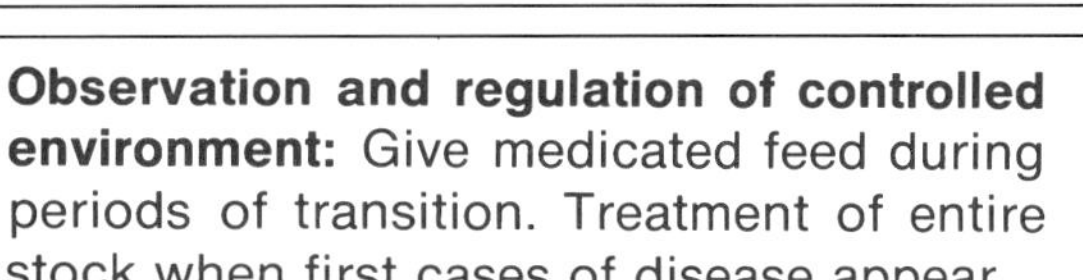 **Observation and regulation of controlled environment:** Give medicated feed during periods of transition. Treatment of entire stock when first cases of disease appear. | |
| 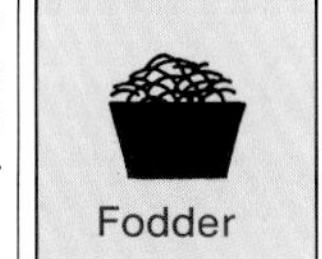 Fodder | **Feeding:** Well-balanced ration; adapted to basic ration and fattening ration. Nutrient substances: minerals, trace elements, vitamins; cf. page 275. | |

*Fig. 293: Treatment schedule for crowding disease.*

*Fig. 294: Separate reception house with straw litter. Cleaning and disinfection before occupation. Health check on housing. Prophylaxis on arrival, placing same age groups together.*

*Fig. 295: Correct weaning requires penning calves individually during the drinking period. This reduces mutual licking and favours the intake of pelleted calf starter feed.*

*Fig. 296: Measures to contain crowding disease.*

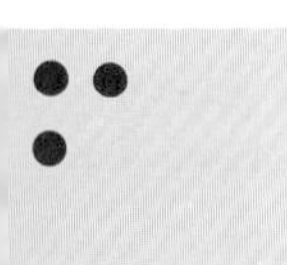

Vaccination

There are two vaccines against crowding disease on the market, which contain different spectra of pathogens: PNEUMOVAC PLUS and BOVIGRIP.

These are combined vaccines containing various kinds and types of viruses. These viruses have been inactivated whereby their pathogenic effect has been largely eliminated. However, they retain sufficient activity to stimulate the formation of antibodies. The injection of a vaccine – like a field infection (droplet infection via the mucosa) – introduces pathogens into the body which then forms antibodies to combat the vaccine viruses, without actually showing signs of disease. Protective vaccination is thus tantamount to a mild latent disease in the stock. It is therefore important that the animals to be vaccinated are healthy. If they are not healthy, the vaccination may in fact provoke and enhance any disease present.

Fig. 297

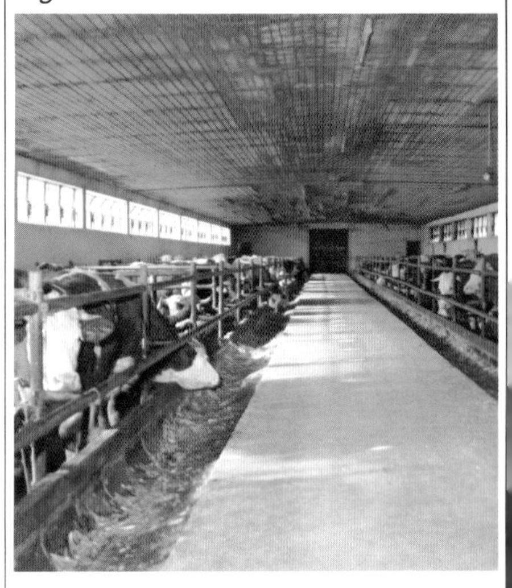

Vaccination against crowding disease does not as yet provide reliable protection, but may be carried out as an additional preventive measure. In our experience, vaccination is not always advisable, for the following reasons:

■ The right time for vaccination is difficult to determine, since only healthy calves should be vaccinated. They should have been on the farm for at least 3 weeks and should be at least 6 weeks old. The vaccination of large groups of animals is problematic, because such groups almost invariably include individual animals with a visible or latent chill or digestive disorder or suffering from mild feverish influenza-like disease. In such animals, the stress of vaccination will aggravate the existing disease.

■ At least 15 different kinds and types of viruses are known today as possible causative pathogens of crowding disease. It is always several viruses or virus types that are involved in an outbreak of crowding disease. However, the vaccines available only protect against some of these pathogens. This explains why cases of virus-induced crowding disease occur, despite vaccination against the disease.

■ Quite frequently, vaccination gives the livestock farmer a false sense of security, and he neglects caution and the necessary observation of the animals. For this reason, chills are not recognised and treated early enough and lead to substantial losses.

*Figs. 297 and 298: Beef oxen in a newly built cattle house with slatted floor. – Fattening bulls in an old cattle house. The type of the cattle house is less important to economy than good management and the preservation of the animals' health.*

*Fig. 299: Crowding disease vaccines available in Germany.*

Fig. 298

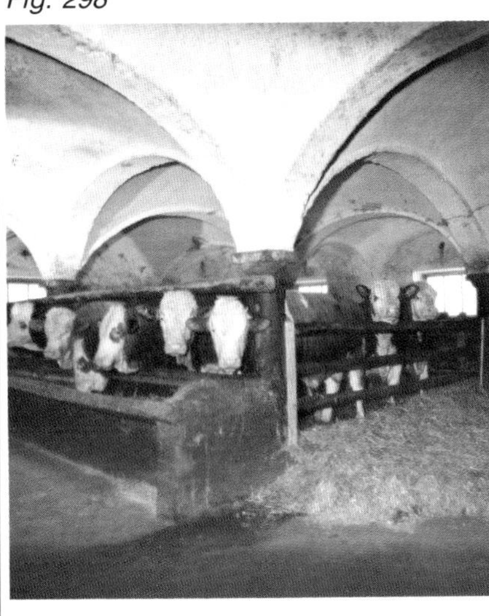

■ Our experience has shown that if vaccination against crowding disease is carried out, it is much more successful, particularly in large animal groups, if additional protection is provided by the administration of medicated feed. From 5 days before until 10 days after vaccination, we give 10 g CHEVIBULL per animal/day. Since vaccination, like a mild infection, may induce a bacterial infection, this method has proved successful. The development of immunity is not affected by this treatment.

■ If the virus of IBR or mucosal disease is demonstrated in the stock, vaccination against these pathogens is necessary (see chapters on IBR and mucosal disease). PNEUMOVAC PLUS contains some inactivated vaccine viruses of mucosal disease and IBR. However, better protection is conferred by specific vaccines against IBR or mucosal disease, which will induce the development of effective immunity.



Fig. 299

| Vaccine | PNEUMOVAC PLUS | BOVIGRIP |
| --- | --- | --- |
| Manufacturer | Hydrochemie | Behringwerke |
| Content of inactivated antigens (viruses) | Parainfluenza III virus<br>Adenovirus, serotype 3<br>Reovirus, serotype 1<br>Infectious bovine rhinotracheitis (IBR-IPV)<br>Virus diarrhoea (BVD-MD) | Parainfluenza III virus<br>Adenovirus, serotype 1<br>serotype 3<br>serotype 5<br>Reovirus, serotype 1<br>serotype 3 |
| Contra-indication | Do not vaccinate sick animals | Do not vaccinate sick animals or calves under 6 weeks old |
| Time of vaccination/vaccination schedule | 1st vaccination: from 10th day of life<br>2nd vaccination: 6th to 8th week of life<br>3rd vaccination: 2 to 4 weeks after second vaccination<br>4th vaccination: 9 to 12 months<br>1st vaccination may be omitted | 1st vaccination: from 6th week of life<br>2nd vaccination: at least 4, but preferably 6 weeks after first vaccination.<br>3rd vaccination: 1 year. |

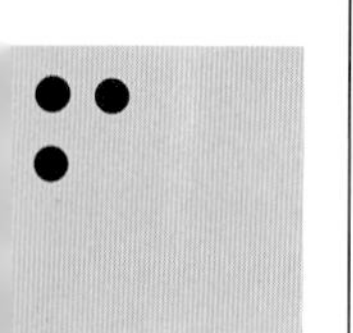

Another possibility of obtaining short-term protection against virus diseases, "interferonisation", is currently being paid increasing attention. It has been found that body cells being attacked by a virus, form some kind of protective substance against other micro-organisms. This protective substance, called interferon, prevents the penetration of other viruses, but also of bacteria, into the cell. If this condition is artificially created, by introducing attenuated, harmless viruses into the body cells, the formation of interferon is induced. In this way, pathogens like crowding disease viruses can be prevented, for a short period (approx. 10 days), from invading the animal body.

**Interferon inducers**

Interferon inducers offer the advantage that they can be used at a time when vaccination cannot yet be carried out, e. g. before transport and on housing.

Since the effect of interferon inducers abates after 7 days, the treatment often has to be repeated. Difficulties following transport and housing usually occur in the second or third week.

There are two products on the market: BAYFERON and PI-III VACCINE. PI-III Vaccine in addition induces the development of immunity against parainfluenza III viruses.

Vaccination against crowding disease and the use of interferon inducers should only be regarded as additional supportive measures in combating this factor disease. The most important pre-condition of avoiding crowding disease is to carry out the preventive measures listed in Fig. 296.

*Fig. 300: IBR: Listless behaviour; reddening of the line of transition from the haired skin to the muzzle. Mucoid/foamy discharge from nose and mouth.*

*Fig. 300*

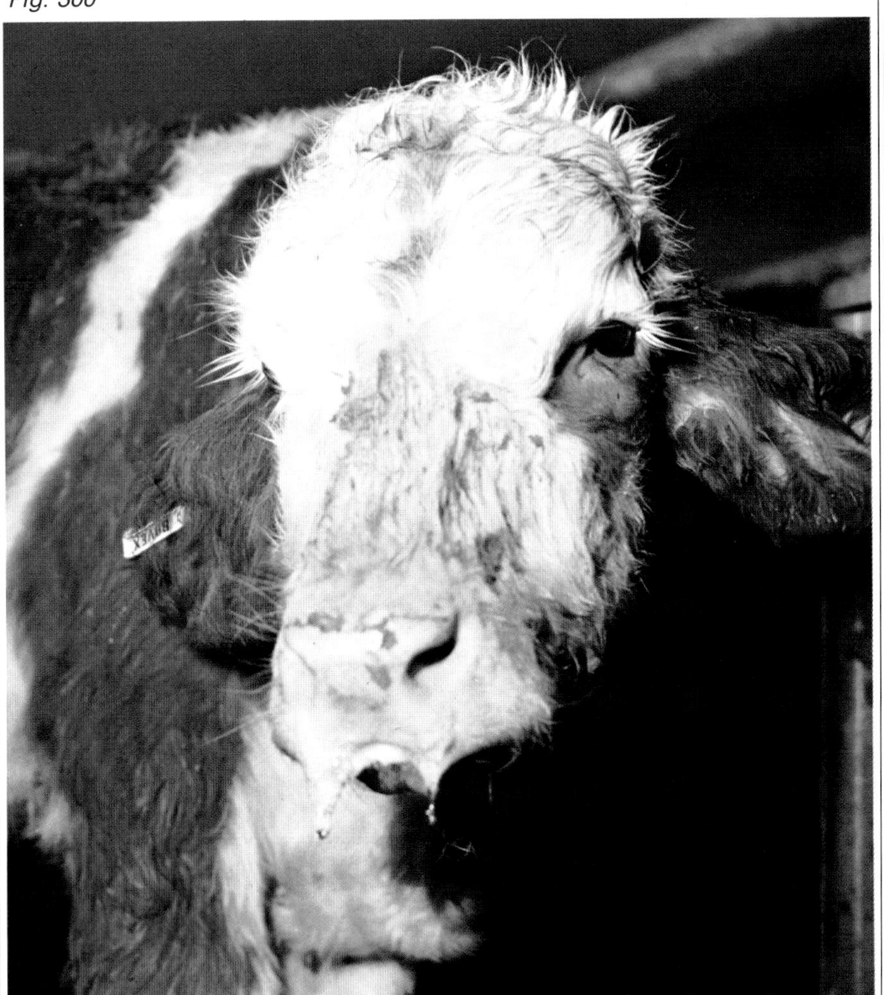

IBR

**Term**

**I**nfectious **b**ovine **r**hinotracheitis (IBR) is caused by a herpes virus. This pathogen also causes **i**nfectious **p**ustular **v**ulvovaginitis (IPV), a vesicular eczema.

**Incidence**

IBR initially manifests itself as a disease of the upper respiratory tract. The clinical picture is aggravated by the supervention of a bacterial infection. In recent times, IBR has increasingly been observed in beef bull stocks with up to 70% of all animals being affected. High losses of cattle aged 6 to 8 months have been recorded.

Fig. 301

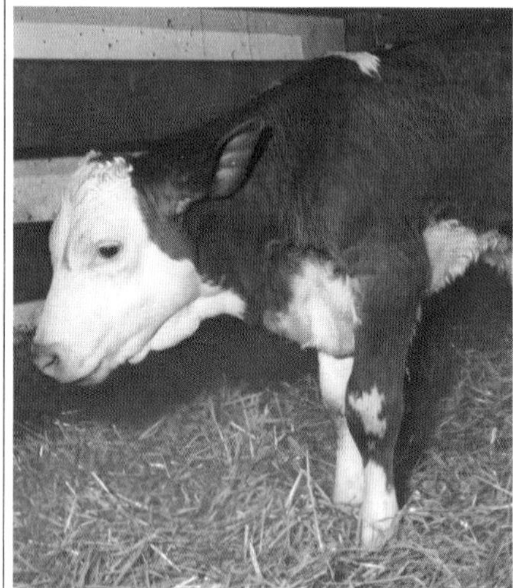

Fig. 302

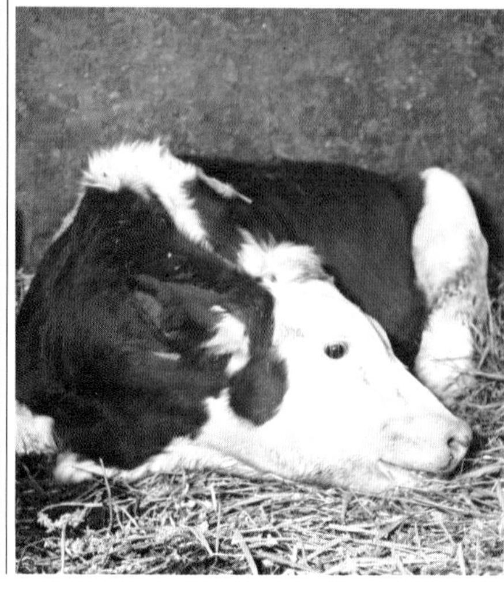

Fig. 303

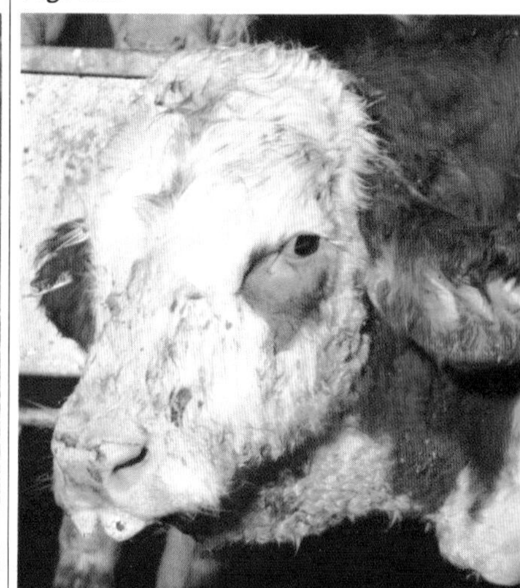

**Importation into the stock**

IBR is often imported into the stock by newly purchased animals. The outbreak of the disease occurs within 4 to 7 days of infection. As a result of its multiplication in an affected animal, the pathogenic effect (virulence) of the virus is enhanced and its infective power and propagatory ability increase with each further case of the disease (animal passage). In stocks with a large number of animals of the same age (6 to 8 months), IBR is therefore particularly severe.

After the initial outbreak of IBR in a stock, the infection usually appears to abate, especially if no further animals are purchased. During this period the virus withdraws into the lymph nodes of the respiratory organs. This condition is called a latent infection. If the animals are then subjected to stress, the IBR viruses again spread to the mucosae, are excreted and may cause a new outbreak of the disease in the same animal or in other animals.

Poor controlled environment (excessively high air humidity and ammonia concentration) accelerate the progress of the disease. Inadequate vitamin supply or poor fodder intake also favour a rapid spread of IBR. This applies particularly to rehousing problems after the purchase of fattening calves, rehousing on slatted floors and the housing of grazing animals. IBR reaches its peak after approx. three weeks. It is at this time that the heaviest losses occur (up to 15%).

*Fig. 301: Initial stage of IBR: dyspnoea.*

*Figs. 302 and 303: Terminal stage of IBR: Resting head, strained look, open mouth, formation of foam at the mouth.*

*Fig. 304: Severe dyspnoea, poor general condition. Head lowered; stretched head and neck posture; drooping ears; white foam at the mouth.*

*Fig. 305: Pulmonary emphysema. In IBR, as a result of the obstruction of the airways with mucus, inhalation and exhalation are impaired. Coughing and physical exertion (rounding up animals) lead to bursting of pulmonary alveoli.*

*Fig. 304*

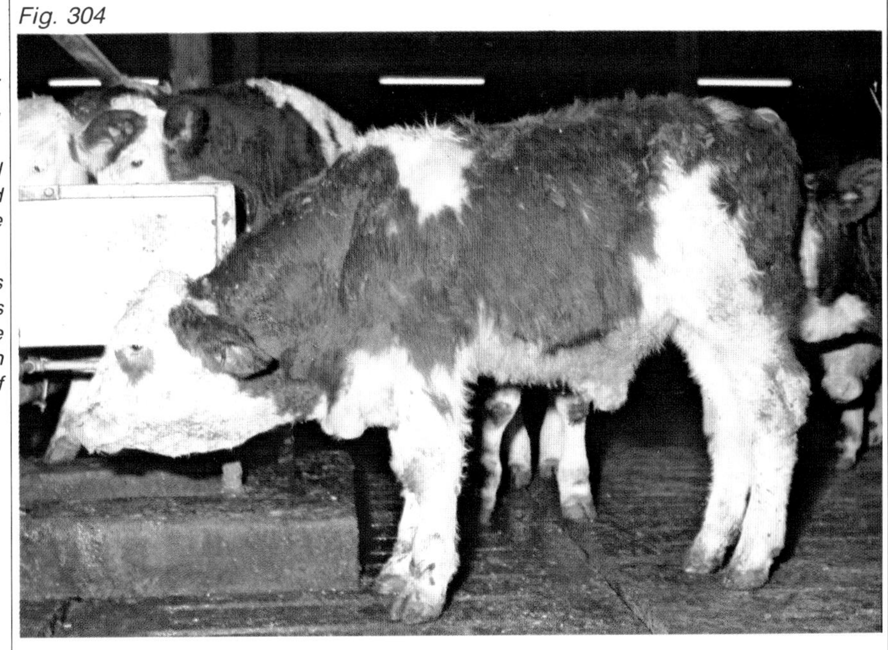

**Symptoms**

Initially the disease manifests itself in reduced appetite, listlessness and an increase in body temperature to 41–42° C within 1 or 2 days. Shortly afterwards salivation, a profuse aqueous or mucoid nasal discharge and an aqueous discharge from the eyes are observed. The muzzle is often bright red, particularly at the point of transition from the skin to the mucosa, hence the name "red nose". With the further progress of the disease, breathing accelerates and has a "pumping" action. The obstruction of the larynx, the windpipe and the bronchi with mucus narrows the airways and mechanically impairs inhalation and exhalation. Impaired exhalation and sudden bouts of coughing result in the bursting of pulmonary alveoli and finally lead to pulmonary emphysema. Due to increased pressure in the thoracic cavity, reduced oxygenation of the blood and pneumonia, congestion with increased extravasation of aqueous (serous) fluid into fissures in the tissue are observed (pulmonary oedema). The animals stand with their forelegs splayed and their heads lowered and are audibly fighting for breath. At this stage white foam appears around the mouth. If the animals show these symptoms, they are critically ill. Severe dyspnoea and refusal to feed quickly weaken the cattle.

*Fig. 305*

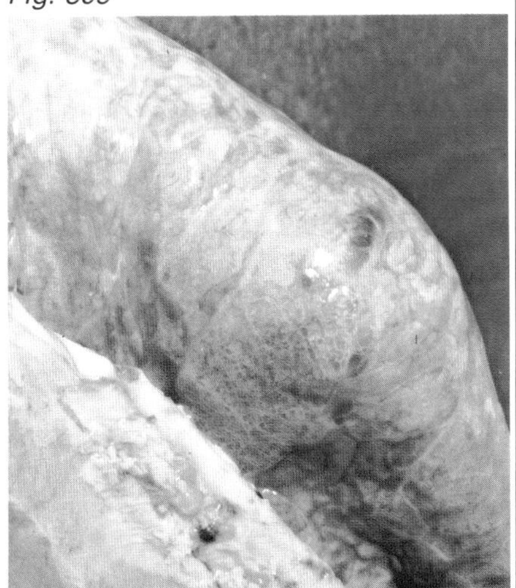

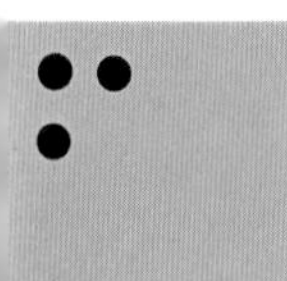

Symptoms

Fig. 306

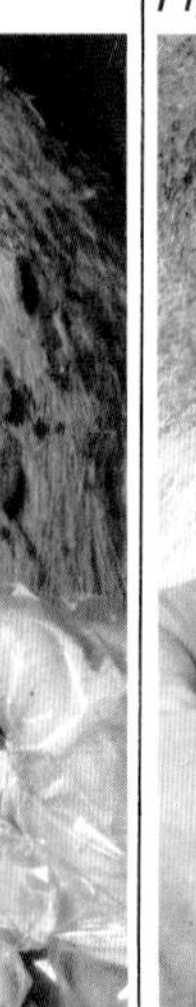

Fig. 307

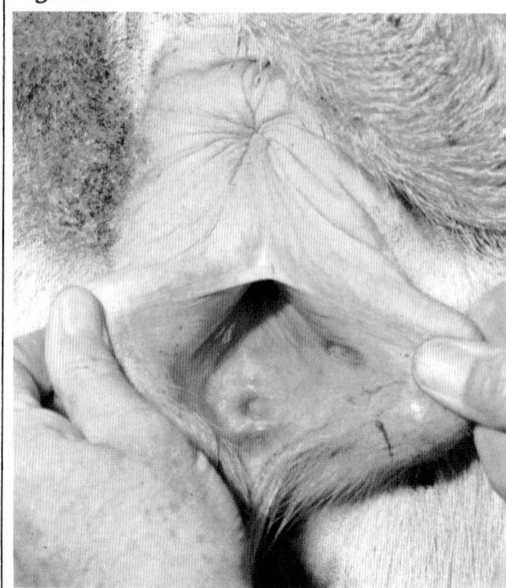

Fig. 308

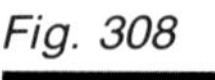

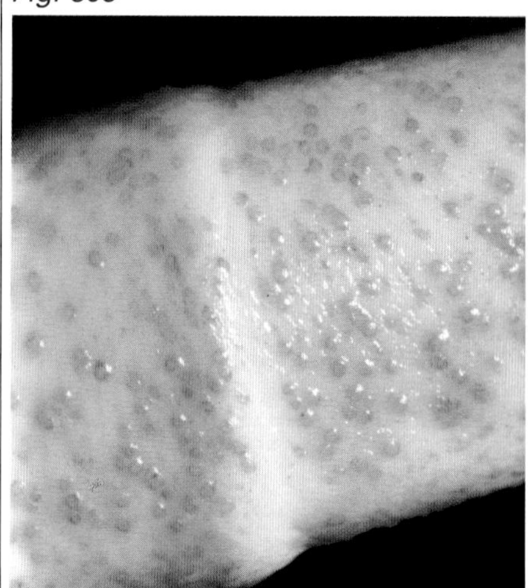

Secondary bacterial infections, mainly due to pasteurellae, produce severe pneumonia.

Virus-induced abortion is possible in cows 4 to 8 weeks after the end of an outbreak of IBR. Intra-uterine death of the calf with subsequent mummification may occur.

Once the disease has been overcome, local tissue immunity develops. This is why an animal that has recovered from the respiratory form of the disease, is unlikely to contract this form again in the near future, although the same animal may contract the genital form (IPV). IBR and IPV do not occur simultaneously in the same animal.

IPV is characterised by small pustules which may become suppurative as a result of the supervention of bacteria. In cows, the pustules are seen on the vulvae, particularly at the point of transition from the outer skin to the vaginal mucosa, and in the clitoral fossa. There is a vaginal discharge which may range from aqueous/mucoid to mucoid/purulent in consistency.

In bulls, the pustules are observed in the region of the urethral orifice and on the glans penis. Following rupture of these pustules, mucosal defects develop which may ulcerate as a result of bacterial infection. Adhesion of the penis to the sheath may occur, totally or partly preventing the protrusion of the penis. A bull suffering from IPV should be excluded from breeding.

Fig. 309

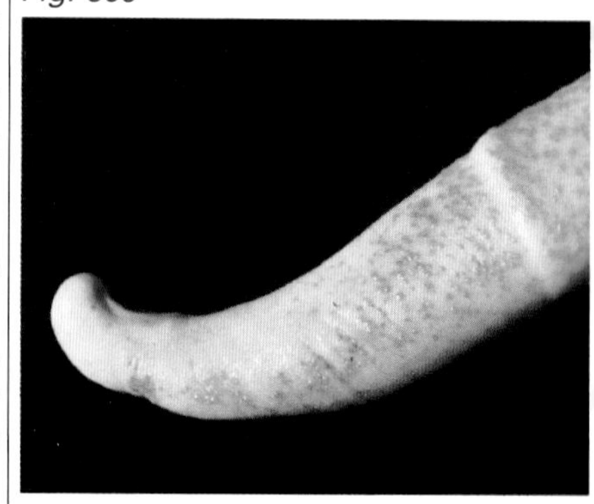

*Figs. 306 and 307: IPV – pustular eruption in the vagina.*

*Figs. 308 and 309: IPV – pustular eruption on the penis.*

*Fig. 310: Similar clinical picture: Mucosal disease. Erosions with furfuraceous crusts on the muzzle and in the nose.*

*Fig. 310*

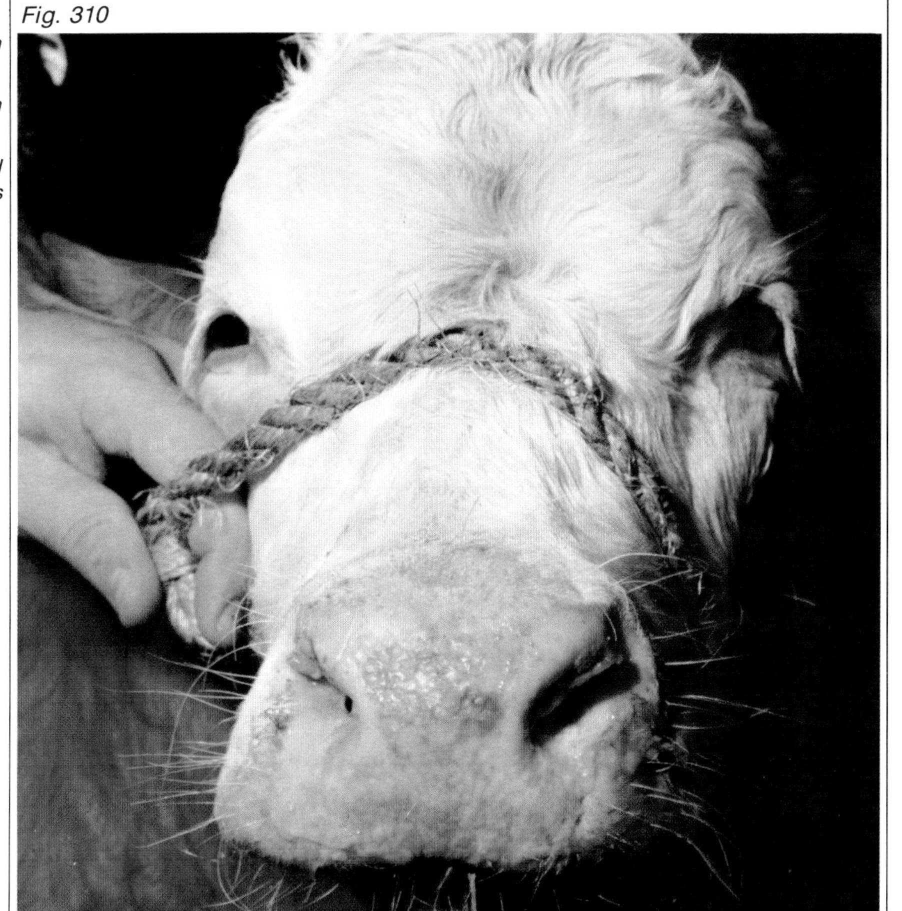

**Similar symptoms**

The manifestations of IBR resemble the respiratory condition which is generally known as crowding disease. A definitive differentiation is possible only by demonstrating the virus in swabs taken from the eye secretion and the nasal mucus. A blood test whereby the level of antibodies to IBR/IPV viruses is determined, can also confirm the diagnosis.

Confirmation of the diagnosis is desirable because, if IBR is present, specific preventive measures can be taken by vaccinating the animals not yet affected.

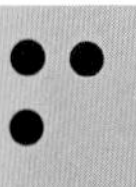

The reddening of the mucosa on the muzzle and in the nose is similar to the erosions seen in mucosal disease. However, with mucosal disease there is almost invariably concomitant severe diarrhoea. Here, too, demonstration of the pathogen is necessary and vaccination is possible.

**Similar symptoms**

Very similar symptoms appear in malignant catarrhal fever where, in contrast to IBR, severe inflammation of the eyes (with the animals shunning light), discharge from the eyes and, at a later stage, corneal turbidity (keratitis) are seen.

**Treatment**

Treatment is confined to combating the secondary bacterial infection. This is done by giving antibiotics, and particularly sulphonamides in high dosage. Mucolytic drugs counteract any obstruction of the windpipe with mucus. The cardiovascular system of the animals should be supported.

*Fig. 311*

| | | |
|---|---|---|
| 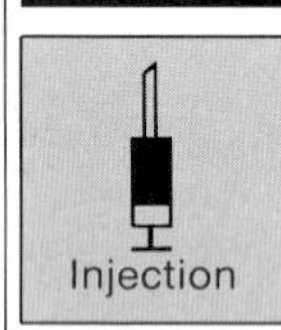 Injection | **Severely affected animals:** 1 ml KELFIZIN/10 kg body-weight; 1 ml BISOLVON/10 kg body-weight; 10 ml VITAMIN-$AD_3$-EC-100/animal; 0.3 ml CAFFEINE (50%)/10 kg. | 1st day |
| 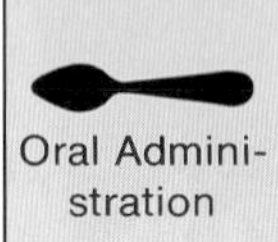 Oral Administration | **All visibly affected animals (with fever):** Give 1 BOVIBOL/150 kg body-weight. | 1st day |
| 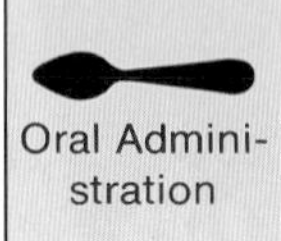 Injection | **Severely affected animals:** 1 ml BISOLVON/10 kg body-weight; 0.3 ml CAFFEINE (50%)/10 kg if necessary; 0.2 ml VOREN/10 kg once on second day. | 2nd and 3rd day |
| 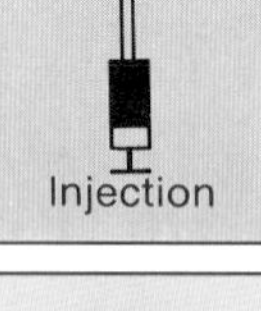 Fodder | **Affected animals and all those at risk:** 10 g CHEVIBULL/animal per day, for at least 3 weeks; if necessary continue treatment with half the dosage. | 1st to 21st day |

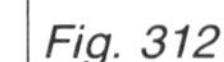

*Fig. 312*

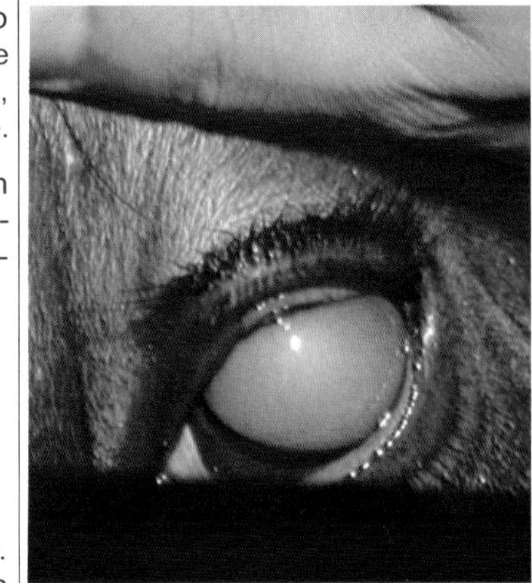

*Fig. 313*

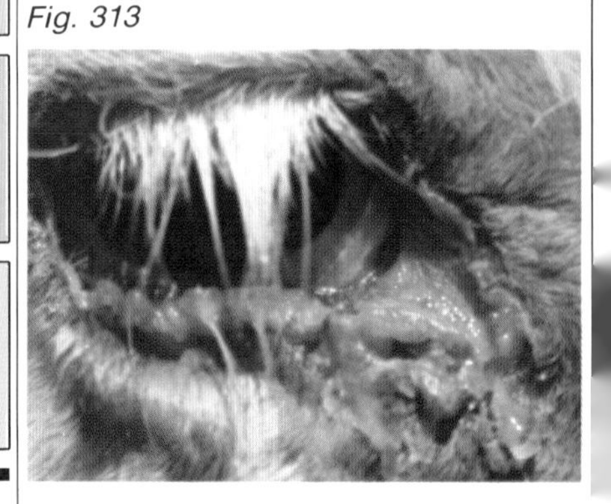

Fig. 314

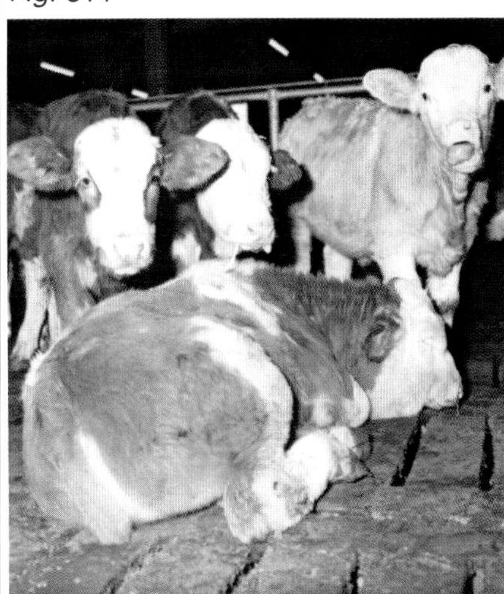

**Treatment**

All visibly affected cattle should be given injection treatment as soon as possible. This treatment needs to be repeated several times. Rounding up the animals in a covered yard always presents particular problems, because the existing dyspnoea is further aggravated by this disturbance. There is the danger of the sudden appearance of a pulmonary emphysema. We therefore prefer to give a sulphonamide bolus (BOVIBOL). The bolus is administered by means of an applicator. It falls into the dorsal sac and dissolves over a period of 4 to 5 days. Each bolus releases 5 g sulphamethazine daily for 4 to 5 days. The active substance passes through the abomasum into the intestine where it is absorbed. This bolus is administered to all severely and slightly affected animals at the start of treatment. Only the severely affected animals need additional injection therapy. The rounding up of these animals is less difficult. It is advisable to keep severely ill cattle together in a "sick pen".

**Prevention**

At present only a mixed vaccine (PNEUMOVAC PLUS) is available for vaccination. Although a specific IBR/IPV vaccine does exist, it can only be used by special permission of the regional authorities in Germany. When crowding disease vaccines are used in livestock that is at risk, it should be ensured that they contain an IBR/IPV component. The first vaccination (basic immunisation) should be followed by a second vaccination (booster) at an interval of 4 weeks. Prior to vaccination, the state of health of the entire stock should be checked. The animals to be vaccinated should have been on the farm for at least three weeks and should be clinically healthy.

Attention should be paid to optimal environmental conditions (controlled environment), hygiene and medicinal prophylaxis. To mitigate the stress on purchase and re-housing, 10 g CHEVIBULL/animal per day should be given for at least three weeks. Here it should be noted that the quantity of 10 g per animal and per day should be given throughout, irrespective of age and body-weight.

We also carry out vaccination under cover of this medication, starting 5 days before the anticipated date of vaccination and completing the course of medicated feed 14 days after the vaccination.

*Fig. 311: Treatment schedule for IBR.*

*Fig. 312: Malignant catarrhal fever: Here, turbidity of the cornea (keratitis) is often observed.*

*Fig. 313: Malignant catarrhal fever: Purulent discharge from the eyes. Hairs of the eyelids are matted with dried pus.*

*Fig. 314: Severely affected young bull. In order to increase the chances of survival with purposeful treatment, it is essential to move affected animals to a "sick pen".*

# Mucosal disease

Fig. 315

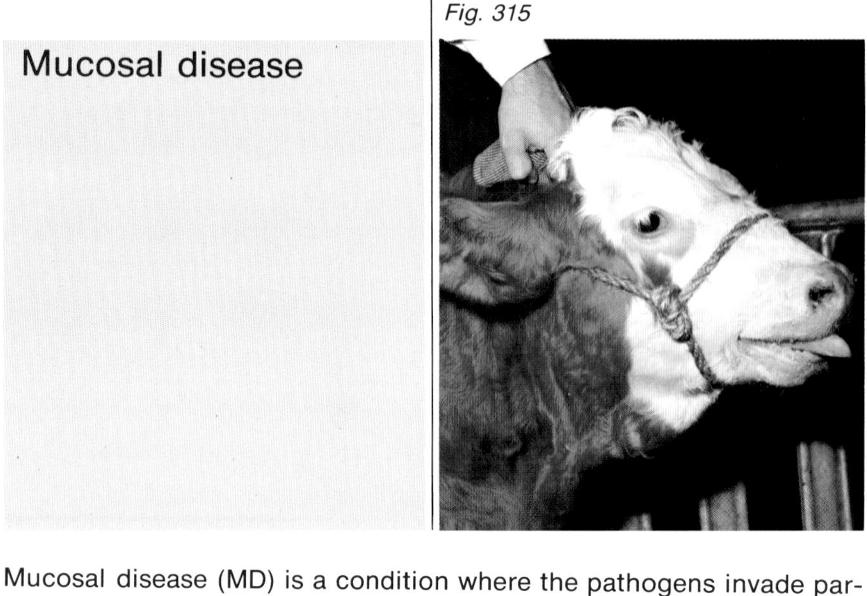

Fig. 316

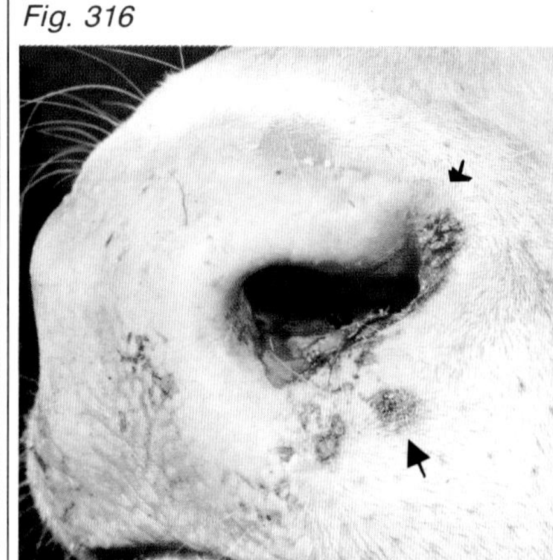

**Term**

Mucosal disease (MD) is a condition where the pathogens invade particularly the mucosae of the digestive tract, but also those of the respiratory tract. The most striking characteristic of the disease is severe intractable diarrhoea which results in death in the majority of cases.

**Incidence**

Investigations in cattle stocks have shown that the virus causing mucosal disease is widely distributed in Germany and that more than half the cattle have been exposed to the pathogen and have formed antibodies against it. We have found that the increase in intensive rearing over the past few years has brought with it a substantial increase in the incidence of the disease. Cattle of all age groups may contract the disease, young animals being particularly at risk.

Fig. 317

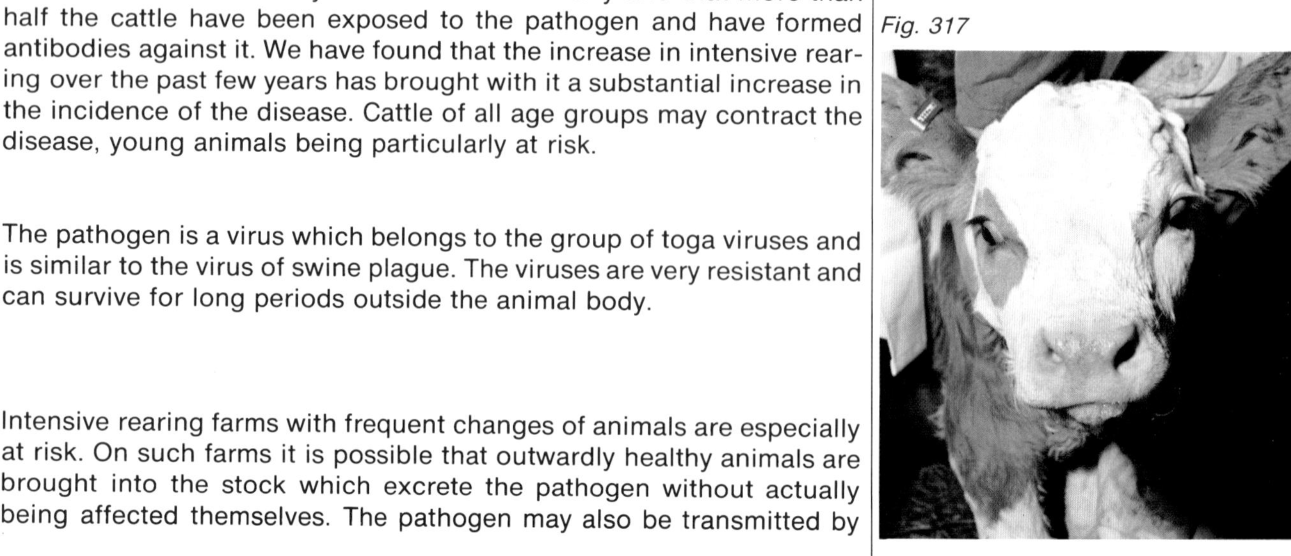

**Pathogen**

The pathogen is a virus which belongs to the group of toga viruses and is similar to the virus of swine plague. The viruses are very resistant and can survive for long periods outside the animal body.

**Importation**

Intensive rearing farms with frequent changes of animals are especially at risk. On such farms it is possible that outwardly healthy animals are brought into the stock which excrete the pathogen without actually being affected themselves. The pathogen may also be transmitted by

*Fig. 315: Mucosal disease: Erosions of the mucosa in the nostrils and involvement of the respiratory tract (coughing).*

*Fig. 316: Furfuraceous crusts and erosions on the mucosa (arrows).*

*Fig. 317: In the newborn calf, a red muzzle and minor mucosal defects should be regarded as normal.*

*Fig. 318: Mucosal disease in a bull weighing 12 cwts: Fluid yellowish brown faeces already containing some blood.*

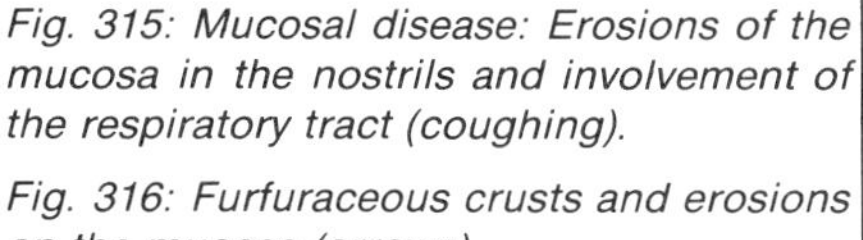

*Fig. 318*

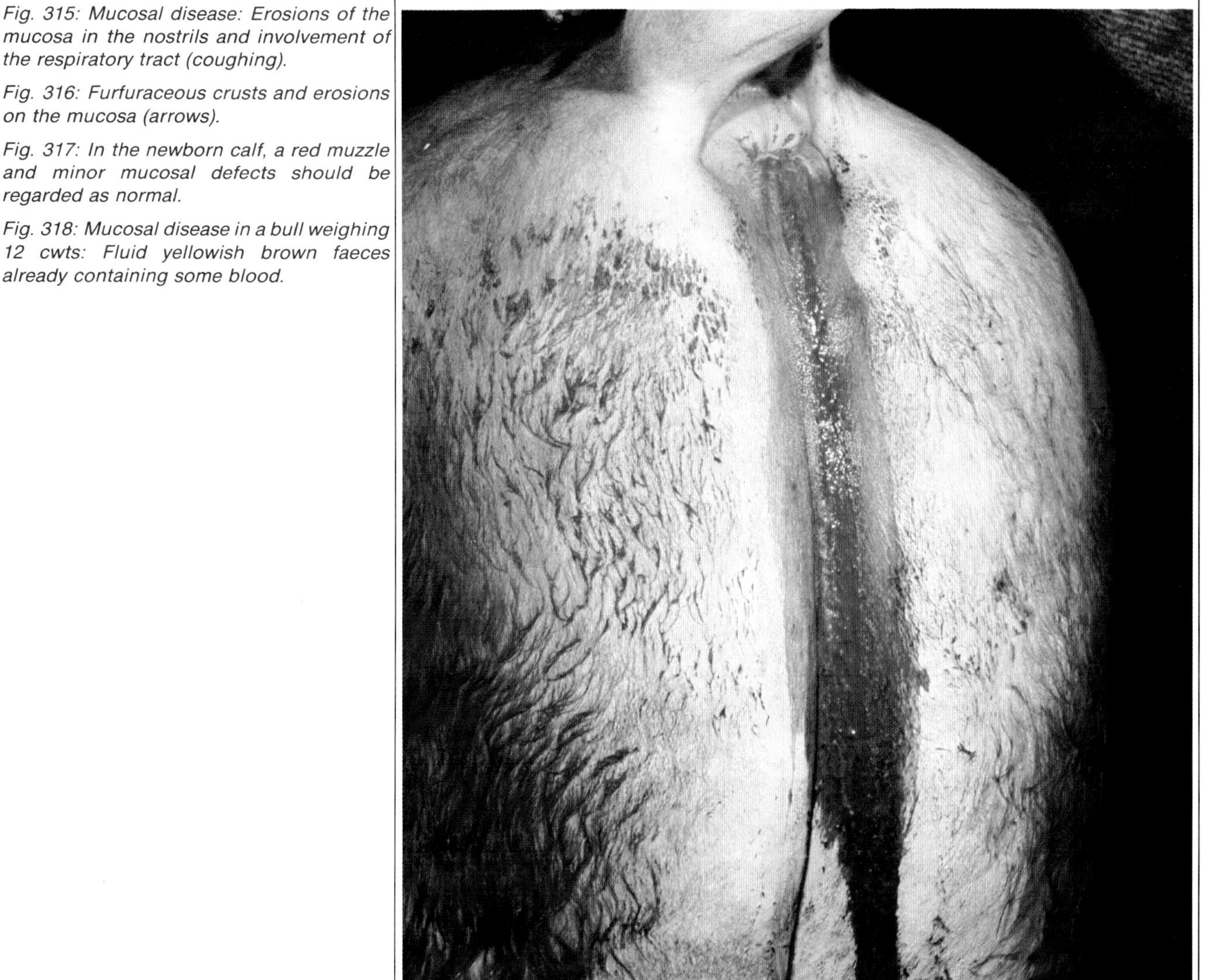

humans, vehicles, clothing etc. from one stock to another, resulting in animals being affected which have not yet formed any antibodies to the disease. The state of health of such animals does not permit the disease to be contained in its latent form, and there is therefore an outbreak of MD. Typically, only some animals at a time show visible symptoms. The disease progresses through the stock over a prolonged period in which cases appear again and again.

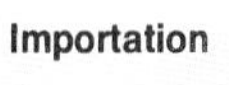

**Importation**

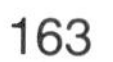

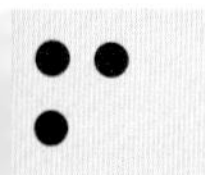

Fig. 319

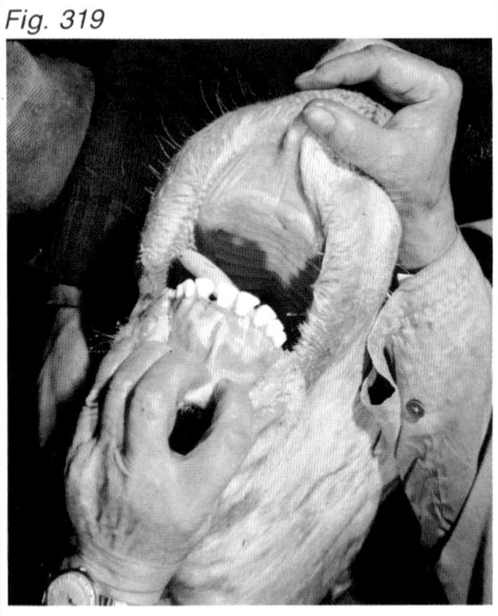

Fig. 320

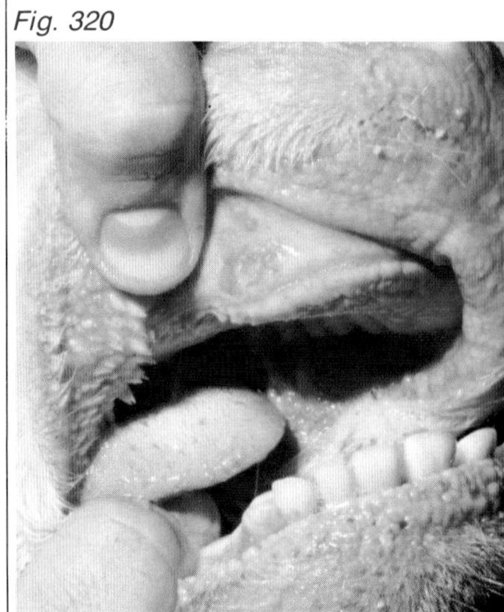

Fig. 321

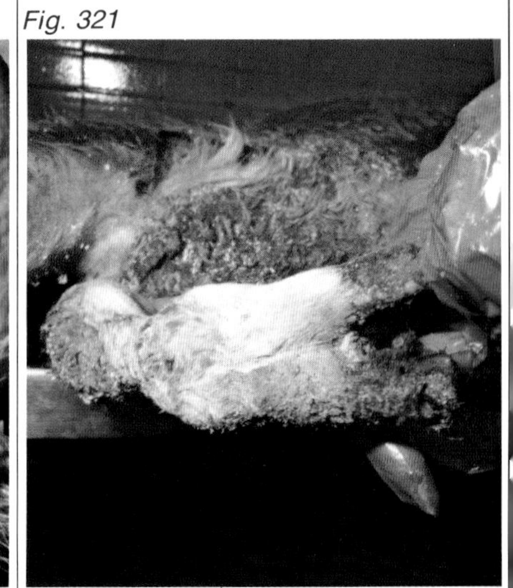

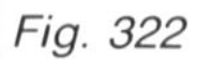

Symptoms

The period from the initial infection to the outbreak of manifest disease is approximately one week. A preceding attack of fever (first viral attack) usually goes unnoticed (see Fig. 322). In the majority of cases the stockman's attention is not attracted until the second viral attack induces high temperature, loss of appetite and dullness. Accelerated breathing, increased aqueous nasal discharge and conjunctival inflammation are observed.

Fig. 322

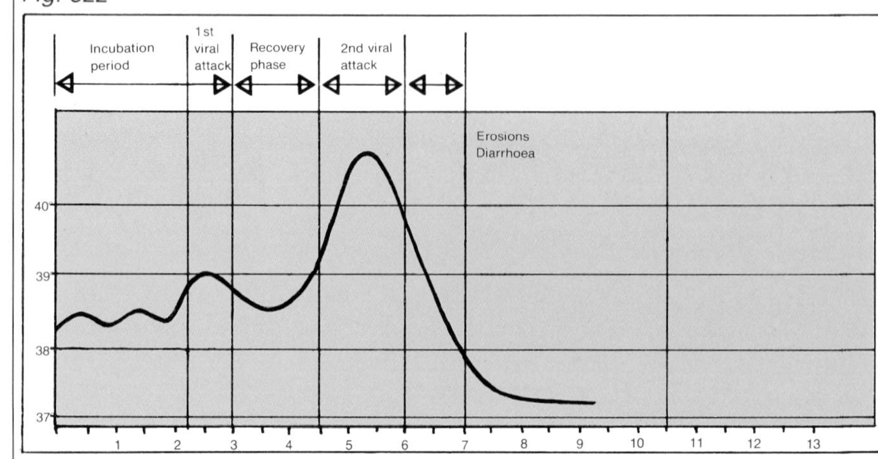

*Fig. 319: Inflammation of the buccal mucosa: The gums, particularly around the neck of the tooth, show a fine, reddened edge.*

*Fig. 320: Severe inflammation of the buccal mucosa with erosions (arrow).*

*Fig. 321: Inflammation of the coronal edge and the space between the claws in mucosal disease.*

*Fig. 322: Mucosal disease starts with a two-stage increase in body temperature. The first temperature increase is small and usually goes unnoticed. The second viral attack raises the temperature to above 40° C. The first symptoms appear with the second temperature peak: erosions on the mucosae of the entire digestive tract, intractable diarrhoea and occasionally manifestations in the respiratory tract.*

*Fig. 323: Mucosal disease in a sucking calf: Inflamed gums may also be observed in rota/corona infection and when the calf cuts its milk teeth.*

*Fig. 323*

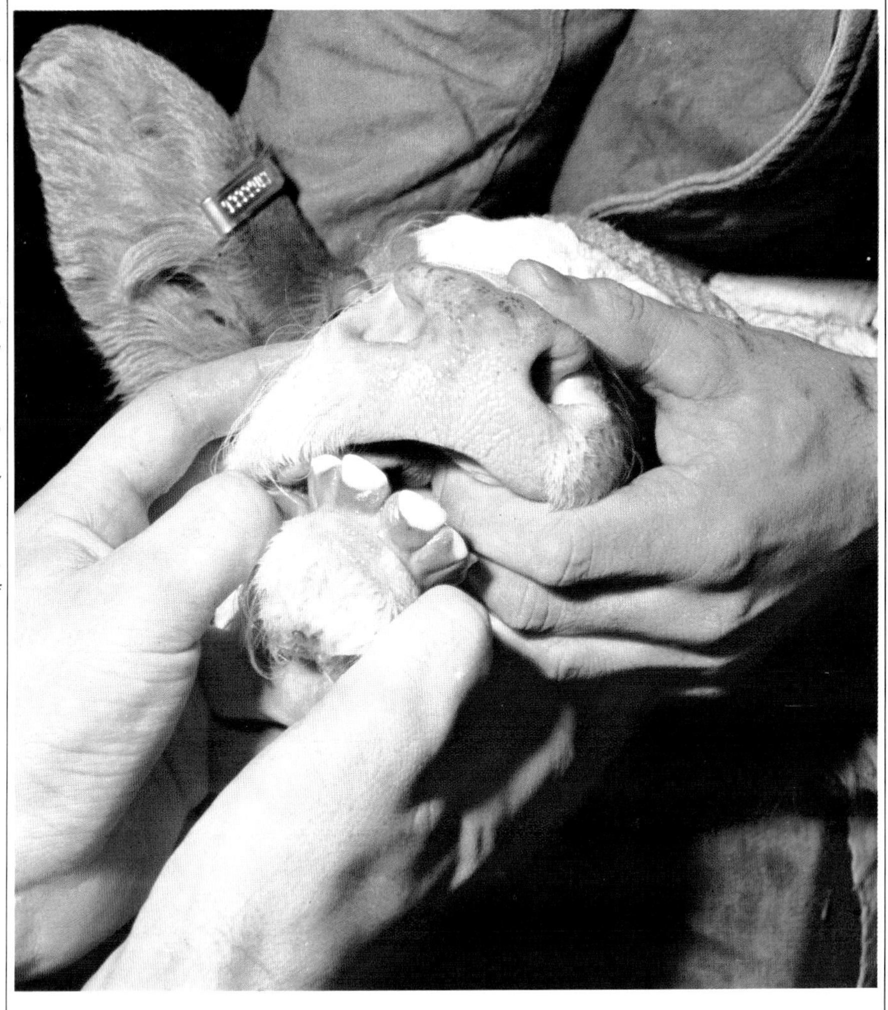

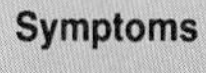

**Symptoms**

Finally, mucosal erosions (superficial losses of tissue on the mucosa) in the nostrils, cheek pouches and tongue lead to a further stage of the disease in which severe diarrhoea occurs very frequently. The faeces are initially very fluid, yellowish brown to greyish green and later on contain blood. As a result of the loss of water, pronounced desiccation of the body with deep-set eyes is observed. Raised skin folds level out slowly. The body temperature decreases to below normal levels.

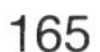

Fig. 324

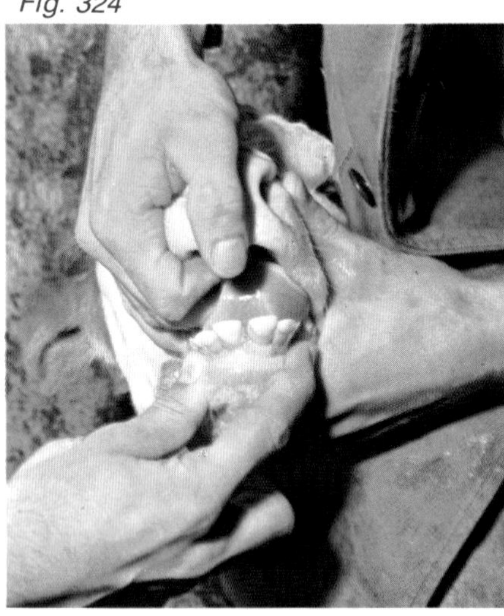

Fig. 325

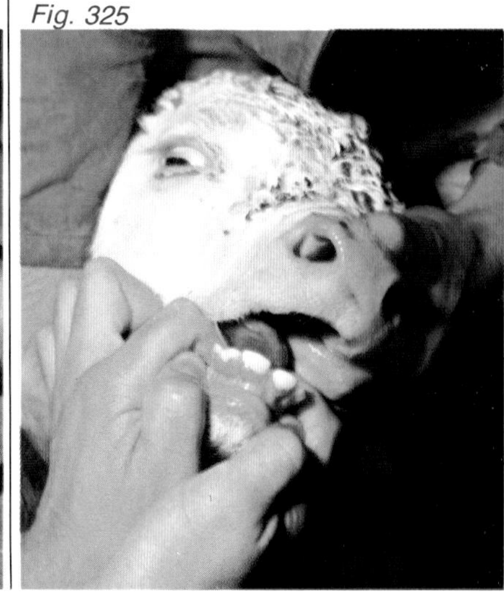

Fig. 326

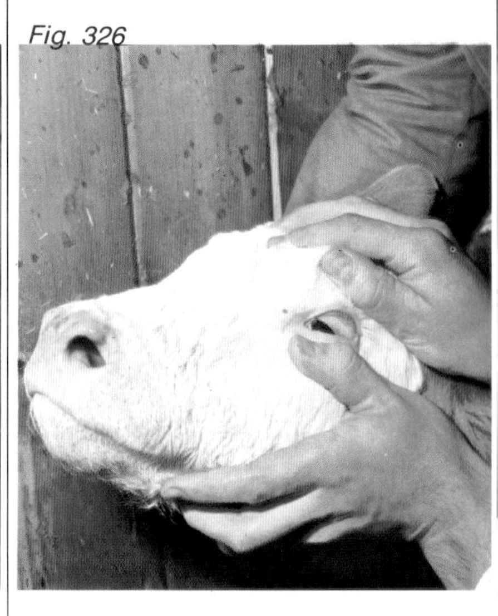

Symptoms

Pregnant cows may abort, particularly during the first three months of pregnancy. Lameness due to inflammation of the coronal edge and the space between the claws, may also occur.

In acute mucosal disease the animals die within 2 or 3 days. Up to 90% of the cattle affected do in fact die.

Apart from the acute form of mucosal disease, there is also an insidious (chronic) form where the animals suffer from diarrhoea over a period of weeks and months with recurrent attacks of fever.

The main economic loss from mucosal disease is no doubt due to the acute form with its high mortality rate. However, the chronic form of the disease with its persistent diarrhoea and recurrent bouts of fever, can also cause significant losses.

Diagnosis

The clinical picture is characterised by intractable diarrhoea. If mucosal changes (erosions and crust formation) on the muzzle and in the nostrils are observed in addition, this points to mucosal disease. An important criterium is inflammation of the buccal mucosa, especially inflammation of the gums where reddened margins are observed.

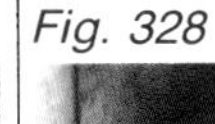

Fig. 327

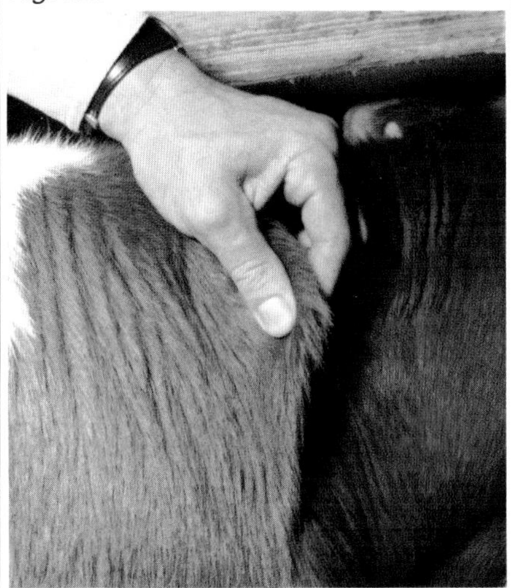

Fig. 328

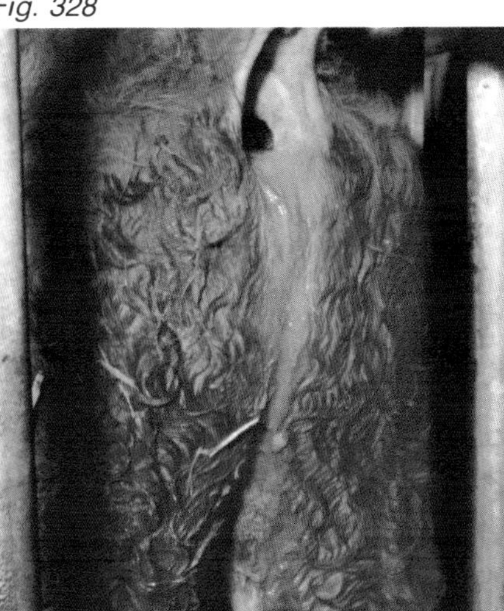

Fig. 329

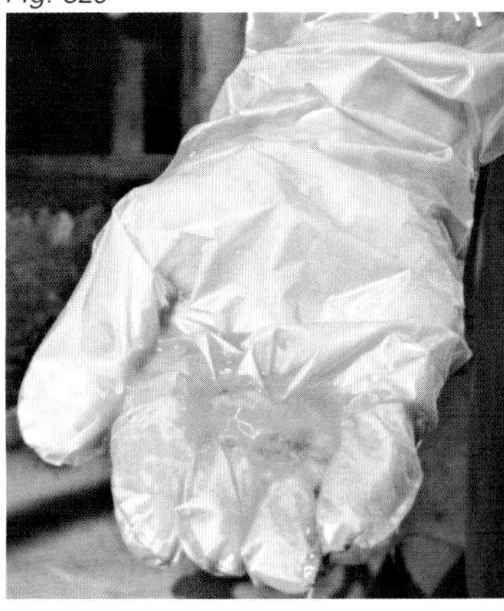

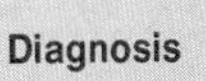

**Diagnosis**

The diagnosis is confirmed by autopsy and by demonstration of the virus. On dissection of the animal body, inflammation, erosions and yellow flocculent crusts (fibrin exudates) are found on the mucosa of the first three stomach compartments and of the entire intestine.

Fig. 330

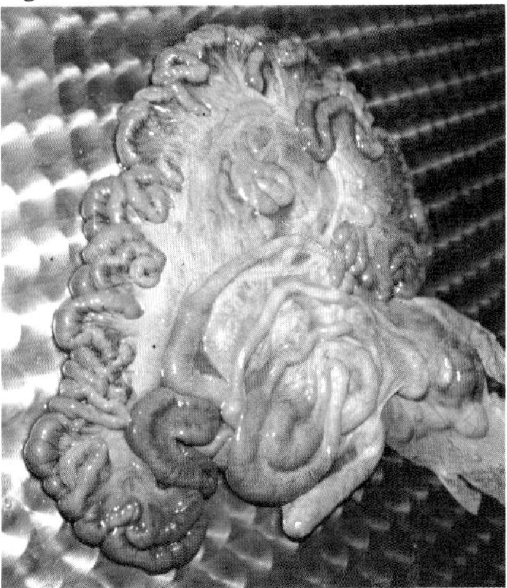

Fig. 331

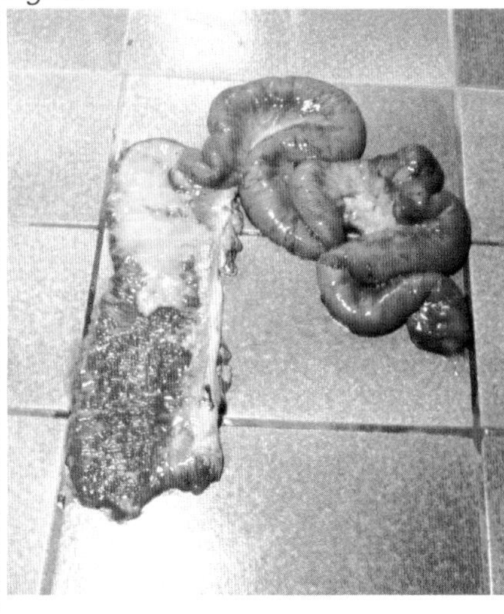

*Fig. 324: Pale pink buccal mucosa and gums in a healthy calf.*

*Fig. 325: Inflamed buccal mucosa in an affected calf.*

*Fig. 326: Incipient inflammation of the internal nasal mucosa and of the palpebral conjunctiva.*

*Fig. 327: Testing the elasticity of the skin. In mucosal disease, intractable diarrhoea leads to life-threatening desiccation of the body within 1 or 2 days.*

*Figs. 328 and 329: Severe aqueous diarrhoea. Flocculent fibrin admixtures. Heavy straining on the part of the animals.*

*Fig. 330: Pronounced (and partly bloody) inflammation of the small and the large intestine with severe swelling of the intestinal lymph nodes.*

*Fig. 331: Severely inflamed and swollen intestinal mucosa with pronounced yellow fibrin exudation.*

The most important distinguishing features of similar diseases are:

**Similar symptoms**

| | |
|---|---|
| ■ Foot-and-mouth disease: | Large blisters (aphthae) on the buccal mucosa, the claws and the udder; hypersalivation; usually no diarrhoea. |
| ■ Malignant catarrhal fever: | Heavy salivation; mucopurulent nasal discharge; turbidity of the cornea (keratitis). |
| ■ IBR: | Diarrhoea seen only in isolated cases; no mucosal erosions; severe dyspnoea; "red nose". |
| ■ Acid burns due to fertilisers or wood preservatives: | Extensive acid burns; central nervous disorders following oral ingestion. |

**Treatment**

The treatment of the acute form of mucosal disease with severe diarrhoea has no prospect of success in virtually all cases. Early slaughter is therefore advisable, so as to save part of the animal's value. In slightly affected animals, the administration of antibiotics and sulphonamides will serve to prevent secondary infections. In addition, high-dosed vitamins (particularly vitamin E to protect the epithelium) will promote the healing of the mucosa and will have a generally supportive effect. In sucking calves we use bovine gammaglobulin.

**Prevention**

Vaccination is the most effective method of combating mucosal disease. Since the disease does not appear suddenly, but over a prolonged period with individual animals being affected in turn, even emergency vaccination may be successful. Both preventive annual vaccinations on livestock farms at risk, and emergency vaccination of affected stocks are therefore possible.

Since resistance to MD is reduced by stress, medicated feed – as in the prevention of crowding disease – should also be given in this condition.

When fattening calves are purchased, on re-housing and at the time of vaccination, we give 10 g CHEVIBULL per animal and per day for 2 or 3 weeks (cf. also preventive measures in crowding disease, page 151).

*Fig. 332: Measures to be taken if mucosal disease appears.*

*Fig. 332*

| | | |
|---|---|---|
| 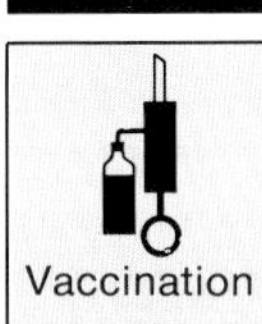 Vaccination | **All animals at risk:** Emergency vaccination with BVD/MD VACCINE | Immediately |
| 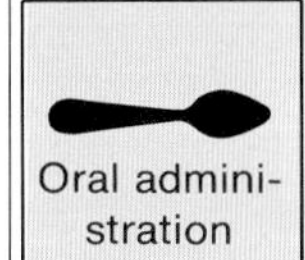 Oral administration | **All animals at risk:** 10 g CHEVIBULL (animals with rumen digestion) or 10 g CHEVICALF (animals fed on milk) per animal and per day for 2 to 3 weeks. | 1st to 21st day |
| 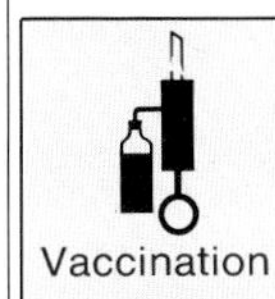 Vaccination | **Revaccination:** Calves which were younger than 3 months at first vaccination. Second vaccination not earlier than 4 weeks after first vaccination. Earliest age: 3 months. | |
| | **Severely affected cattle with severe diarrhoea:** Treatment usually hopeless. Early slaughter. Slaughter of sick animals. | Immediately |

**Treatment**

**Legal provisions***

Mucosal disease must be notified to the authorities. It is incumbent upon the veterinary surgeon who diagnoses the disease to notify the local veterinary officer.
Official measures are not usually taken, since notification is only intended to inform the veterinary authorities of the extent of the disease.

* Valid in W. Germany

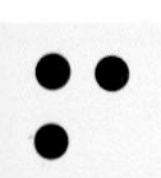

# Foot-and-mouth disease

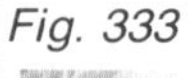

Fig. 333

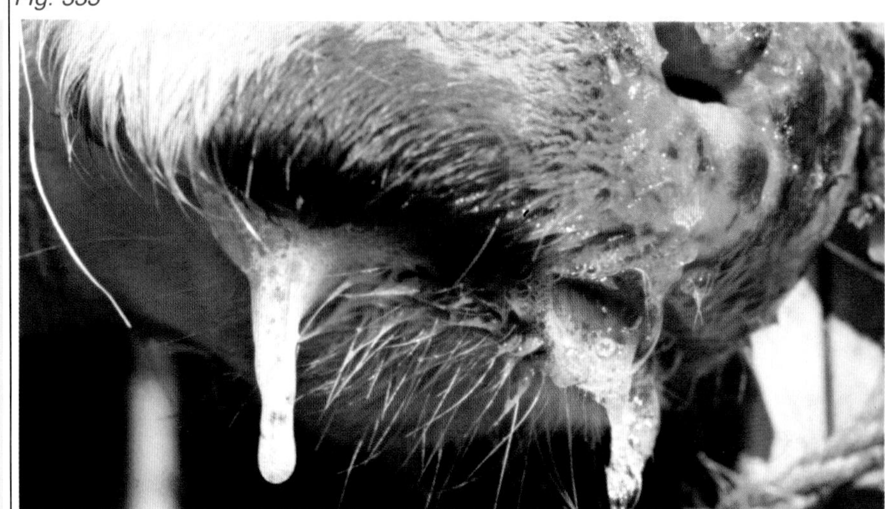

**Term**

Foot-and-mouth disease (FMD) is a highly contagious virus disease.

**Incidence**

Apart from cattle, the disease may occur in all cloven-hoofed animals, and in rare cases also in man.

**Pathogen**

FMD virus belongs to the group of picorna viruses. The types O, A and C occur in Central Europe.
The period from the time of infection to the outbreak of the disease (incubation period) is 2 to 7 days.

**Symptoms**

Fever (up to 42° C) is the first symptom and lasts for a maximum of two days. Several animals or the entire stock may be affected simultaneously. Initially, vesicles filled with virus-containing fluid (primary aphthae) form on the buccal mucosa. From there the virus reaches the various organs via the blood stream. After a few days further vesicles (secondary aphthae) form in the buccal cavity, on the udder and on the edge of the claws. In the mouth, apart from the aphthae, the buccal mucosa is inflamed causing salivation. The inflammation on the edge of the claws leads to a festinating unsteady gait and possibly to lameness. After 1 to 3 days the aphthae burst and heal within approx. 14 days if there is no secondary infection.
After surviving the disease, the animals are immune to the virus type to which they have been exposed, for at least one year.

*Fig. 333: Hypersalivation in FMD. The aphthae on the muzzle and in the nose have already burst and have become secondarily infected with bacteria.*

*Fig. 334: Formation of aphthae on the tips of the teats in FMD.*

*Fig. 335: Cardiovalvulitis and degeneration of the heart muscle in FMD. The heart muscle looks as if it has been boiled.*

Fig. 334

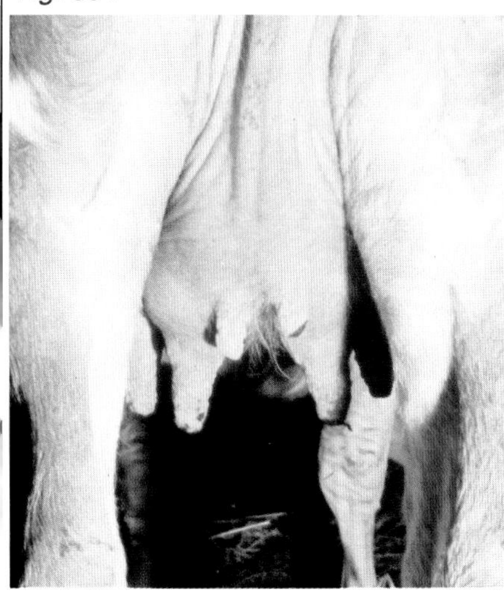

**Diagnosis**

FMD may be suspected from the rapid spread and the characteristic changes on the visible mucosae, the udder and the edge of the claws. Even the suspicion of FMD must be notified to the authorities. The necessary differentiation of virus types will then be carried out by government laboratories without delay*.

**Similar symptoms**

- Malignant catarrhal fever shows similar manifestations in the initial stage, but no formation of vesicles. Increased body temperature is observed for prolonged periods.
- In mucosal disease, severe intestinal inflammation with aqueous diarrhoea is observed in addition. No formation of vesicles, although erosions are seen.

**Treatment**

Any type of treatment is prohibited. The veterinary authorities will order the destruction of the stock*.

**Prevention**

Vaccination is possible. Annual revaccinations provide good protection against FMD.

**Danger to other animals**

The disease may be transmitted to all cloven-hoofed animals.

**Legal provisions***

Any suspicion or the outbreak of the disease must be notified to the local veterinary officer. This notification is incumbent upon all persons that have a professional or occupational connection with the animals concerned, e. g. stockmen attending to the animals' claws, milking staff, cattle dealers or butchers. Until the official diagnosis has been established, the animals must not be moved, nor may any new animals be added to the stock. After the official diagnosis of FMD, the authorities will order quarantine measures to be taken:

- No cloven-hoofed animals may be moved from or taken to the affected farm and the **quarantine area.** Grazing cattle must be housed **(house quarantine).** The veterinary authorities will order the destruction of the entire stock of cloven-hoofed animals on the affected farm.
- Since man, solipeds, poultry, dogs and cats must also be regarded as carriers, movement is greatly restricted **(quarantine for humans and animals).**
- In the **observation area** which usually comprises adjoining communities, and in the **protective zone** (10 mile radius), transport of cattle and cattle markets are prohibited or restricted.

Fig. 335

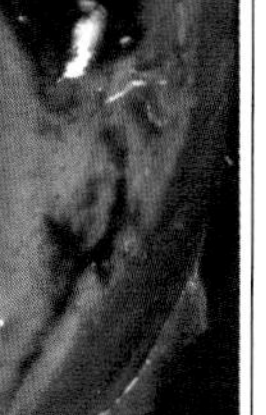

* Valid in W. Germany

# Hypersomnia of bulls ISTME

Fig. 336

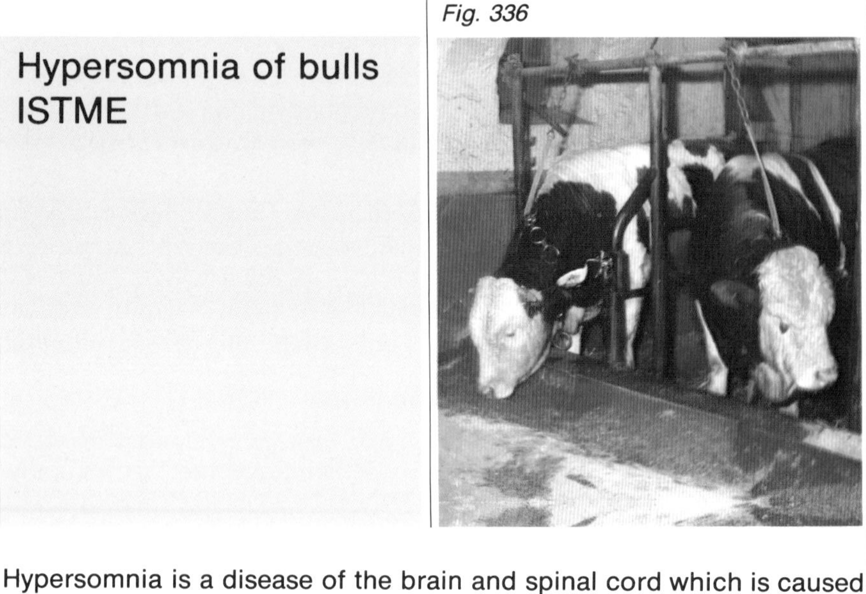

*Fig. 336: Initial stage of ISTME in a one-year-old bull: sleepy, listless behaviour; shunning light.*

*Fig. 337: Hypersomnia, advanced stage II: Fixed look; the animals lie on the side with stretched or slightly bent legs.*

**Term**

Hypersomnia is a disease of the brain and spinal cord which is caused by bacteria. Its scientific name is **i**nfectious **s**epticaemic **t**hrombosing **m**eningo**e**ncephalitis – ISTME.

**Incidence**

The disease is observed particularly in the autumn and winter and mainly in beef cattle weighing 200 to 400 kg. Stress conditions like transport, re-housing, crude fibre deficiency and vitamin $B_1$ deficiency favour the appearance of the disease. Approx. 2 to 4% of the cattle in the stock are affected. 90% of the affected animals die of the disease.

**Pathogen**

The causative organism (haemophilus somnus) is present in many beef cattle stocks, but the disease only appears through the effect of stress factors. The pathogen can be isolated from the brain or cerebrospinal fluid of animals that have died.

**Symptoms**

The clinical symptoms and the progress of the disease depend on the site and the extent of the brain damage and therefore differ from case to case. The disease appears in two stages:

■ Stage I

Affected animals can be recognised from their reduced fodder intake and from the way they stand about sleepily. They appear to be tired, stand listlessly in the pen, tend to lie down or wander about restlessly.

Fig. 337

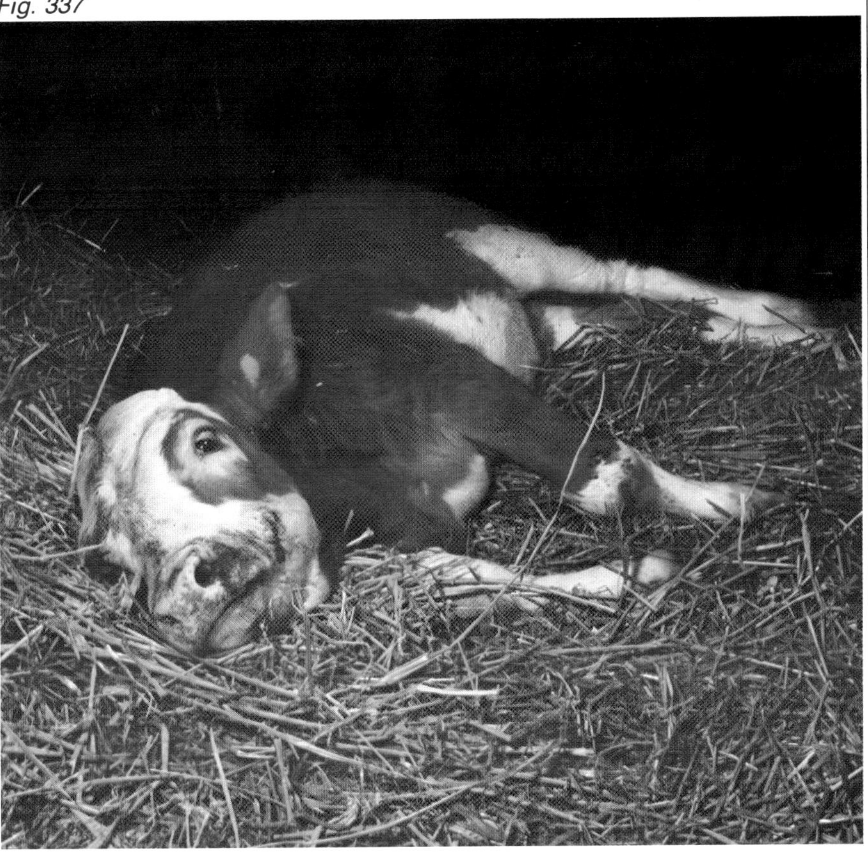

Symptoms

Aqueous nasal discharge and bouts of coughing may be observed in some bulls. The body temperature is within or slightly above normal limits.

■ Stage II

After 10 to 36 hours the animals lie down all the time showing central nervous symptoms. Initially, the bulls lie on the chest with one or both forelegs stretched forward, the head turned sideways and the eyes half closed.

In the advanced stage, the animals lie on the side with stretched or slightly bent legs. The body temperature of the animals lying down permanently is below normal (36–37° C). Paralysis of the tail, the anus and the rectum is observed. The mortality rate is very high (in excess of 90%).

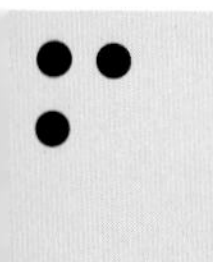

**Diagnosis**

The deficiency symptoms of the locomotor system, the somnolence of the bulls and the appearance of disease in the higher weight groups point to the presence of ISTME. Cerebrospinal fluid is withdrawn by spinal puncture at the back of the head. Because of the inflammation, the spinal cord is under increased pressure. This is why the cerebrospinal fluid escapes spontaneously on puncture. The fluid shows yellowish white turbidity and coagulates after a short period. The protein content is increased to above 300 mg/100 ml (Normal animal: 10 to 40 mg/100 ml).

At autopsy, the typical changes caused by the disease – thromboses – are found in the brain.

*Figs. 338 to 340: Changes in the meninges and the brain in ISTME.*

*Fig. 338: Meninges congested with blood (arrow).*

*Fig. 339: Pronounced meningeal haemorrhage. The zones showing greyish discoloration indicate necrotic areas of the brain, caused by thrombosis.*

*Fig. 340: As Fig. 339: Section of necrotic areas (arrow).*

*Fig. 341: Treatment schedule for ISTME.*

*Fig. 342: Summary of notifiable, but rare diseases (pages 176 and 177).*

**Similar symptoms**

The central nervous disorders seen with ISTME are also observed in vitamin $B_1$ deficiency, listeriosis, warble-fly infestation and phosphoric acid ester poisoning. The most important distinguishing characteristics are:

- Vitamin $B_1$ deficiency: Unsteady gait with splayed legs; head raised upwards and backwards ("star-gazing"). Early treatment with vitamin $B_1$ produces rapid improvement.
- Listeriosis: Raised body temperature; animal wandering about in circles; the head is always turned to the **same** side. The animals die within 4 to 14 days.
- Lameness due to warble-fly infestation: Migrating warble-fly larvae (December to February) in the vertebral canal may cause lameness in the hindlegs. At autopsy, warble-fly larvae are found in the spinal canal.
- Poisoning with phosphoric acid esters: Phosphoric acid esters are used for the treatment of mange and warble-fly infestation. In cases of overdosage, diarrhoea with admixture of blood and colic occur 2 to 24 hours after treatment. Frequent micturition and salivation are typical.

*Fig. 338*

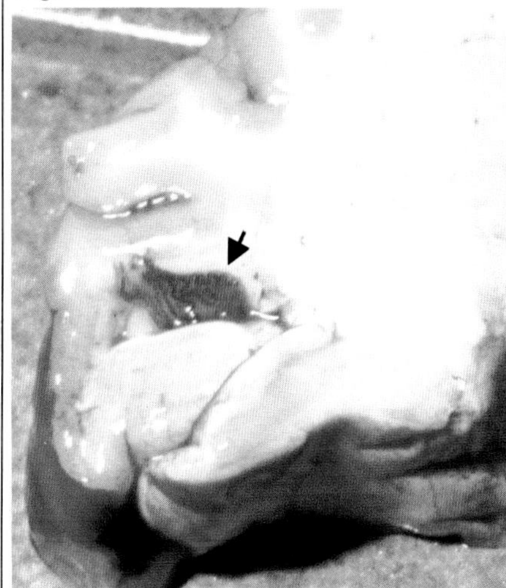

*Fig. 339*

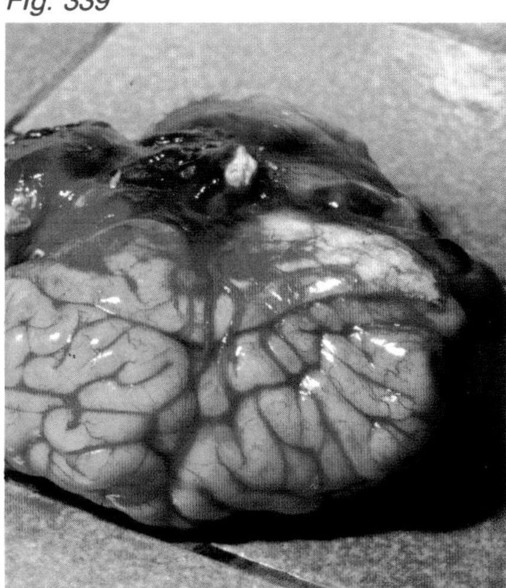

*Fig. 340*

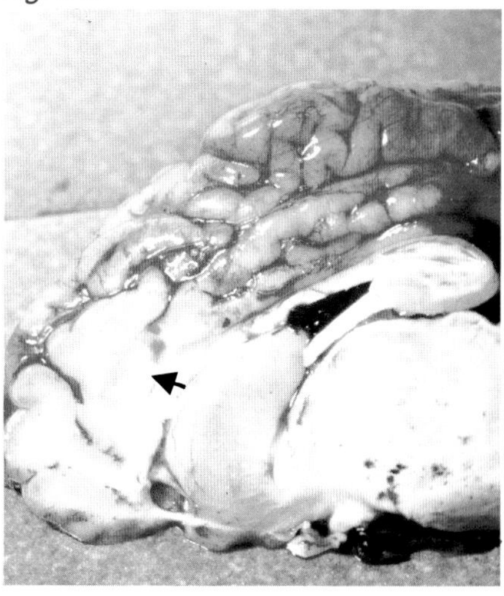

**Treatment**

Once the animals lie down all the time, treatment is unlikely to be successful. In the early stage of ISTME, Ampicillin is given in high dosage, supplemented by injections of vitamin B.

Since the disease is obviously precipitated by stress factors and as animals in groups of the same age are affected successively, treatment of the stock would appear to be indicated. Good results have been obtained with the administration of a long-acting sulphonamide bolus and medicated feed.

*Fig. 341*

| | | |
|---|---|---|
| 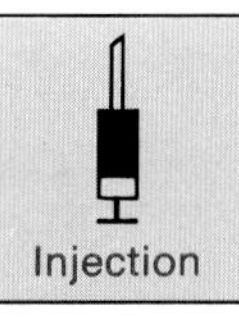 Injection | **Affected animals:** 3 ml PENBROCK/10 kg. 4 intramuscular injections at intervals of 12 hours. Plus: 1 i. m. injection of 2 ml HEPASTON/10 kg. | 1st and 2nd day |
| 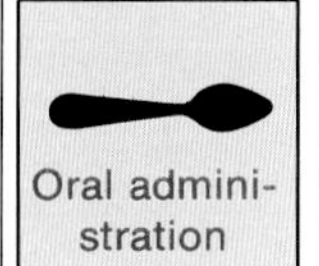 Oral administration | **Animals of the same age in the stock:** 1 bolus of BOVIBOL/150 kg body-weight to be given by mouth. | 1st day |
|   Fodder | **Follow-up treatment of animals of the same age in the stock:** 10 g CHEVIBULL per animal and per day, for 3 weeks. | 1st to 21st day |

## Important, but rare diseases

Fig. 342

| | 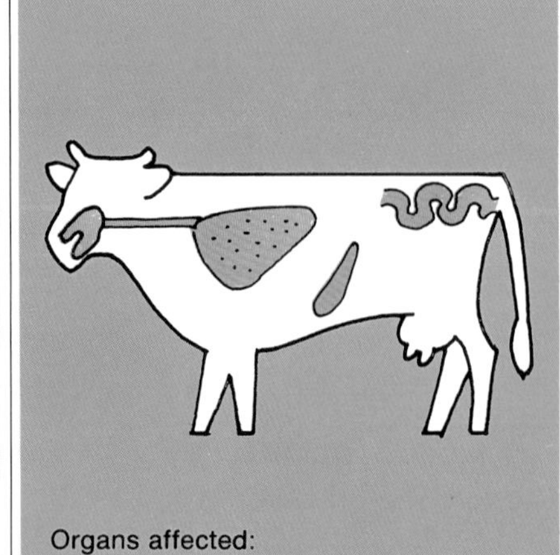 Organs affected: Lungs, intestine, spleen | 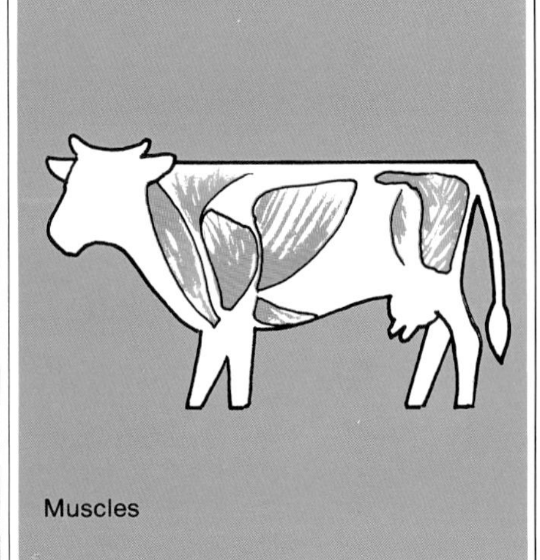 Muscles |
|---|---|---|
| Disease | Anthrax | Blackleg |
| Pathogen | Bacillus anthracis | Clostridium feseri |
| Route of infection | The permanent forms (spores) of the pathogen are extremely resistant; may survive in the soil for decades. Oral ingestion of the spores with fodder and water (especially after floods). | The spores of the pathogen are extremely resistant. Blackleg occurs only in certain areas (blackleg areas). Small wounds are the points of entry, often on second dentition. |
| Symptoms | Bleeding from all orifices of the body; dark, poorly coagulating blood; spleen discoloured reddish black and severely swollen. Inflammation of the intestine. | Painful swellings which crackle on palpation are seen in muscular parts of the body of mainly young grazing animals. Death ensues within 1 to 3 days. |
| Legal provisions* | Notification obligatory. Slaughter strictly prohibited. Do not bleed dying animals. Do not open up dead animals. | Notification obligatory, even on suspicion. Slaughter prohibited. Do not open up dead animals. Vaccination in blackleg areas. |
| Danger to the livestock holder | Highly contagious, life-threatening. Anthrax of the skin, intestine or lungs, depending on route of infection. | |

* Valid in W. Germany

| 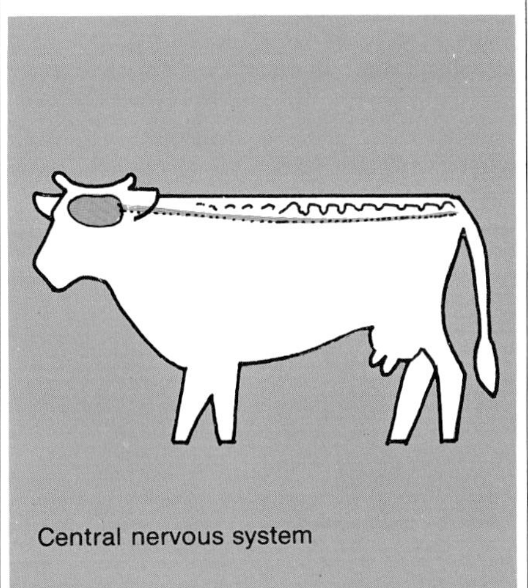 Central nervous system | 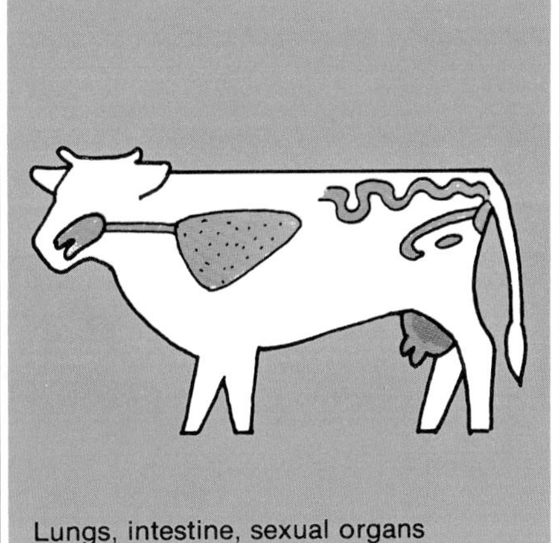 Lungs, intestine, sexual organs | 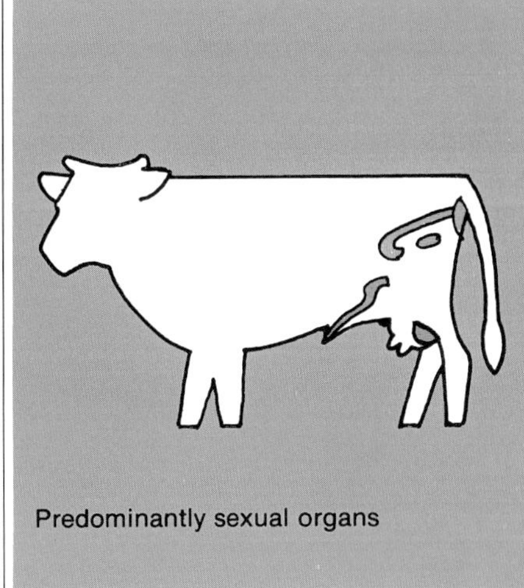 Predominantly sexual organs |
|---|---|---|
| Rabies | Tuberculosis | Brucellosis |
| Rhabdo virus | Mycobacterium bovis | Brucella abortus |
| Transmission through bites. The saliva contains the pathogen. | The pathogens are carried into the respiratory tract (lungs) in bacteria-containing dust or by droplet infection. Oral infection by ingestion of raw milk. | Only sexually mature animals contract the disease. Oral infection after licking aborted foetuses. Transmission also possible through raw milk. |
| Abnormal behaviour; difficulty in swallowing, tympany; running against obstacles; sudden collapse; the animal then rises again and shows normal behaviour. | Varying course of the disease, depending on the animals' physical condition: Cough, pneumonia, mastitis, metritis. | Epidemic abortion (6th to 8th month). Retention of after-birth. Premature calving. Swollen foetal membranes with yellowish slimy covering. Testitis. |
| Notification obligatory. Suspect animals to be kept in quarantine. Treatment and slaughter of affected animals prohibited. | Notification obligatory. Official measures: Carriers are traced by the tuberculin test and eliminated. | Notification obligatory. Official measures: Carriers are traced by periodic blood tests and eliminated. |
| Immediate vaccination after contact with rabid animals. Life-threatening disease leading to death in excruciating pain. | Contagious protracted disease which is difficult to treat. | Contagious protracted disease. Undulating fever. Caution with retention of after-birth after abortion. |

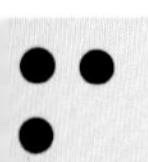

# Disturbed micturition

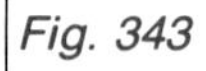

Fig. 343

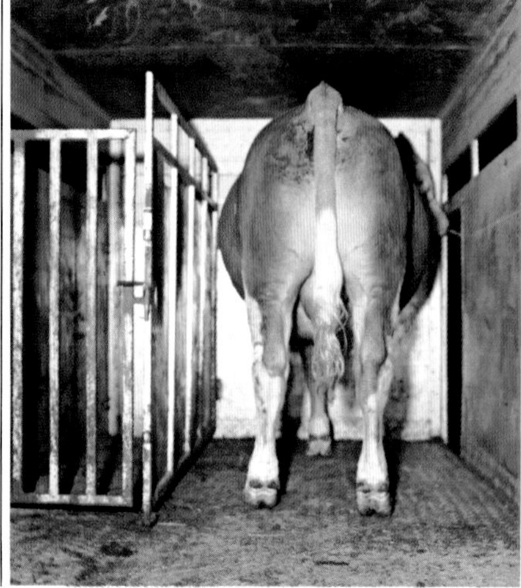

Fig. 344

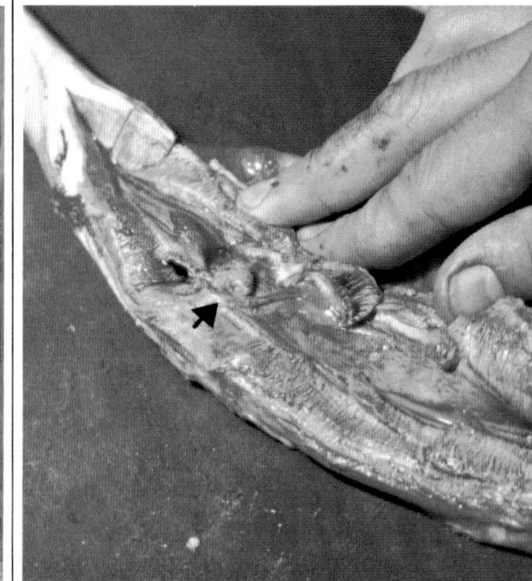

**Term**

A disturbance of urine flow is observed almost exclusively in male cattle. The main causes are **urinary stones** or **injuries** causing an obstruction of the urethra and congestion of the bladder and the kidneys with urine, resulting in uraemia.

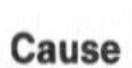

**Cause**

## Formation of urinary stones

In cattle, urinary stone formation is mainly induced by inappropriate composition of the fodder. The condition is rarely due to inflammatory causes. A change in the equilibrium of the body salts excreted in the urine may be regarded as the starting point of stone formation. A shift in the solubility ratio and the degree of acidity of the urine leads to the precipitation of small crystals to which further crystals attach themselves. In the course of weeks or months, these crystals grow to the size of visible urinary stones, reaching a diameter of 1 to 5 mm. They are called "urinary gravel" and may differ in colour (white, yellow, brown, grey). Their hardness depends on their composition. In the majority of cases, the stones consist of silicate, carbonate, phosphate or oxalate, or of a mixture of salts. They constantly irritate the mucosa of the bladder (inflammation) and thus promote the formation of further stones.

Fig. 345

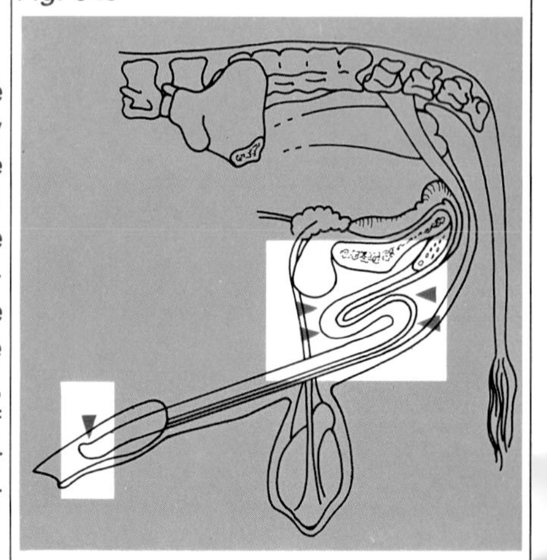

Fig. 346

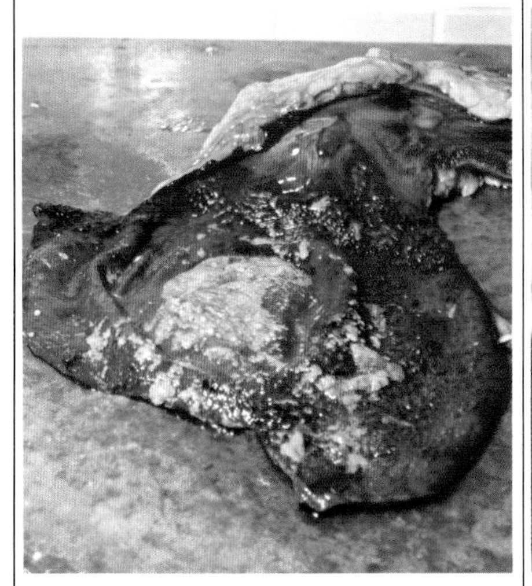

Fig. 347

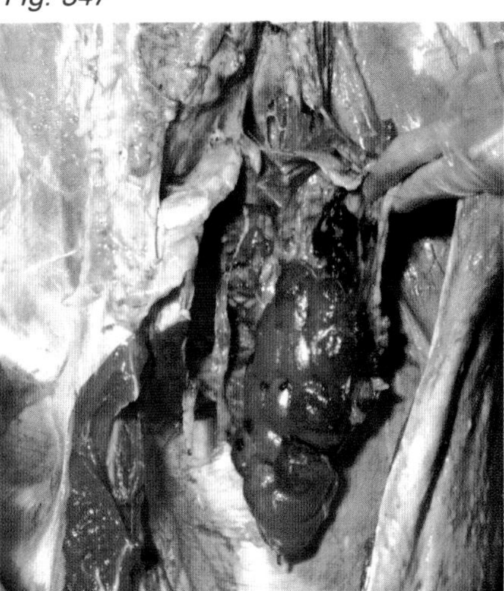

Fig. 348

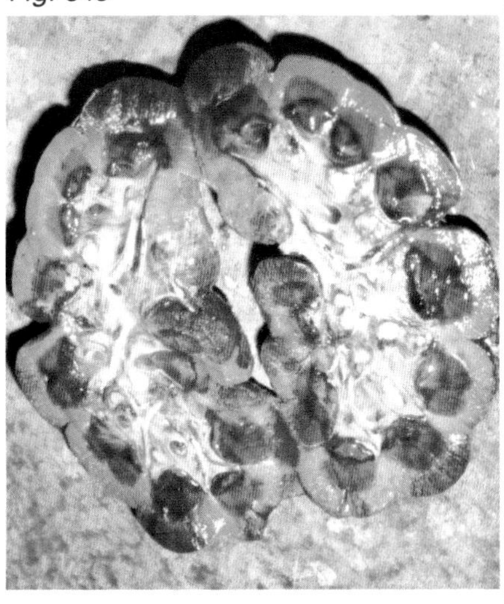



If unduly large or sharp-edged stones pass into the urethra, they may become wedged in the S-shaped curve of the penis (see Fig. 345) or in the tip of the penis. Local irritation may then lead to spasms of the urethral muscles. The stones become even more firmly lodged and a complete blockage of the urethra may result. In such cases, urination decreases initially to a trickle and then stops altogether. Congestion of the urinary tract with urine leads to overdistention or rupture of the bladder and to uraemia.

*Fig. 343: Bull with ruptured bladder due to urethral stone. The abdominal cavity was filled with 50 litres of urine.*

*Fig. 344: Occlusion of the urethra by a stone being lodged in the sigmoid curve (arrow).*

*Fig. 345: The S-shaped curve and the tip of the penis are preferred sites where urethral stones may become wedged.*

*Fig. 346: Severe bloody inflammation of the bladder due to urinary gravel.*

*Figs. 347 and 348: Severe kidney damage. Obstruction of the urethra by stones caused congestion of the kidneys with urine.*

*Fig. 349: Rupture of the bladder.*

*Fig. 350: Peritonitis and inflammation of the greater omentum due to extravasation of urine.*

Fig. 349

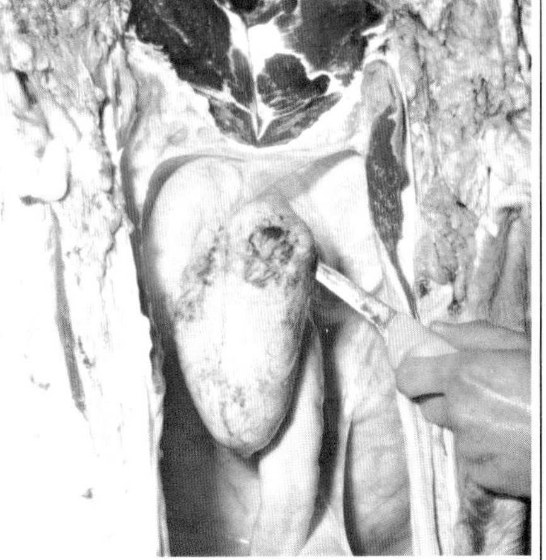

Fig. 350

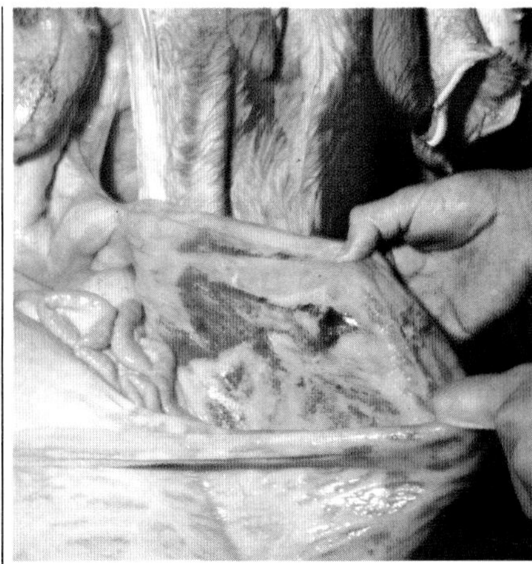

Fig. 351

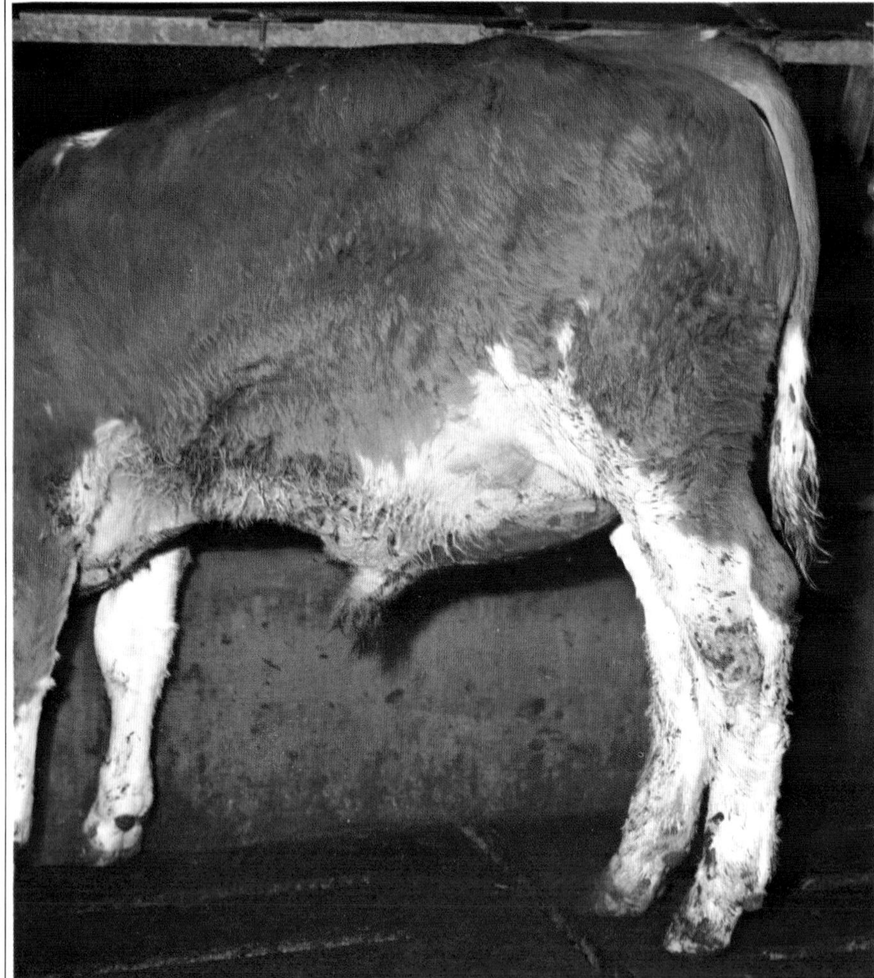

Fig. 352

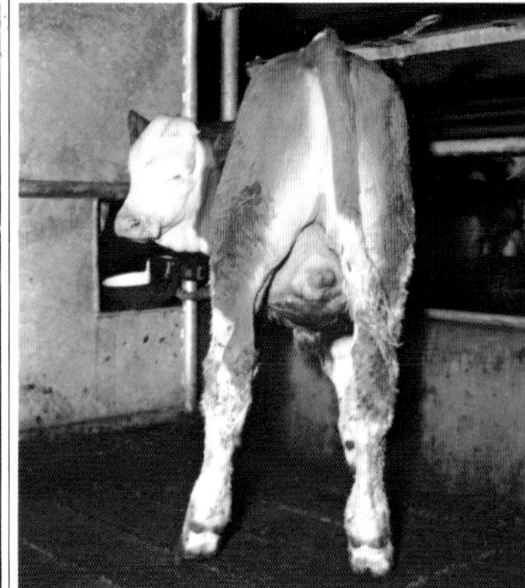

Fig. 353

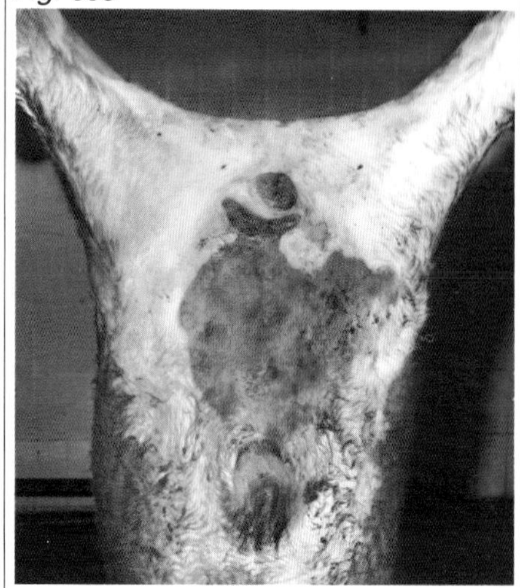

**Cause**

## Injuries due to kicks

Sudden restlessness in overcrowded pens sometimes results in injuries to the penis caused by kicks, which may be followed by disturbed micturition. Such injuries may occur if some bulls suddenly jump up while others remain lying down. This is frequently the case with fatigued animals after prolonged transport. The prepuce and the tip of the penis are particularly at risk from injuries.

Figs. 351 to 353: The connective tissue of the abdomen is congested with urine. Skin discoloured bluish black in this region. Scrotum barely visible. Cause: Laceration of the penis through injury caused by kicking. The urethra is blocked by fibrin adhesions, so that the urine was able to penetrate into the connective tissue.

Fig. 354: Injury caused by kicking with laceration of the urethra. The urine seeped into the subcutaneous connective tissue causing congestion with urine. Lacerated, blood-soaked and some necrotic tissue can be seen.

Fig. 355: Laceration of the urethra through injury caused by kicking, with pronounced fibrin plug which obstructed the urethra.

Fig. 355

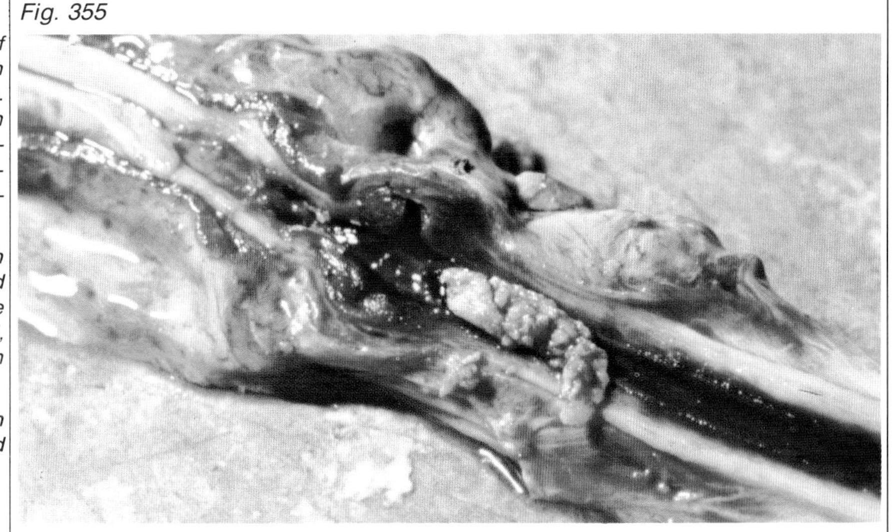

Fig. 354

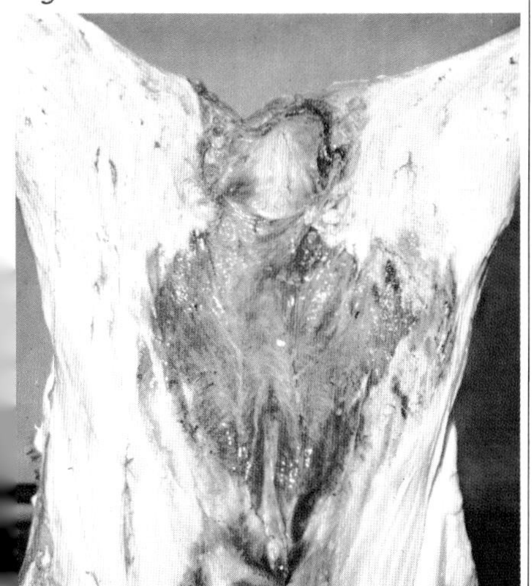

**Symptoms**

Laceration of the urethra may occur as a result of injuries caused by kicking. A large haemorrhage appears at the site of the injury. Blood components (fibrin) form adhesions in the region of the wound and block the urine flow. The urine seeps into the loose connective tissue below the skin. On the underside of the abdomen the connective tissue is congested with urine, forming an indentable pasty mass which is cold to the touch. In this area the skin shows a bluish black discoloration. However, the urinary bladder remains tightly filled since the urine can only extravasate into the connective tissue under pressure. The animals refuse their fodder and die within a few days from uraemia.

**Diagnosis**

Both conditions are characterised by congestion of the bladder with urine. Rectal examination reveals the tightly filled bladder. With urethral injuries as a result of kicking, a pronounced swelling on the lower abdomen and bluish black discoloration of the skin are observed.

The condition appears suddenly. The animals suffer attacks of severe colic and are restless. They refuse to feed, but still drink water. The animals die within a few days from rapidly progressing uraemia.

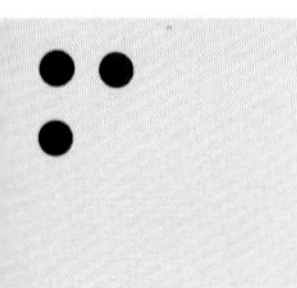

In the advanced stage, treatment is usually impossible. If urethral stones are recognised early, they can be removed surgically.

**Treatment**

In stocks where urinary stones occur frequently, the stones must be examined chemically to determine their composition. On the basis of the chemical examination and a calculation of the composition of the ration, feeding can be corrected accordingly.

Fig. 356

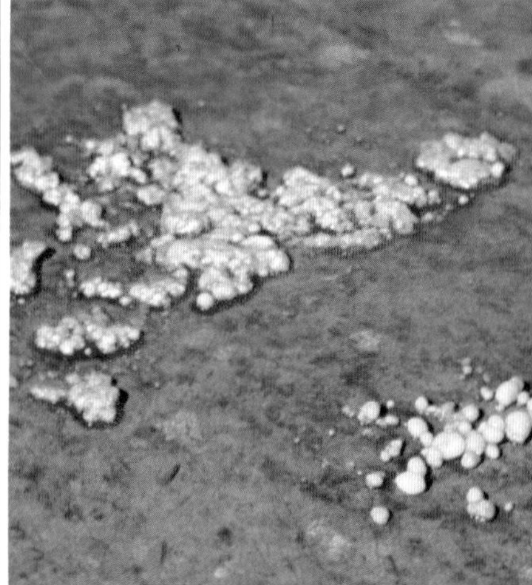

Fig. 357

| | | |
|---|---|---|
| Surgery | In valuable animals and provided the condition is recognised at an early stage, surgery is possible. | Immediately |
| Laboratory | Examination of the urine, pH determination, chemical examination of urinary stones. | |
| Fodder | Checking fodder ration: Weighing fodder components actually ingested (basic ration and supplements) | |
| Laboratory | Determination and calculation of dry substance (content and structure), crude fibre and mineral substances. | |
| Fodder | Change of feeding according to the result of the examination of the urinary stones and the feedstuffs. | |

Fig. 358

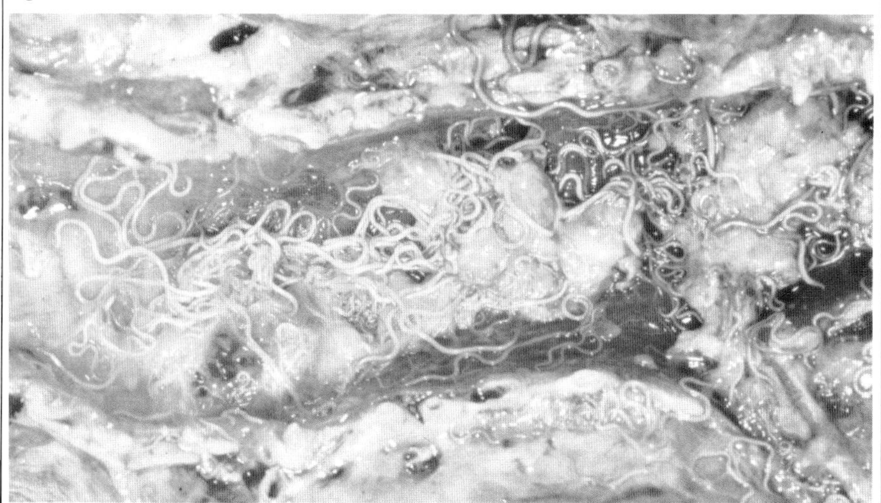

# Lungworm infestation

**Term**

Lungworms are greyish white worms of the thickness of sewing cotton. Their sexually mature forms live in the bronchi and the windpipe. In cattle, mainly the large lungworm, Dictyocaulus viviparus, is found.

**Incidence**

The infestation occurs particularly on moist pastures. Since such pastures also offer favourable conditions for other parasites, the same cattle usually harbour gastrointestinal worms in addition.

**Pathogen**

**Life cycle**

The female lungworms lay a large number of eggs in the bronchi and the windpipe, from which larvae are hatched in the windpipe. The larvae migrate to the larynx and are expectorated or swallowed and excreted in the faeces. By the action of rain water or by active intrinsic movements, they leave the faeces and reach the grass. Moist pastures, rank patches and frequent rainfall extend the viability of the larvae. Drought will destroy them. If hay dries on the ground it is free from lungworm larvae, because they migrate into the moist ground. If infective larvae are ingested with the fodder, they shed their protective cover, penetrate into the mucosa of the small intestine and reach the lungs via the blood stream. In the lungs they mature within 20 to 25 days. The life-span of sexually mature lungworms is approx. 2 months.

*Fig. 356: Urinary gravel from the bladder. The larger stones cannot pass through the urethra and obstruct the urine flow.*

*Fig. 357: Measures to be taken in stocks with increased incidence of urinary stone formation.*

*Fig. 358: Severe lungworm infestation of the bronchi: Irritation of the bronchial mucosa causes profuse mucopurulent secretion.*

Life cycle

Fig. 359

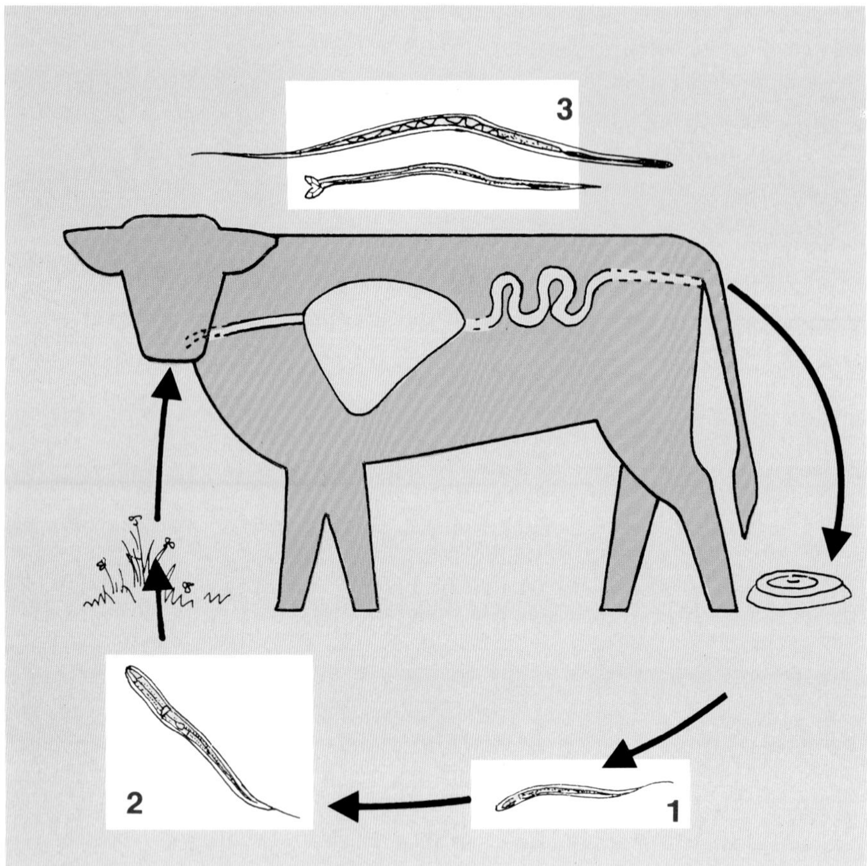


*Fig. 359: Life cycle of lungworms. Lungworm larvae are expectorated or swallowed and excreted in the faeces.*

*1 Free lungworm larva.*

*2 Infective lungworm larvae are ingested during grazing.*

*3 Ingested larvae penetrate into the mucosa of the small intestine and pass into the lungs via the blood stream. In the lungs they develop into sexually mature lungworms.*

Dead lungworms are swallowed or expectorated. At normal winter temperatures, larvae living in the open air will perish. During the winter the development of larvae ingested by cattle in the autumn, lies dormant.

These larvae do not develop into sexually mature worms until the spring when the cattle again excrete larvae in the faeces.

Fig. 360

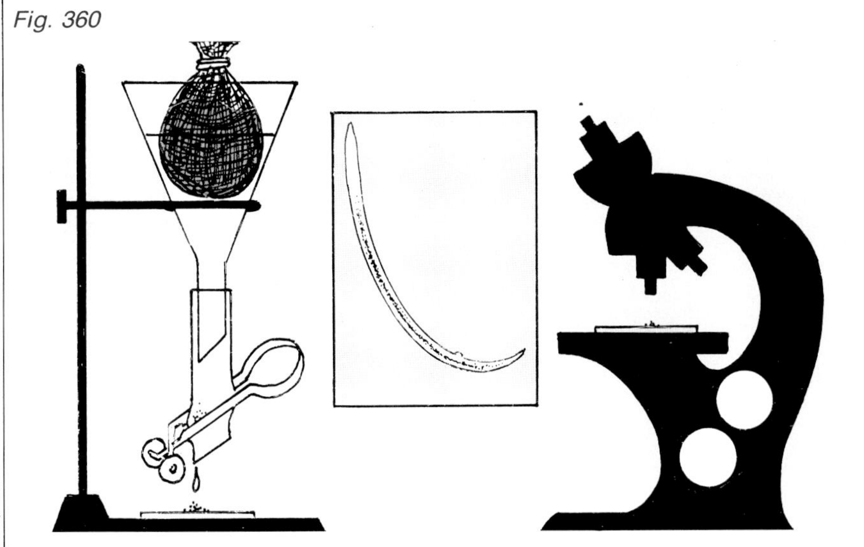

*Fig. 360: Parasitological examination of the faeces using the migration method (funnel method). A gauze bag filled with faeces is suspended in a funnel. This funnel is extended by means of a tube approx. 7 cm long, enabling a tube clamp to be applied. The funnel is filled with water to a point where the faeces are only partly immersed. The larvae contained in the faeces migrate into the water and sink towards the tube clamp. 6 hours after immersing the faecal sample, the clamp is opened carefully. The first drop of water which contains numerous larvae, is caught on a slide and studied under the microscope.*

*Fig. 361: With severe lungworm infestation the bronchi are obstructed, giving rise to inflammatory changes of the bronchial mucosa. Wet cough with mucoid sputum is observed.*

**Symptoms**

The first signs of lungworm infestation usually appear 4 weeks after the animals have been put out to graze. The cattle begin to cough and breathe heavily. With acute infestation, loss of appetite, dullness, nasal discharge and fever up to 41° C may occur.

Worm infestation, particularly with lungworms, leads to debility of the animals, which in turn may induce other diseases. If cattle are brought in from the pasture in the autumn and housed for fattening, lungworm infestation may easily lead to bacterial pneumonia and crowding disease.

Fig. 361

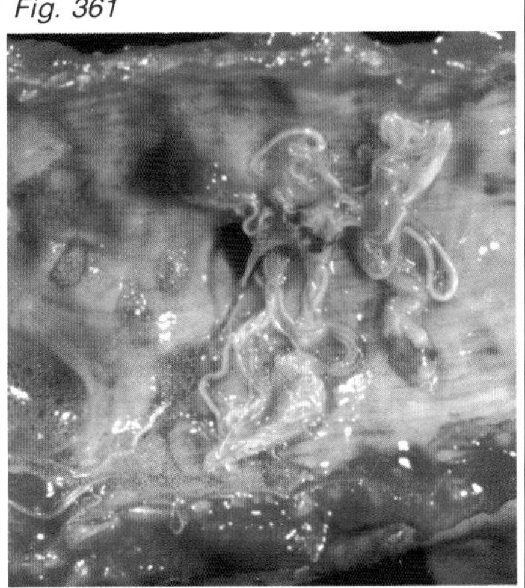

**Diagnosis**

The faeces of grazing animals that cough and show poor development, should be examined for lungworm larvae. For this purpose, the migration method according to Baermann/Wetzel is used, taking advantage of the characteristic of the larvae to migrate from the faeces into the water. The larvae can then be observed under the microscope. During the dormant stage in the winter, the demonstration of larvae in the faeces is uncertain. Dissection of the lungs reveals masses of thread-like greyish white worms in the respiratory tract.

Treatment

Treatment of individual animals, de-worming treatment of the entire stock and treatment of the pasture all help to exterminate the lung-worms in the cattle and to prevent re-infection on the pasture. We use CITARIN-L, which is injected subcutaneously, to kill eggs, larvae and sexually mature worms. For pour-on treatment we use CITARIN-L SPOT-ON. The dosage is adjusted to the body-weight and must be strictly adhered to.

*Fig. 362*

| | | |
|---|---|---|
| 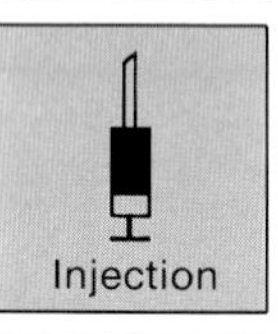 Injection | **De-worming:** Injection of 5 ml CITARIN-L 10%/100 kg body-weight. Not more than 10 ml per injection site and not more than 20 ml per animal. | Imme-diately |
| 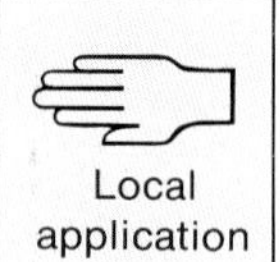 Local application | **De-worming:** Instead of the injection: Pour on 10 ml CITARIN-L SPOT-ON/100 kg body-weight. Maximum: 40 ml. | Imme-diately |
| 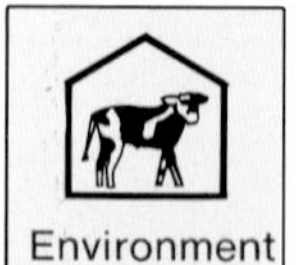 Environment | **Housing** of infested animals. Parasitological examination. | Imme-diately |
| 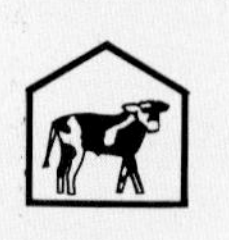 Environment | **Preventing infestation by taking prophy-lactic measures on the pasture:** Mowing grass on infested pastures; making hay. Larvae migrate from drying grass into the moist soil. Separate young from old cattle. | At the start of grazing period |
| 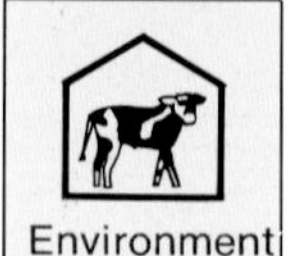 Environment | Arrange drinking troughs to avoid contact with faeces. Change pasture every 5 days. Divide pasture into grazing sections. De-worm animals in the spring. | At the start of grazing period |

Fig. 363

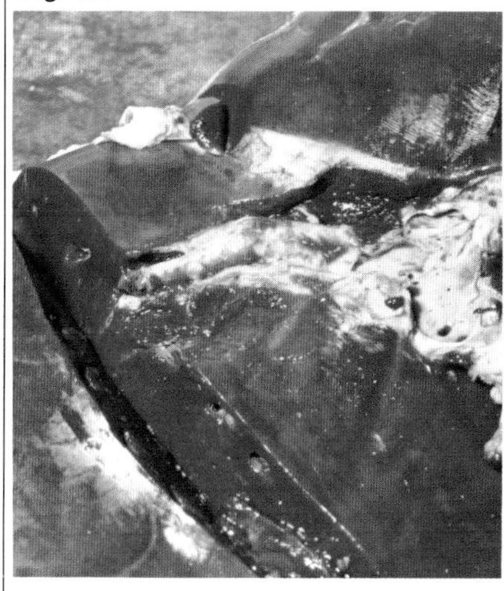

Fig. 364

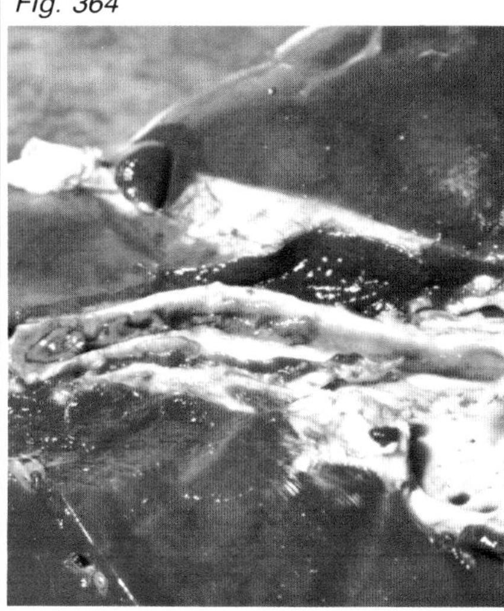

# Liver fluke infestation

**Term**

Liver flukes live as parasites in the bile ducts of the liver. They damage the liver itself and cause changes in the bile ducts.

**Incidence**

Liver fluke disease is a problem in areas where the cattle are kept on moist pastures. The disease therefore occurs especially in low-lying regions. The animals are particularly at risk during the first grazing period.

**Pathogen / Cause**

Liver flukes belong to the group of trematodes which are included among the flatworms. In Central Europe it is almost exclusively the large liver fluke (Fasciola hepatica) which causes damage, whereas the small liver fluke (Dicrocoelium lanceatum) is only seen in isolated cases. For its development the large liver fluke needs an intermediate host, the dwarf snail Limnaea truncatula which measures approx. 0.8 cm. This so-called liver fluke snail lives along the banks of shallow, stagnant or slow-flowing waterways and on moist pastures. They can survive months of drought in the mud. However, only 5 to 10% of the snails survive the winter. For this reason there are only few infected snails in the spring that can infect the grazing cattle. As a result of continual excretion of eggs in the faeces of the cattle and the consequent increase in the snail population, the risk of infection steadily increases from the summer until the autumn.

*Fig. 362: Treatment schedule in lungworm infestation.*

*Fig. 363: Liver invaded by liver flukes. The bile ducts are distended and thickened.*

*Fig. 364: This section of the bile ducts shows the liver flukes. The wall of the bile ducts shows callous thickening.*

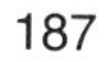

**Life cycle**

Fig. 365

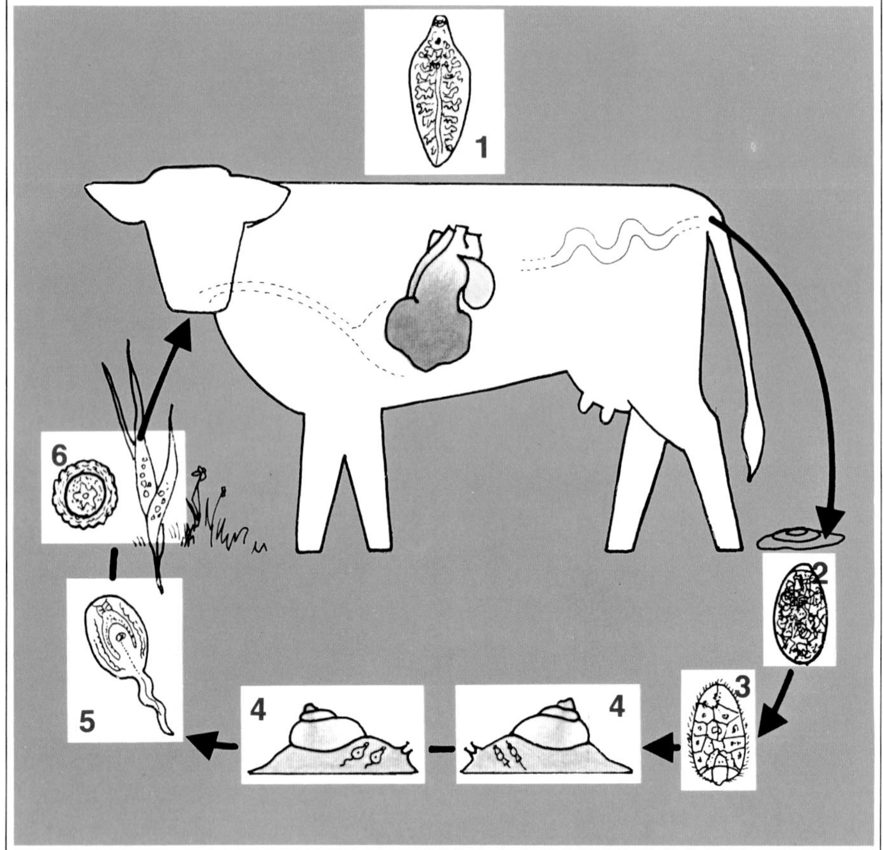


*Fig. 365: Life cycle of the large liver fluke.*
*1 Mature liver fluke*
*2 Egg of liver fluke*
*3 Miracidium*
*4 Dwarf snail with miracidia and caudate larvae*
*5 Caudate larva (metacercaria)*
*6 Encapsulated larva (metacercarial cyst)*

*Fig. 366: When an incision in the liver is made, the liver flukes ooze out from the bile ducts.*

The life cycle of the large liver fluke comprises two stages:

- Development in the environment and in the intermediate host: In a moist environment, the fluke eggs excreted in the faeces develop into miracidia within 3 to 4 weeks. These larvae penetrate through the skin into the snails where they multiply asexually. One miracidium produces up to 250 caudate larvae (cercariae) which leave the snail, attach themselves to wet grass and form encapsulated larvae.
- Development in cattle:
  The cattle ingest the encapsulated larvae with the grass or hay. The capsule is dissolved in the small intestine; the larvae (metacercariae) are released and penetrate the intestinal wall.

Fig. 366

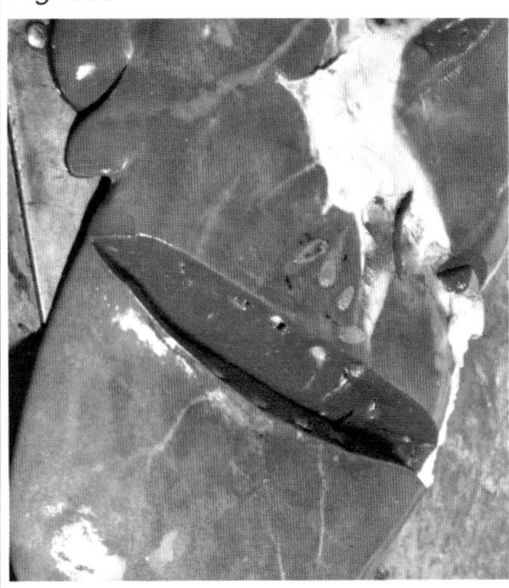

The larvae pass into the abdominal cavity and migrate to the liver. They penetrate the liver capsule and invade the liver. Young liver flukes move about the liver for 6 to 8 weeks and then invade the bile ducts where they become sexually mature and parasitise for approx. 1 year.

**Life cycle**

One liver fluke lays 5,000 to 10,000 eggs daily which pass into the intestine with the bile and are excreted in the faeces. The small liver fluke needs two intermediate hosts for its development, snails and ants.

If the larvae released from the capsules migrate into the liver veins, they may be carried into other organs (e.g. uterus) and mature there. These are called "vagrant" or "errant" liver flukes and provide an explanation of the fact that even calves as young as a few weeks old may be carriers of liver flukes (prenatal invasion).

**Importation / Route of infection**

Infection with infective encapsulated larvae occurs mainly by ingestion on the pasture. Since the larvae survive in the hay for up to 6 months, infection in the cattle house is possible. Importation into a stock previously free from liver fluke, is usually due to the purchase of infested cattle.

**Symptoms**

Migrating liver fluke larvae which penetrate through the intestinal wall into the abdominal cavity may cause peritonitis presenting symptoms not unlike those caused by foreign bodies in the first three stomachs. The young flukes penetrating the liver capsule and migrating in the liver cause inflammation of the hepatic tissue and hepatitis. Dullness, anaemia and increased body temperature (up to 41° C) are the result. Doughy swellings (oedemas) are observed on the lower abdomen and the neck.

The liver flukes parasitising in the bile ducts cause irritation and inflammation of the bile duct walls. At these sites, granulation and eventually calcification lead to a narrowing of the bile ducts and may even occlude them. The resulting bile engorgement may cause jaundice which manifests itself by yellow discoloration of the mucosae.

Bile acids are necessary for fat digestion. Disturbed bile flow leads to intermittent diarrhoea and changing appetite. Dullness, rough coat and emaciation are therefore also an indication of liver fluke disease.

Fig. 367

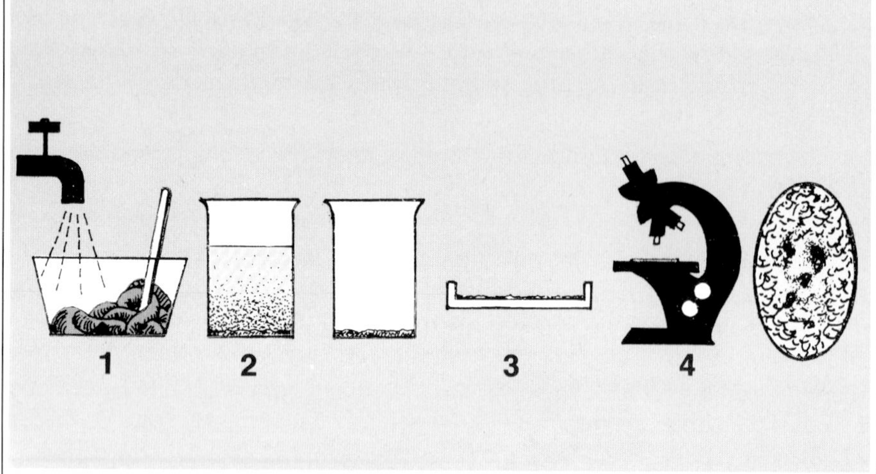


Fig. 368

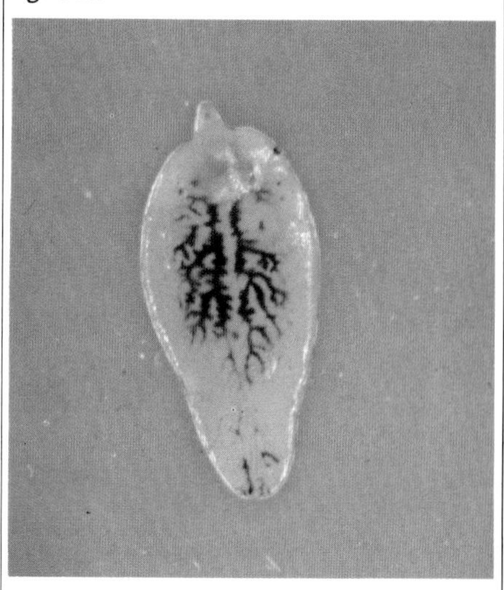

**Diagnosis**

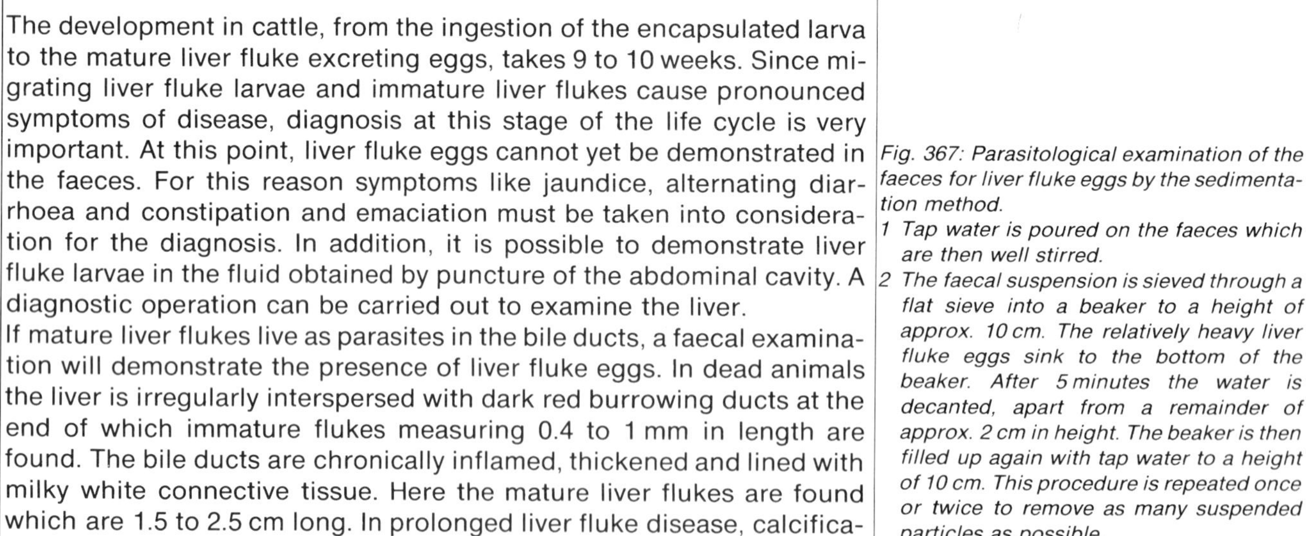

The development in cattle, from the ingestion of the encapsulated larva to the mature liver fluke excreting eggs, takes 9 to 10 weeks. Since migrating liver fluke larvae and immature liver flukes cause pronounced symptoms of disease, diagnosis at this stage of the life cycle is very important. At this point, liver fluke eggs cannot yet be demonstrated in the faeces. For this reason symptoms like jaundice, alternating diarrhoea and constipation and emaciation must be taken into consideration for the diagnosis. In addition, it is possible to demonstrate liver fluke larvae in the fluid obtained by puncture of the abdominal cavity. A diagnostic operation can be carried out to examine the liver.

If mature liver flukes live as parasites in the bile ducts, a faecal examination will demonstrate the presence of liver fluke eggs. In dead animals the liver is irregularly interspersed with dark red burrowing ducts at the end of which immature flukes measuring 0.4 to 1 mm in length are found. The bile ducts are chronically inflamed, thickened and lined with milky white connective tissue. Here the mature liver flukes are found which are 1.5 to 2.5 cm long. In prolonged liver fluke disease, calcifications are formed in the bile ducts which make a crunching noise when an incision is made.

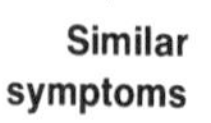

**Similar symptoms**

Liver fluke infestation is an insidious disease. Its most important symptom is the stunting of the cattle. All diseases associated with stunting (e. g. worm infestation, late sequelae of crowding disease) show a similar clinical picture.

*Fig. 367: Parasitological examination of the faeces for liver fluke eggs by the sedimentation method.*

1 *Tap water is poured on the faeces which are then well stirred.*

2 *The faecal suspension is sieved through a flat sieve into a beaker to a height of approx. 10 cm. The relatively heavy liver fluke eggs sink to the bottom of the beaker. After 5 minutes the water is decanted, apart from a remainder of approx. 2 cm in height. The beaker is then filled up again with tap water to a height of 10 cm. This procedure is repeated once or twice to remove as many suspended particles as possible.*

3 *After the last decanting the sediment is poured into a flat Petri dish.*

4 *The yellow liver fluke eggs can now be seen under the microscope. To make them more visible, the eggs can be stained by adding a few drops of methylene blue solution.*

*Fig. 368: Mature liver fluke. One liver fluke lays 5.000 to 10.000 eggs in the bile ducts every day.*

*Fig. 369*

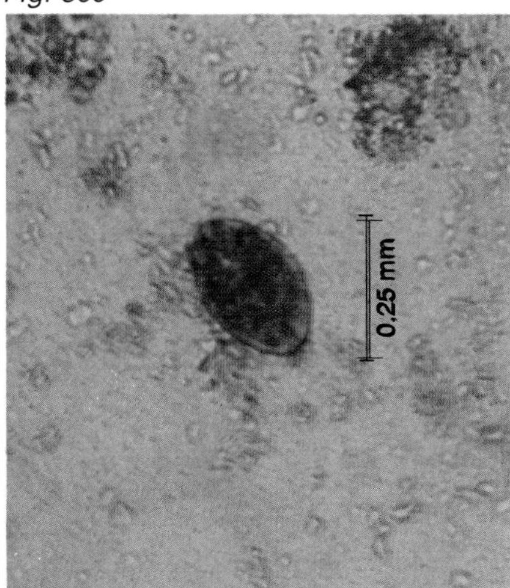


*Fig. 370*

| | | |
|---|---|---|
| 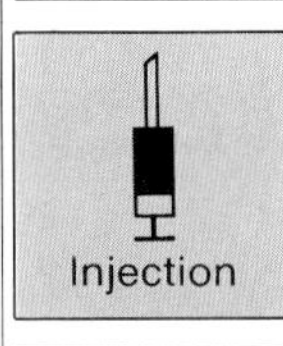 Injection | **Injection treatment:** 1 ml DOVENIX/25 kg subcutaneously into the neck. If the dosage exceeds 15 ml, divide and give several injections into separate sites. | Immediately |
| 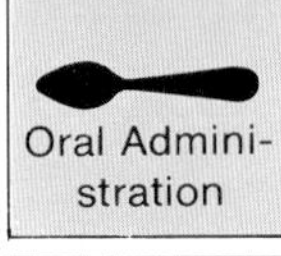 Oral Administration | **In lieu of injection treatment:** 3 ml RANIDEN 2.5%/10 kg body-weight to be given by mouth. | Immediately |
| 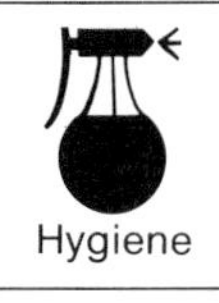 Hygiene | **Additional hygienic measures:** Housing of affected cattle, or at least change of pasture. Combat snails. | At the start of grazing period |

Combined treatment to combat liver flukes in cattle and the dwarf snails harbouring the larvae as intermediate host, should be carried out annually over a period of several years.

*Fig. 371*

| Combating liver flukes in cattle | Combating the dwarf snail |
|---|---|
| All cattle over 4 months old:<br>Injection treatment with DOVENIX or oral administration of RANIDEN.<br>■ Ist treatment: 6 weeks after housing the animals in the autumn, following the end of the grazing period.<br>■ 2nd treatment: End of March. | **Indirect measures:**<br>■ Drain wet pastures<br>■ Fence in swampy sites<br>■ Keep drinking troughs on the pasture clean and reinforce watering sites.<br>■ Movable drinking troughs.<br>**Direct measures:**<br>Before the growing season:<br>■ Treat pasture with 300–400 kg calcium nitrate/hectare.<br>■ Apply 300 to 500 g of Frescon (snail poison) per hectare. |

*Fig. 369: Liver fluke egg, microphotograph.*

*Fig. 370: Treatment schedule in liver fluke disease.*

*Fig. 371: Combating the liver fluke and its intermediate host.*

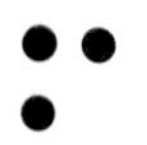

# Gastrointestinal worm infestation (Trichostrongylides)

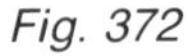

*Fig. 372*

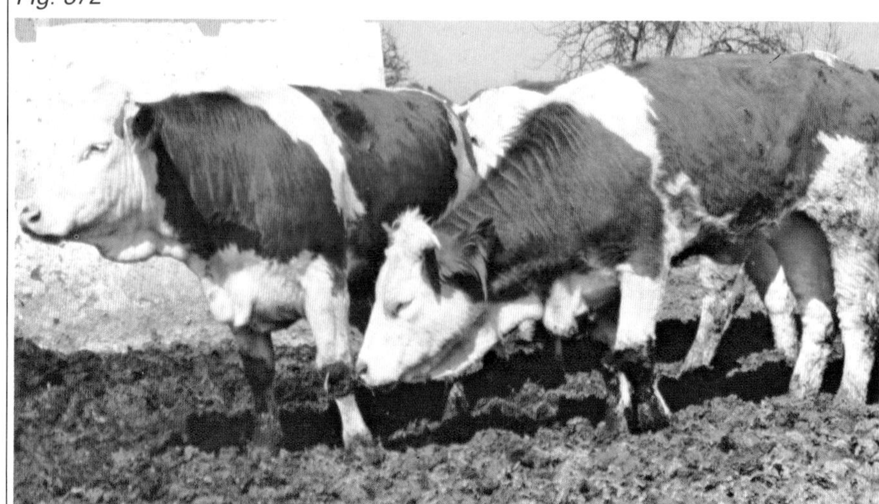

**Term**

Trichostrongylides are small worms as fine as hair, living predominantly in the abomasum and in the anterior sections of the small intestine. The most important species occurring in cattle in our regions are Haemonchus, Ostertagia, Trichostrongylus, Cooperia and Nematodirus.

**Incidence**

Grazing cattle virtually always show slight infestation with gastrointestinal worms. Because of the delayed development (hypobiosis) of the worms in the winter, the animals suddenly start to excrete many worm eggs in the spring. Young cattle are particularly affected.

**Pathogen**

**Life cycle**

Larvae are hatched within 15 to 20 hours from the eggs excreted in the faeces. These larvae shed their skins twice and, depending on weather conditions, will develop into invasive third-stage larvae within 2 to 4 weeks. They are washed from the faeces by the rain or migrate from the faeces and creep up the grass blades with which they are ingested by the grazing cattle. They mature via two further skin changes in the rumen, the abomasum and the small intestine. The larvae of the species Ostertagia, Trichostrongylus and Cooperia lie dormant in the intestinal mucosa from the autumn to the spring. This halts their further development, and the worm eggs are not excreted in large numbers until the animals are put out to graze. Young cattle being put to pasture for the first time are particularly susceptible to infection with the larvae hatched from these eggs and with larvae that have hibernated on the pasture. For this reason young cattle excrete large numbers of gastrointestinal worm eggs when the worms have reached sexual maturity.

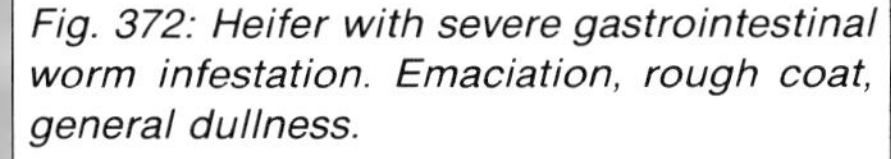

*Fig. 372: Heifer with severe gastrointestinal worm infestation. Emaciation, rough coat, general dullness.*

*Fig. 373: Life cycle of gastrointestinal worms:*
*1 Mature worms in the stomach and intestine of cattle.*
*2 Worm egg excreted in the faeces.*
*3 Larva hatched from the egg.*
*4 Having shed its skin several times, the larva becomes invasive, creeps up the grass blades and is ingested by the cattle.*

*Fig. 373*

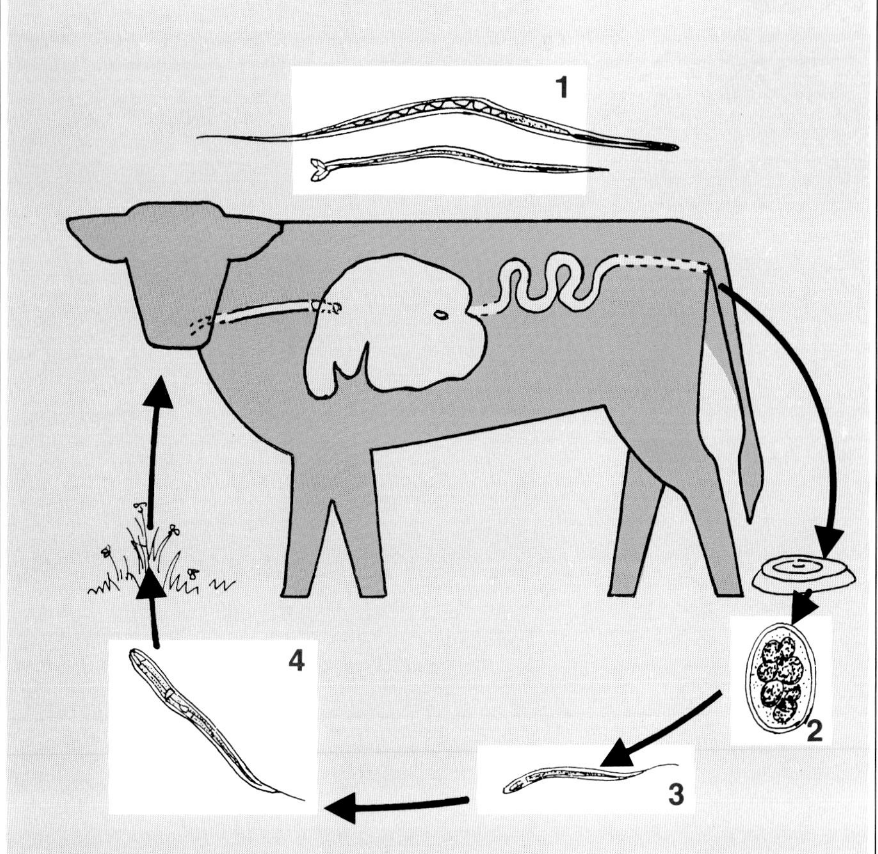


**Life cycle**

**Symptoms**

In late August and early September, worm infestation of cattle is most pronounced. Rough coat despite excellent fodder, retarded growth, emaciation, diarrhoea and debility are the most striking symptoms.
The eggs of the parasites can be demonstrated by an examination of the faeces.

**Treatment and preventive measures**

All animals of a grazing group are given anthelmintic treatment at the end of June. 2 or 3 days later, these animals are put on a pasture on which cattle have not yet grazed in that year, and where the grass has been mown (hay). If only infested pastures are available (i. e. where cattle have already grazed in that year), the young cattle should be put on those pastures where cows have been grazing, because worm infestation and excretion of worm eggs is much less pronounced in older cattle than in young cattle.

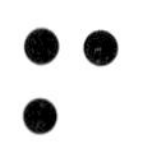

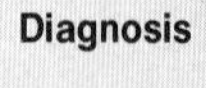

Diagnosis

Fig. 374

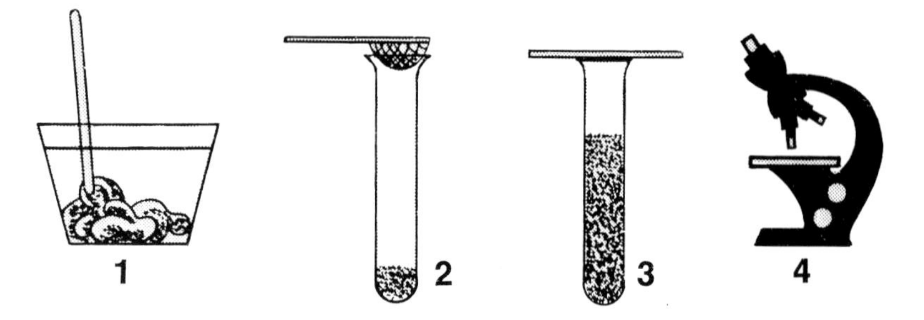


*Fig. 374: Parasitological examination of the faeces using the enrichment method:*

1. *Suspend faeces in saturated sugar or saline solution.*
2. *Pour through a fine-meshed sieve into a test tube. The test tube is filled to the brim so that it has a slightly vaulted surface.*
3. *A cover-glass is placed on the test tube and is in full contact with the surface of the fluid. The saturated solution makes the worm eggs and coccidial oocysts rise and adhere to the cover-glass.*
4. *After 10 to 20 minutes the cover-glass is placed on a slide and examined under the microscope.*

*Fig. 375: Diagrams of different worm eggs.*

1. *Nematodirus*
2. *Haemonchus*
3. *Ostertagia*
4. *Trichostrongylus*
5. *Coccidial oocyst*
6. *Tapeworm egg (moniezia)*
7. *Strongyloides*
8. *Ascaris*

Fig. 375

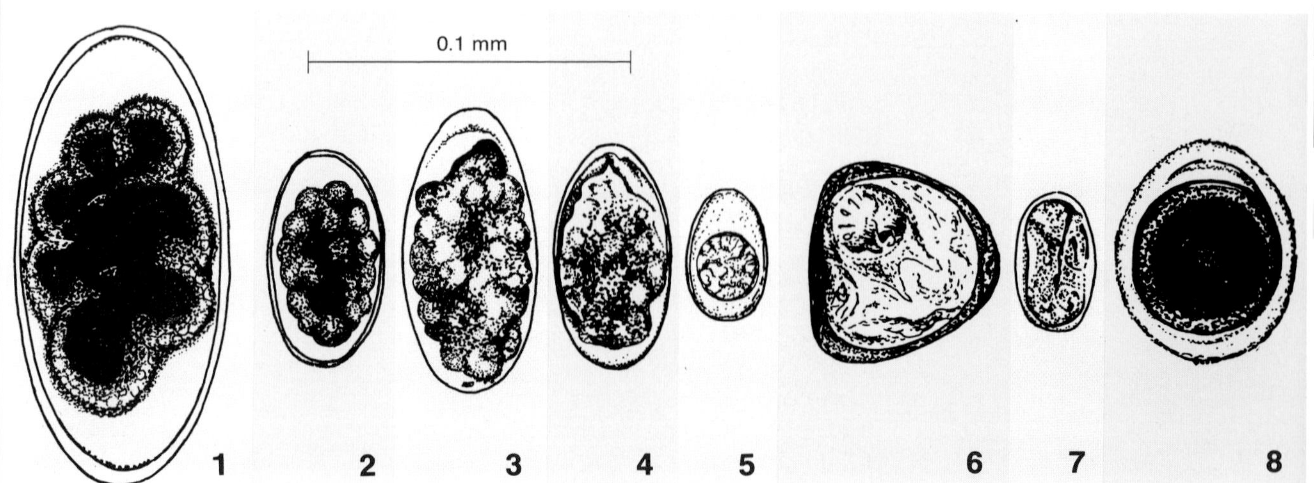

**Treatment and preventive measures**

Regular de-worming of all young animals before putting them out to graze and repeating this treatment two or three times from June to October, are also beneficial. After housing the animals in the autumn, it is advisable to carry out a parasitological examination of the faeces, in order to determine the extent of infestation with gastrointestinal worms and lungworms (see chapter on lungworm infestation). In gastrointestinal worm infestation we use an anthelmintic product containing Thiabendazole and Piperazine. With concomitant lungworm infestation we give CITARIN-L.

*Fig. 376*

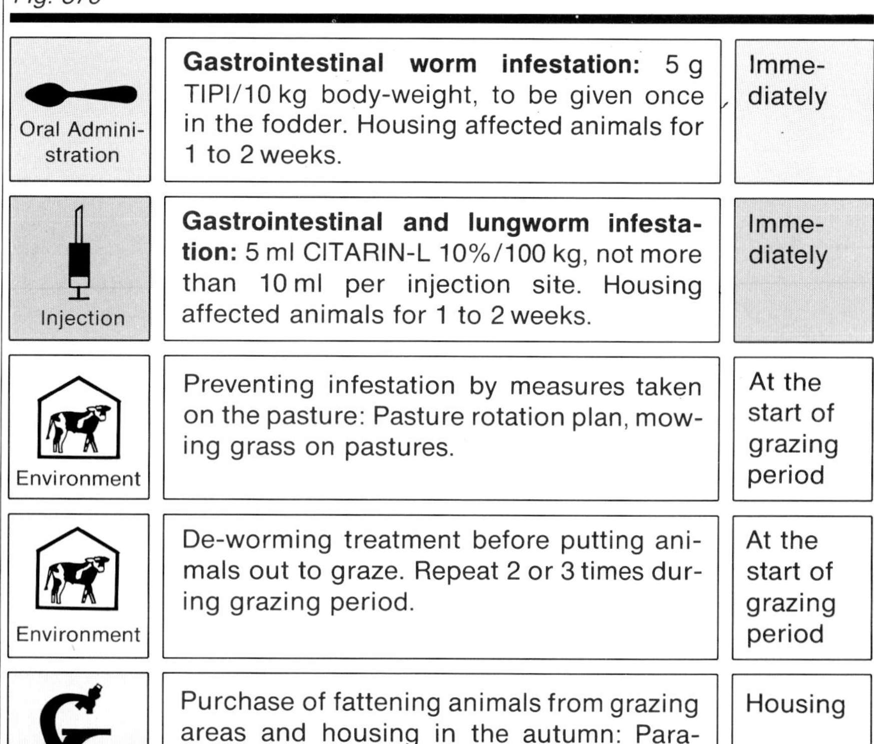

| | | |
|---|---|---|
| Oral Administration | **Gastrointestinal worm infestation:** 5 g TIPI/10 kg body-weight, to be given once in the fodder. Housing affected animals for 1 to 2 weeks. | Immediately |
| Injection | **Gastrointestinal and lungworm infestation:** 5 ml CITARIN-L 10%/100 kg, not more than 10 ml per injection site. Housing affected animals for 1 to 2 weeks. | Immediately |
| Environment | Preventing infestation by measures taken on the pasture: Pasture rotation plan, mowing grass on pastures. | At the start of grazing period |
| Environment | De-worming treatment before putting animals out to graze. Repeat 2 or 3 times during grazing period. | At the start of grazing period |
| Laboratory | Purchase of fattening animals from grazing areas and housing in the autumn: Parasitological examination. De-worming treatment after diagnosis. | Housing |

*Fig. 376: Treatment schedule for gastrointestinal worm infestation.*

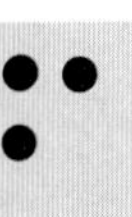

## Warble-fly infestation

Fig. 377

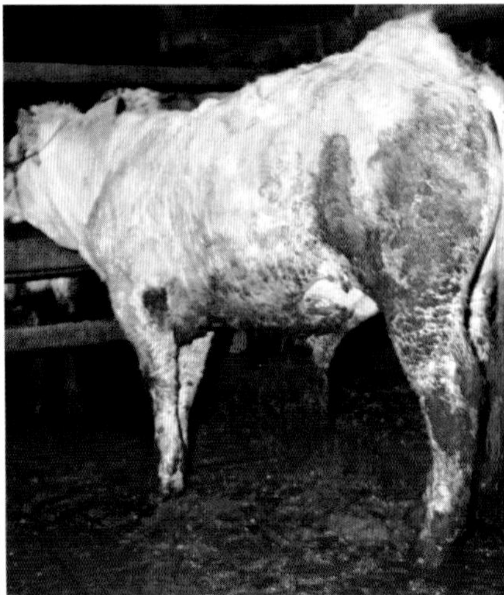

Fig. 378

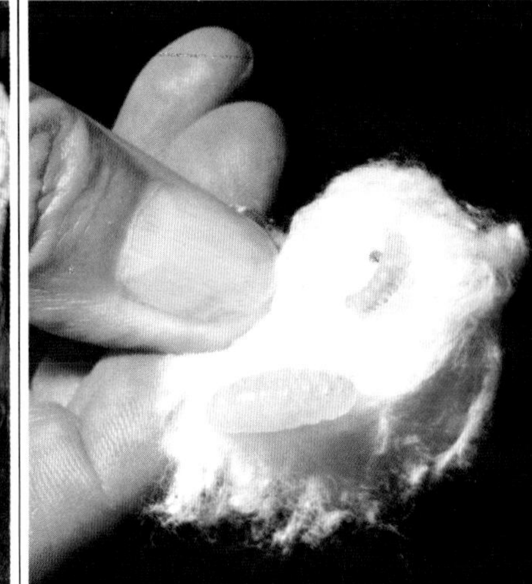

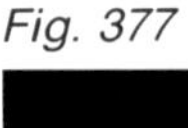

**Term**

Warble-fly infestation manifests itself in the spring by boil-like swellings on the backs of affected cattle. In these boils ("warbles") the larvae of warble-flies live as parasites.

They cause substantial economic damage:

- Reduced weight gain
- Emergency slaughter because of lameness
- Losses on slaughter, because the meat around the warbles must be excised and cannot be used (particularly the valuable back parts)
- Reduced value of hides (holes, scars).

**Incidence**

The disease only occurs in cattle which have been grazing in the summer. Young cattle in the first or second grazing period are particularly affected. Apart from cattle, other wild-living ruminants are infested by various types of warble-fly, although sheep and goats are less frequently affected.

**Pathogen**

Warble-fly infestation is caused by larvae of the small warble-fly (Hypoderma lineatum) and of the large warble-fly (Hypoderma bovis) which penetrate the skin of the animals. The flies are 10 to 15 mm long and resemble bumble-bees. Their larvae grow to a size of 25 mm in the animal body. In normal weather conditions, the life span of mature flies is 2 to 7 days.

*Fig. 377: Warbles. Swellings the size of a child's fist along the animal's back.*

*Fig. 378: Expressed warble-fly larvae at different stages of maturity.*

*Fig. 379: Life cycle of the large warble-fly:*
*1 Larva being hatched from the warble*
*2 Pupation in the grass*
*3 Warble-fly*
*4 Egg attaching to a hair. The hatched larvae are ingested by licking or penetrate the skin.*
*5 Migration through the body to the vertebral canal.*

*Fig. 379*

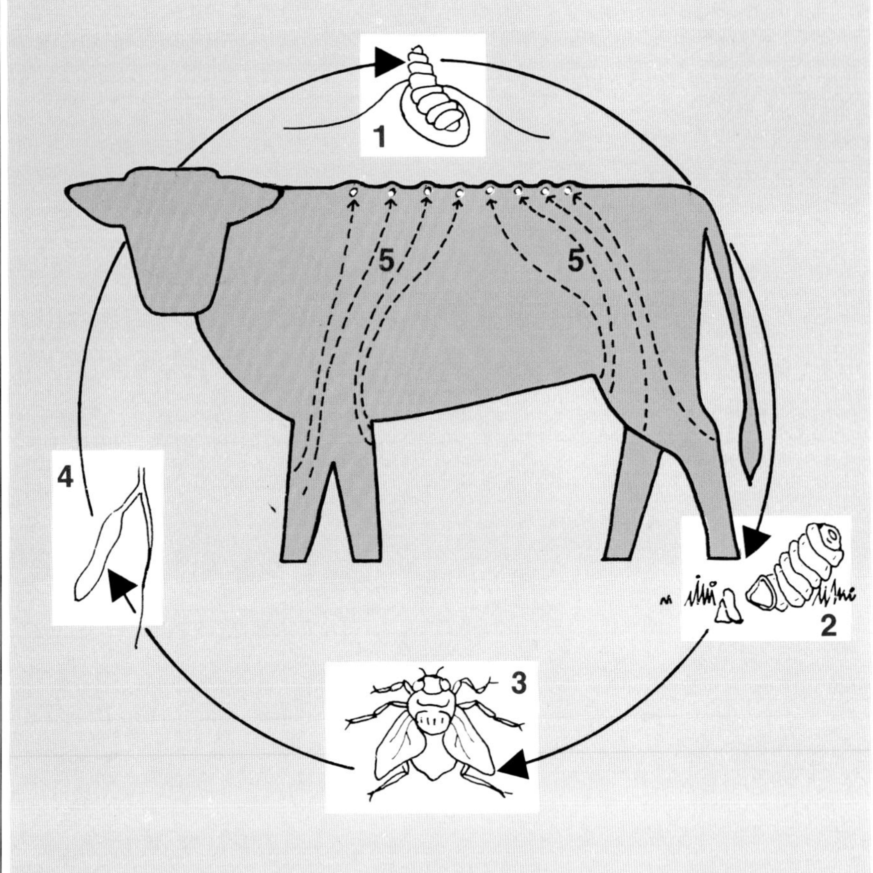


**Life cycle**

From June to September, warble-flies lay their eggs (size: 0.5 to 1 mm) on the coat of grazing animals. Preferred sites are the extremities, abdomen, flanks and chest.
One female lays up to 800 eggs. Larvae are hatched from approx. 30% of these eggs and penetrate the skin. The larvae of the large warble-fly (H. bovis) migrate along the nerve tracts direct to the vertebral canal. The larvae of the small warble-fly (H. lineatum) are deposited on the chest and legs. From there the larvae penetrate the skin and migrate to the gullet muscles. Larvae from eggs deposited on the legs may also be ingested by licking. In this way they are directly introduced into the gullet and migrate to the gullet muscles.

Fig. 380

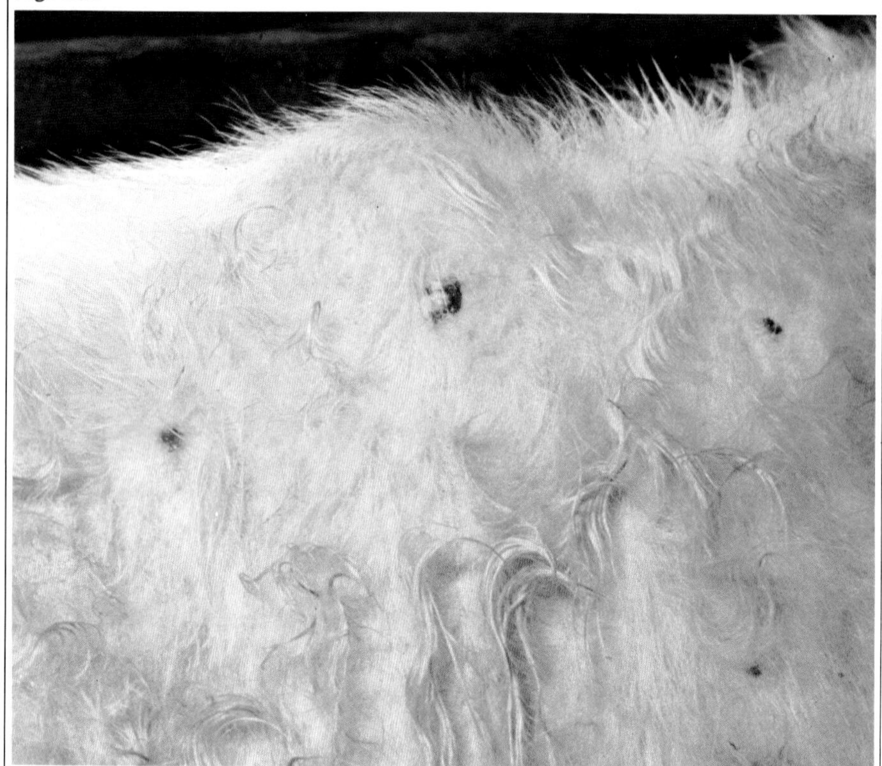

*Fig. 380: Warbles. Each warble has a breathing-hole which is sometimes covered by a scab.*

*Fig. 381: Seasonal course of warble-fly infestation and treatment: 1–12 = January to December.*
*I Eggs are deposited by the flies*
*II Larvae migrate to the vertebral canal*
*III Larvae in the vertebral canal; later under the skin.*
*IV Hatching of the larvae. Pupation.*
*A Sexual maturity of the warble-flies and deposition of eggs.*
*B Migration of the warble-fly larvae to the vertebral canal. Appropriate period for treatment.*
*C Warble-fly larvae in the vertebral canal. No treatment.*
*D Warbles under the skin on the back. Possibly late treatment.*
*E Hatching of larvae and pupation on the ground.*

*Fig. 382: The frequent practice of expressing warbles is not advisable (suppuration due to invading bacteria).*

**Life cycle**

After 7 to 9 months (February/March) the larvae of both types have reached the subcutis of the animal's back. There they drill a breathing-hole into the skin and develop to pupation stage. Typical warbles are caused by inflammatory changes in the subcutaneous tissue which reacts sensitively to the "foreign body" and to the metabolic products of the larva. After a few weeks the larvae leave the warbles through the breathing-hole, fall to the ground and pupate in the grass. Depending on the external temperature, mature warble-flies are hatched from the pupae within 20 to 50 days.

**Symptoms**

Warble-fly infestation rarely causes generalised symptoms in cattle. When the larvae penetrate into the vertebral canal, this may result in lameness of the hindlegs and cause the animals to lie down all the time. Severe warble-fly infestation leads to loss of appetite, emaciation and itching. The animal's back is painful to the touch.

Fig. 381

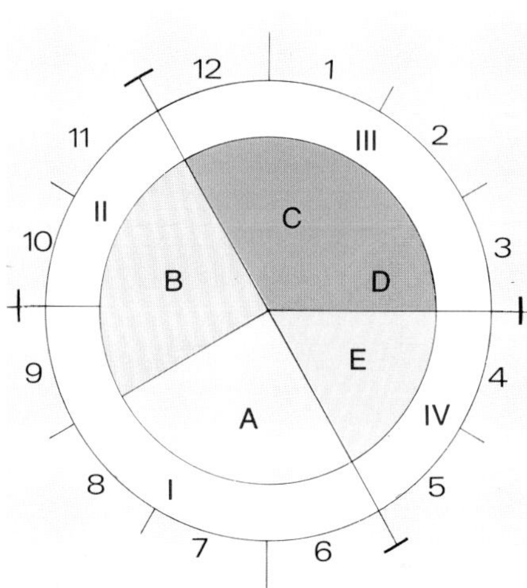


Fig. 382

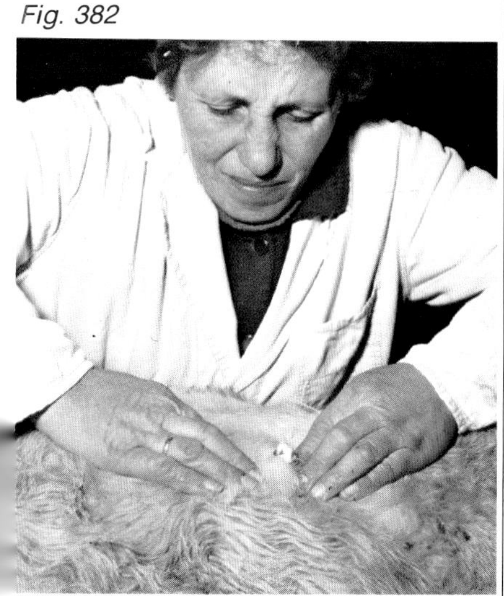

The typical warbles on the back of the animal, which may range in size from a cherry to a fist, are a definite indication of warble-fly infestation. On close inspection, one can see the breathing-holes which are often covered by a scab.

**Diagnosis**

Treatment aims to destroy all larvae in the animal body as early as possible. For this purpose, drugs are required which are well absorbed and pass into all regions of the body, in order to ensure that all larval stages are killed off. Phosphoric acid ester products are now used for treatment in a dosage that is precisely adapted to the body-weight. We use TIGUVON which is poured onto the animal's back. Dosage: 100–200 kg body-weight: 50 ml; 200–300 kg body-weight: 75 ml; 300–400 kg body-weight: 100 ml; 400 kg body-weight and above: 125 ml. Both over-dosage and underdosage should be avoided.

**Treatment**

Treatment should be completed by the end of November at the latest. By that time the larvae have not yet reached the vertebral canal. No treatment should be carried out from the beginning of December until March, because during this period there is a danger of spinal paralysis if the larvae migrating in the vertebral canal are killed.

In exceptional cases treatment may not be possible before 1st December (purchase of grazing cattle from infested regions). In such cases, late treatment may be carried out from the beginning of March to mid-May.

Here it must be accepted that the skin and the back muscles may already be damaged, and that in the event of severe infestation, the larvicidal treatment may cause foreign protein shock in the cattle.

**Legal provisions***

There are legal provisions for the treatment of warble-fly infestation. The stockholder is required to carry out warble-fly treatment at his own expense. Completed warble-fly treatment and the product used must be notified to the local veterinary officer. Even if only one animal shows warble-fly infestation, the treatment of all animals put out to pasture in the previous year, is obligatory. In areas particularly at risk, the veterinary authorities may order treatment to be carried out.

**Prevention**

In the autumn, young cattle are frequently purchased from infested grazing areas. Experience has shown that these animals are warble-fly carriers (e. g. Charolais, Limousine). Warble-fly treatment by the end of November is therefore advisable.

---

* Valid in W. Germany

# Mange

Fig. 383

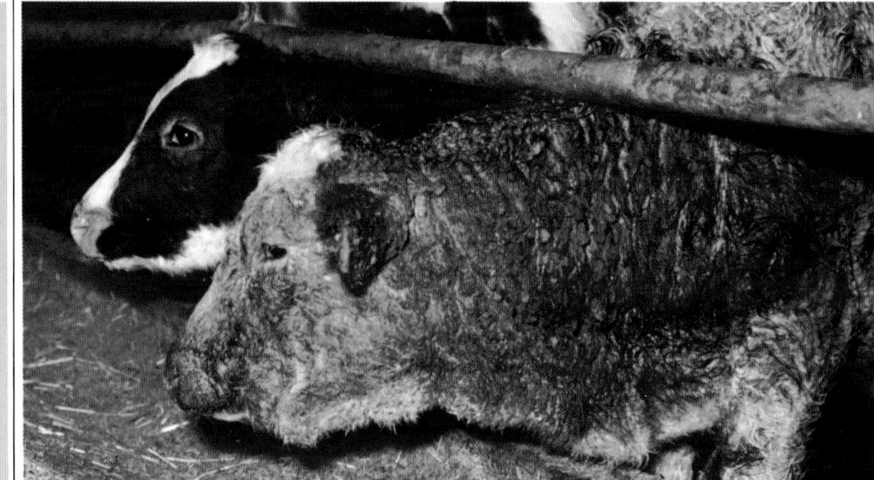

**Term**

Mange is a skin disease associated with intense itching, loss of hair and scab formation. It is caused by parasites (mange mites).

**Incidence**

The disease has been observed with increasing frequency during the past 3 or 4 years. We have found massive mange infestation of entire stocks where young grazing animals had been purchased. Without treatment, some of the animals died.

Slight infestation with mange mites is unimportant in grazing cattle. Since there are no changes of the skin or coat, the condition is not recognised on purchase. It is only 3 to 6 weeks after housing the animals that the first symptoms of the disease may be observed. A change-over from grazing to high-density housing and changed feeding conditions enable the mites to multiply with great speed.

Fig. 384

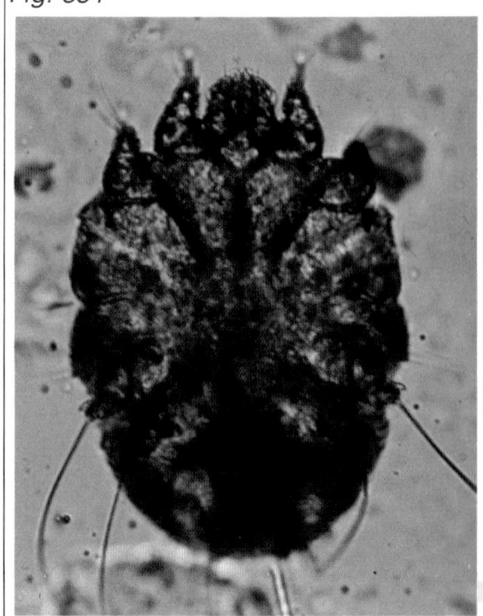

**Pathogen**

Mange mites which belong to the species Arachnida, live in or on the skin where they multiply. They measure only 0.3 to 0.8 mm and are barely visible to the naked eye. There are three types of mange mites occurring in cattle, each of them with somewhat different habits and different preferred sites of settlement:

*Fig. 383: Bull with severe mange. The coat on the whole body is covered with greasy crusts having a stale, sweetish smell.*

*Fig. 384: Mange mite, microphotograph.*

*Figs. 385 and 386: Bull with sarcoptic mange. Bald patches on the back with chafed skin areas.*

*Fig. 385*

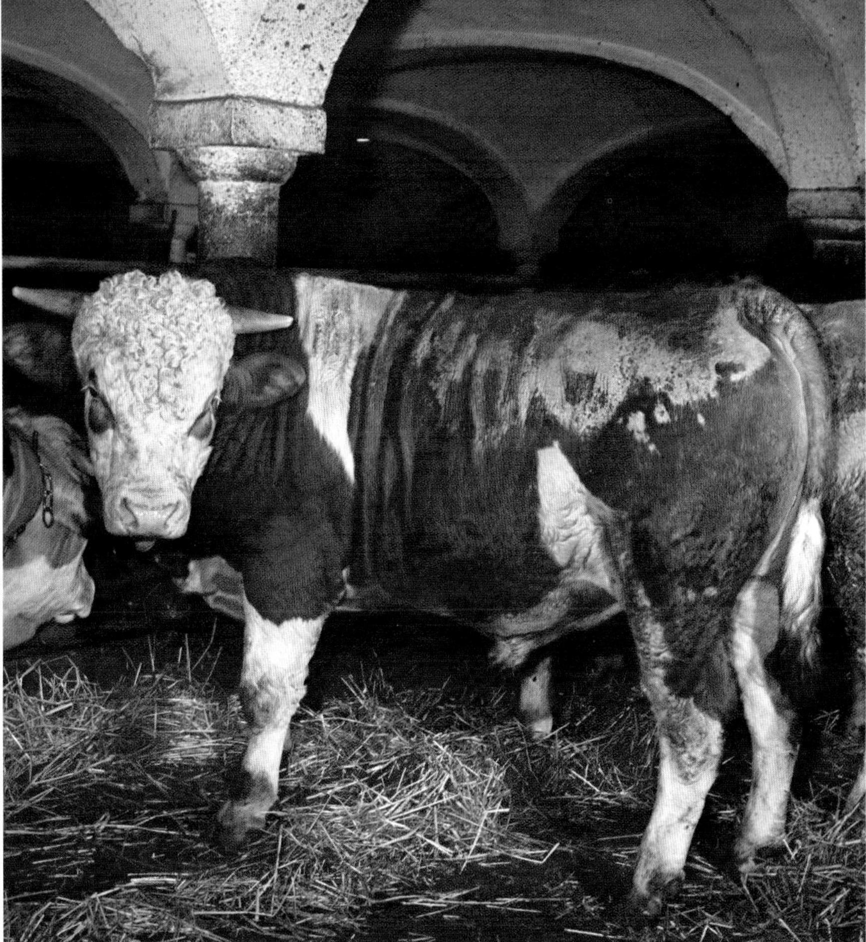

*Fig. 386*

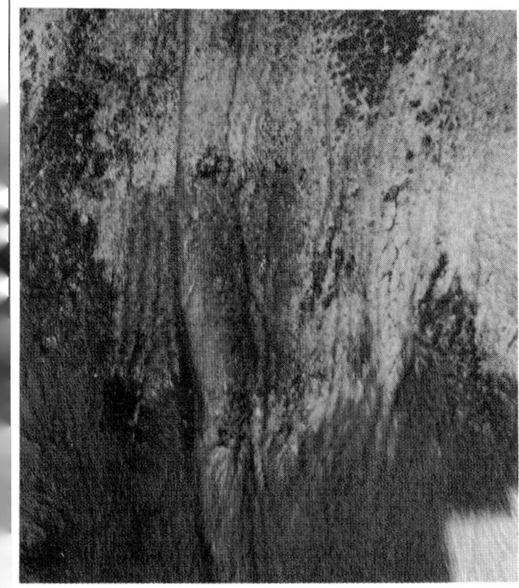

Pathogen

- Sucking mites (Psoroptes) mainly along the dorsal line, at the withers, the sacrum and the base of the tail.
- Burrowing mites (Sarcoptes) on the head, neck and in the sacral region.
- Gnawing mites (Chorioptes) on the tail fold, the rear fetlock joint and the croup.

*Fig. 387*

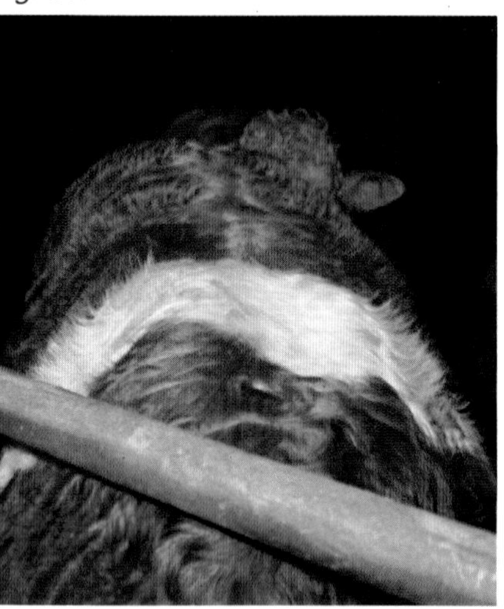

*Fig. 388*

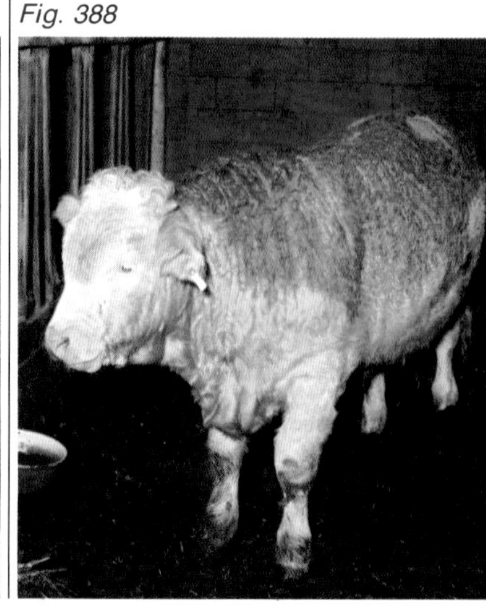

*Fig. 389*

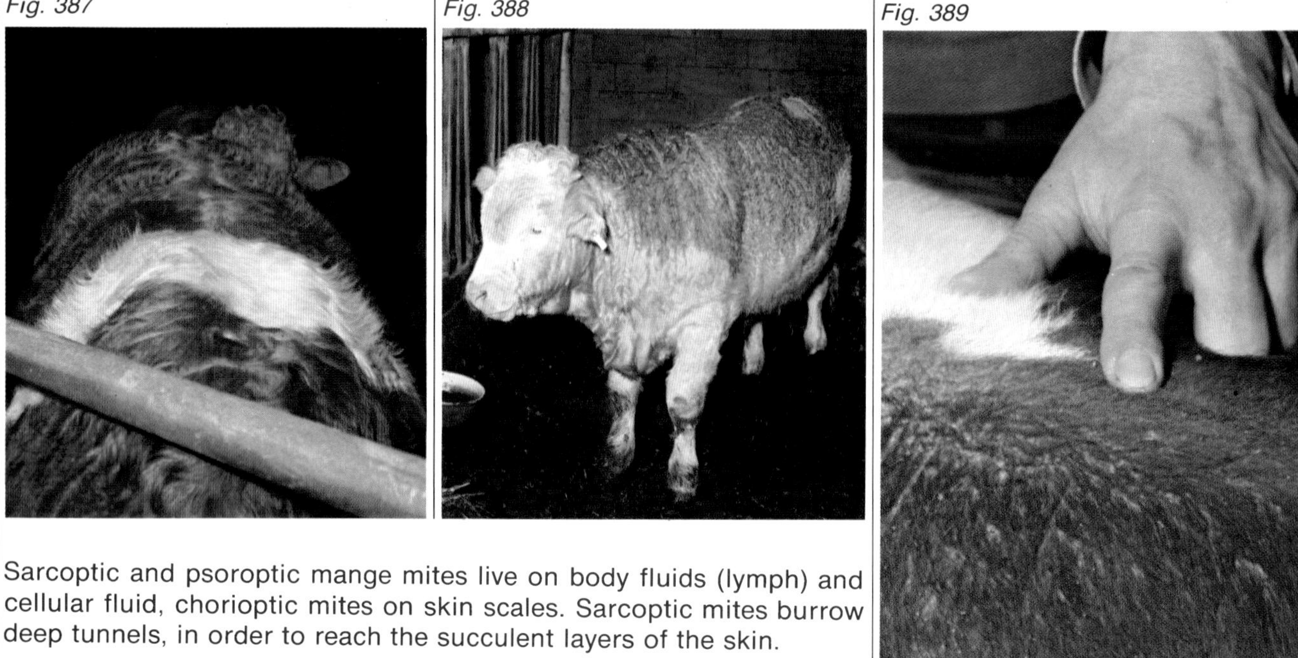

**Pathogen / Life cycle**

Sarcoptic and psoroptic mange mites live on body fluids (lymph) and cellular fluid, chorioptic mites on skin scales. Sarcoptic mites burrow deep tunnels, in order to reach the succulent layers of the skin.

One female lays up to 100 eggs. Larvae are hatched from the eggs and pass through several development stages until they become mature mites. The duration of development from the egg to the mature mite varies. For sarcoptic mites it is 14 to 21 days, for Psoroptes it is 9 and for Chorioptes 11 days. This period of development is important for the effective treatment of mange. Because of their resistant shells, the eggs are not killed by the drugs used, and it is therefore necessary to repeat the treatment several times at intervals of 10 days. It is only by this repeated treatment that the hatched and growing mites are killed.

**Importation / Route of infection**

Mites are transmitted by contact between the animals, and – less commonly – indirectly via cattle house implements or equipment and farmhands.

Mange mites are imported into the stock by the purchase of infested animals which need not necessarily show any visible skin changes.

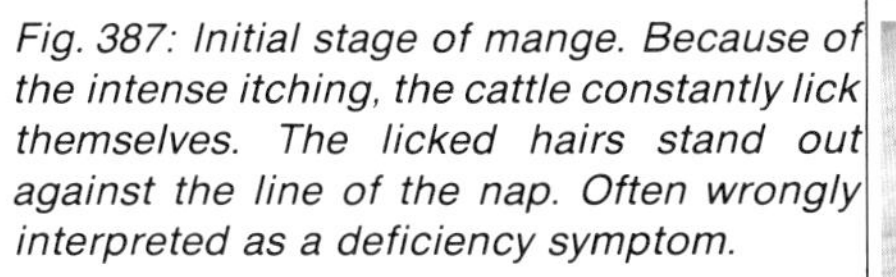

*Fig. 387: Initial stage of mange. Because of the intense itching, the cattle constantly lick themselves. The licked hairs stand out against the line of the nap. Often wrongly interpreted as a deficiency symptom.*

*Fig. 388: Mange in a grazing animal after housing. Formation of crusts and scabs with weeping skin areas.*

*Fig. 389: Incipient mange. Formation of pustules, with hair standing on end at the changed sites.*

*Fig. 390: Transition from normal to mangy skin. Thickened skin with formation of folds in the mangy area.*

*Fig. 391: Common starting point of mange: base of the tail.*

*Fig. 391*

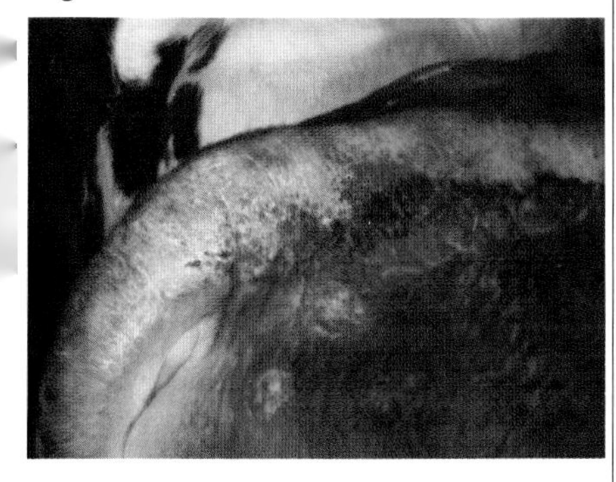

*Fig. 390*

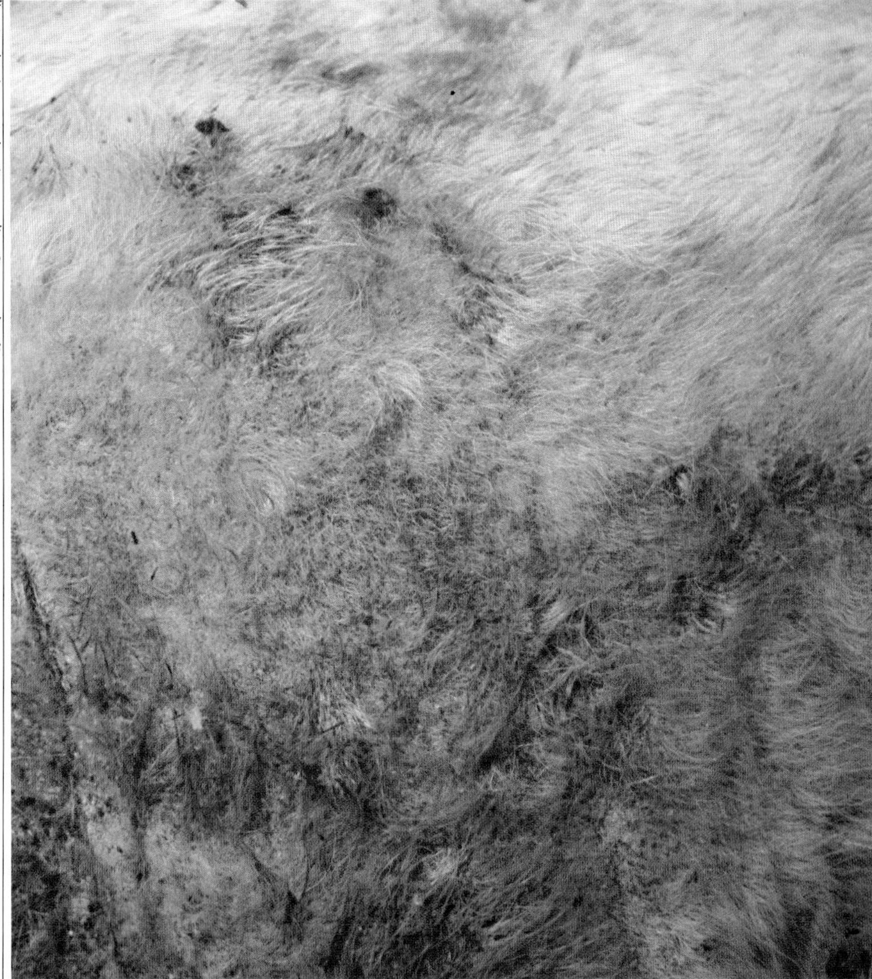

**Symptoms**

The condition is mainly caused by the burrowing, boring, sucking and gnawing action of mites. The mites also excrete noxious substances which provoke defence reactions by the skin.

The first sign of mange is restlessness which is due to intense itching and manifests itself in frequent scratching, rubbing and licking. The skin shows small nodules and pustules. Hairs fall out or break off. The skin becomes dry, chapped and wrinkled. Scabs and crusts form. Continued intense itching leads to chafing.

*Fig. 392*

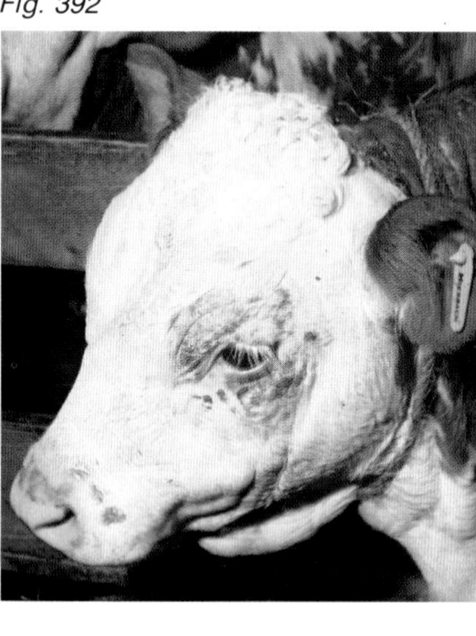

*Fig. 393*

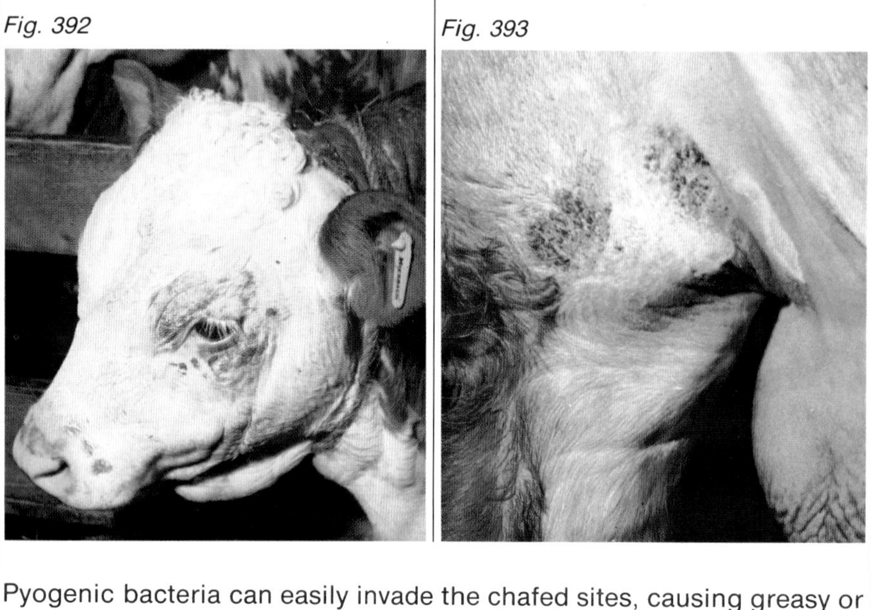

*Fig. 394*

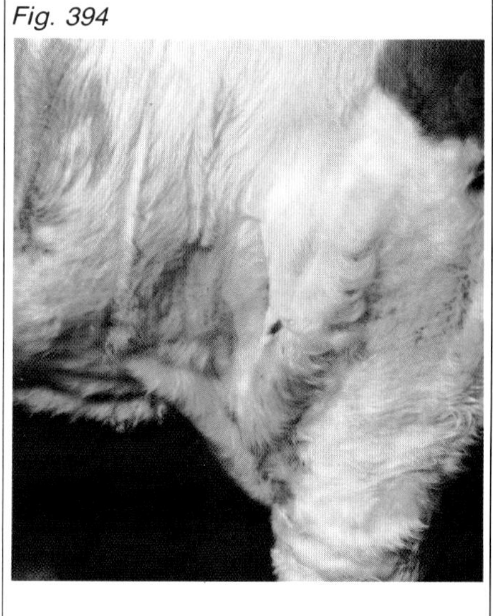

**Symptoms**

Pyogenic bacteria can easily invade the chafed sites, causing greasy or weeping suppurative inflammations with a stale, sweetish odour. Infestation of large skin areas leads to severe generalised disease. Destroyed skin tissue that is not shed, has to be broken down by the animal organism. This may cause auto-intoxication. Death may ensue in particularly severe cases.

**Diagnosis**

Mange can be easily recognised from the typical skin changes. For the demonstration of the pathogen, skin scrapings are collected from the edge of the lesions and are examined under the microscope (cf. Figs. 397 and 398).

**Similar symptoms**

Mange may well be confused with severe infestation with lice or biting lice. These conditions are frequently associated with mange.

Ringworm (trichophytosis) with its typical circular, bald patches is clearly distinguishable from mange. Mixed infestation with mange mites, lice and ringworm is also possible.

*Fig. 392: Incipient head mange in a calf.*

*Figs. 393 and 394: Chorioptic mange in the articular space, and in the elbow and upper arm regions.*

*Figs. 395 and 396: Mange in a milk calf. Incipient loss of hair behind the ears and on the neck. The skin is thickened and forms folds. Hairs sticking together with greasy crusts.*

*Figs. 397 and 398: Collecting skin scrapings in mange. Cutting off the hair at the line of transition from healthy to mangy skin. Using a scalpel or a sharp spoon, the skin is scraped until there is a seeping haemorrhage. The skin scrapings are examined for mites in the laboratory.*

*Fig. 399: Same bull as Fig. 390, 14 days after treatment. The skin is recovering and the hair is slowly growing again.*

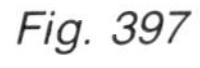

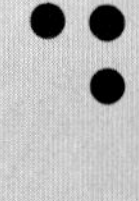

*Fig. 395*

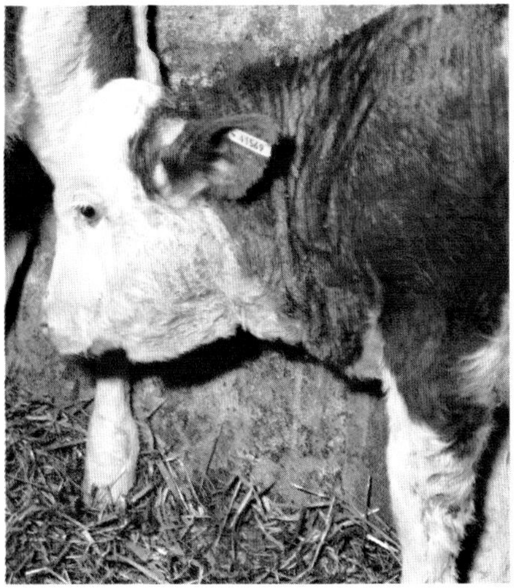

*Fig. 396*

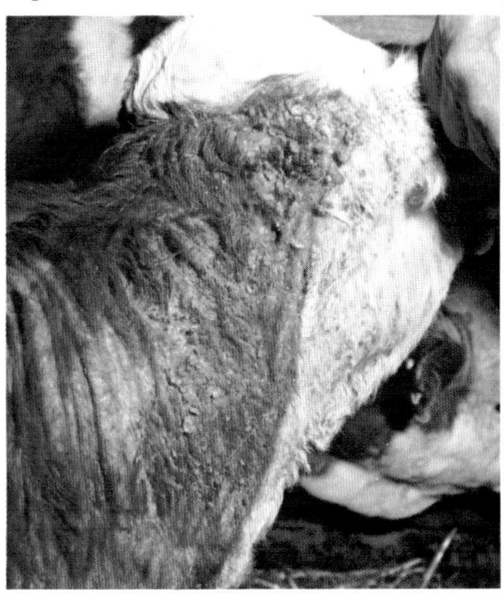

*Fig. 397*

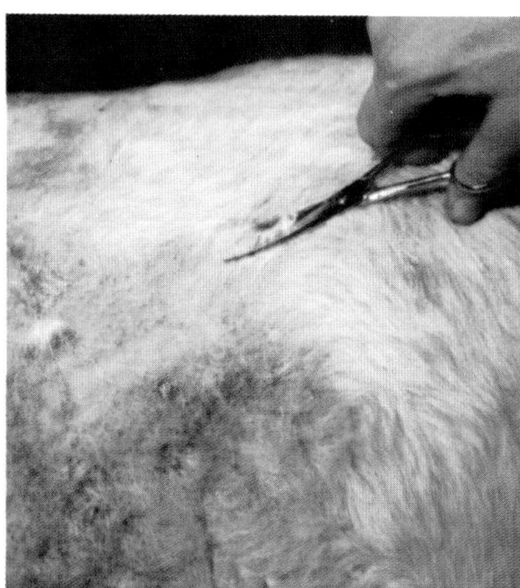

*Fig. 398*

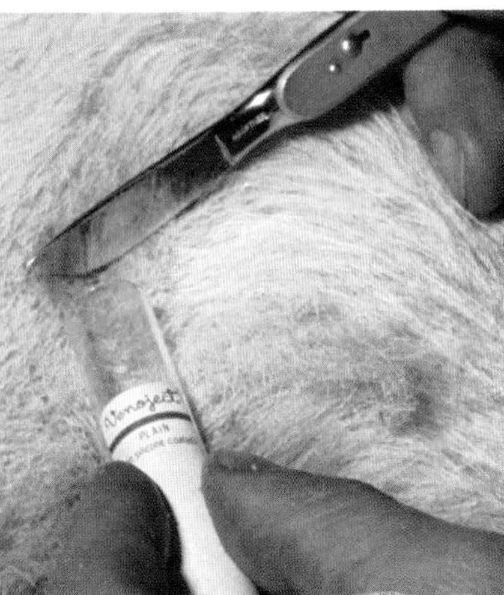

*Fig. 399*

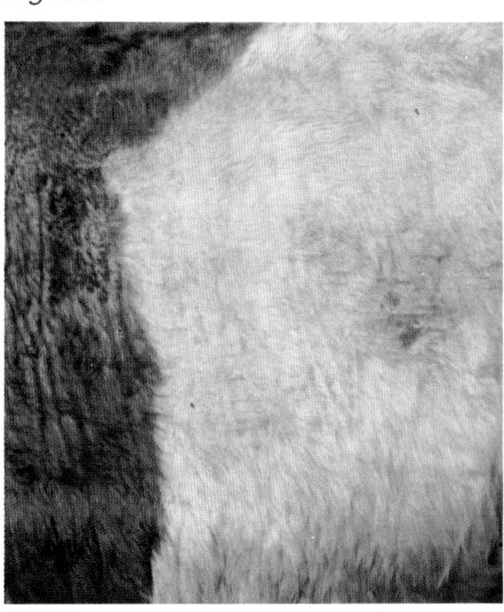

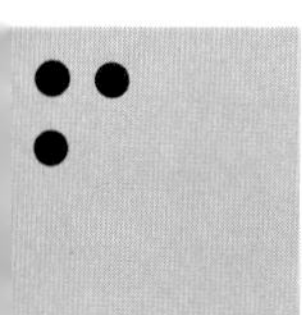

**Treatment**

Treatment is carried out with contact insecticides. Halogenated hydrocarbons and phosphoric acid ester products have proved effective.

All animals of the stock are washed completely, brushed or sprayed to run-off.

During the cold season there is a danger that the animals may catch a chill. For this reason the cattle house should be heated with a fan heater or some other suitable means until the animals are dry.

With severe skin changes involving large areas, it is advisable to confine the first treatment to part of the body, since the animal is already under heavy stress due to the skin changes (kidney and liver damage). After 4 or 5 days, the remaining areas can be treated.

Fig. 400

| | | |
|---|---|---|
| 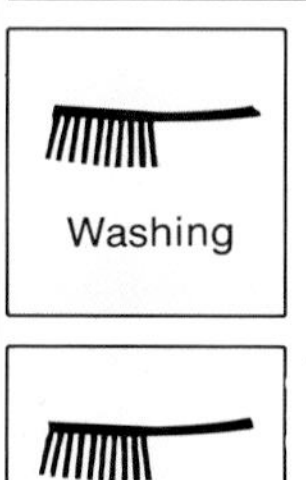 Washing | **All infested animals:** 60 ml EKPAROL in 10 litres of water. Approx. 3 litres of solution per animal, to be applied three times at intervals of 10 days. Wear gloves! | 1st, 10th and 20th day |
| Washing | **Animals with extensive skin lesions** (as Fig. 383): Wash only one half of the body; second half after 5 days. Total wash after 10 and 20 days. | 1st and 5th day. 15th and 25th day |
| 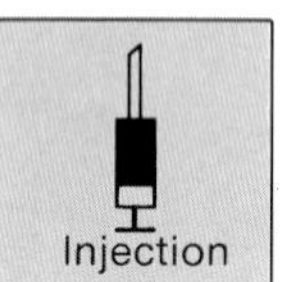 Injection | **Protection of the liver in severely affected animals:** 200 ml HEPAMUGOL/animal intravenously; 20 ml PERLACAR/animal subcutaneously; 20 ml VITIN/animal s.c. | 1st day |
| 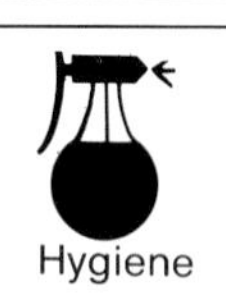 Hygiene | **Disinfection:** Cleaning and spraying cattle house (walls of pens) and implements (curry-combs, brushes) with the anti-mange agent used. | 1st day |
|  Washing | EKPAROL may be replaced by: ALUGAN, DIAZINON, ASUNTOL or NEGUVON. | |

Fig. 401

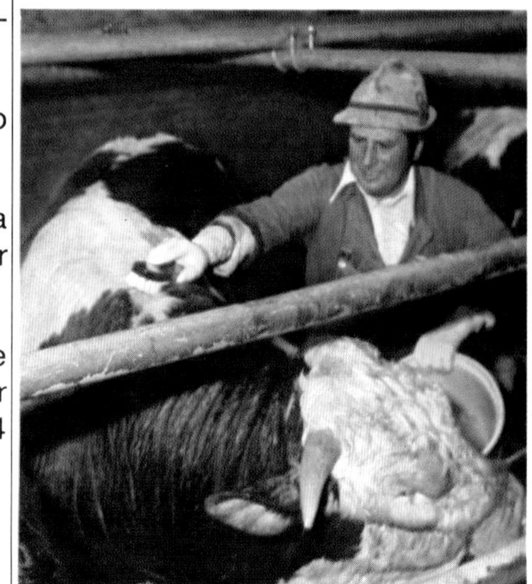

Fig. 402

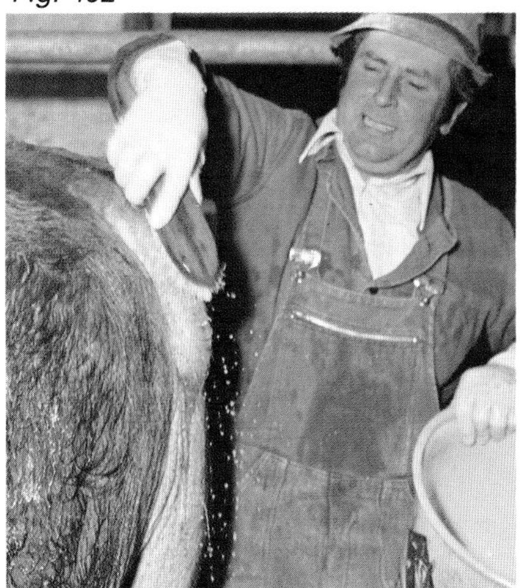

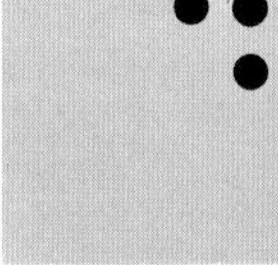

During treatment, the killed mites and the insecticides used have to be broken down by the animal organism. Severely affected cattle should additionally be given liver-protecting products, high-dosed vitamins and excitometabolic drugs. Since the eggs of the mites are not killed by insecticides, the washing of the animals should be repeated at least twice at intervals of 10 days, in order to kill newly hatched mites.

**Treatment**

Because of the formation of residues in the milk and the meat, the waiting times laid down for the various drugs (see page 246) should be observed after treatment. Pens, edges against which the animals rub themselves, and equipment should also be treated with the same insecticide.

**Danger to the livestock farmer**

Mange mites, particularly Sarcoptes, are also transmitted to man, causing unpleasant skin irritation. According to our own observations, mites also multiply on the human skin.

Fig. 403

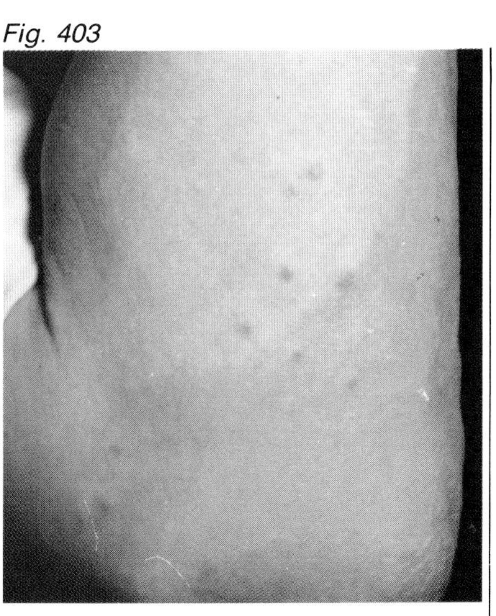

Fig. 404

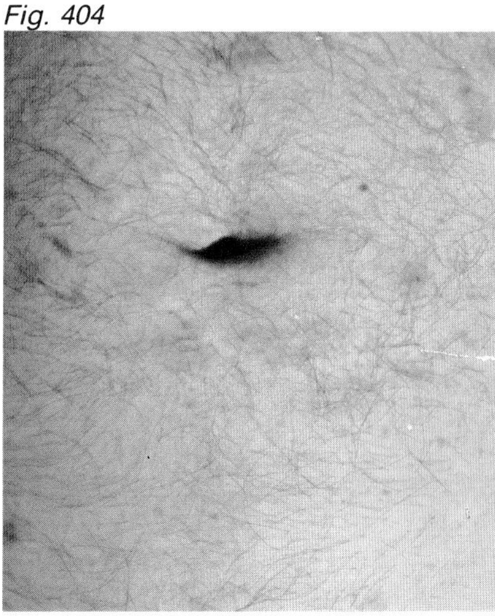

*Fig. 400: Treatment schedule for mange.*

*Figs. 401 and 402: Brushing in the insecticide is the most effective form of applying the anti-mange product. The wearing of gloves is necessary since the active ingredients are absorbed by the human skin.*

*Figs. 403 and 404: Bovine sarcoptic mange in man. Transmission occurs during the treatment of cattle. The first pustules occurred at the elbow where contact with the animal was intensive. After approx. 7 days the mites had multiplied and spread over the whole body (Fig. 404).*

# Lice

Fig. 405

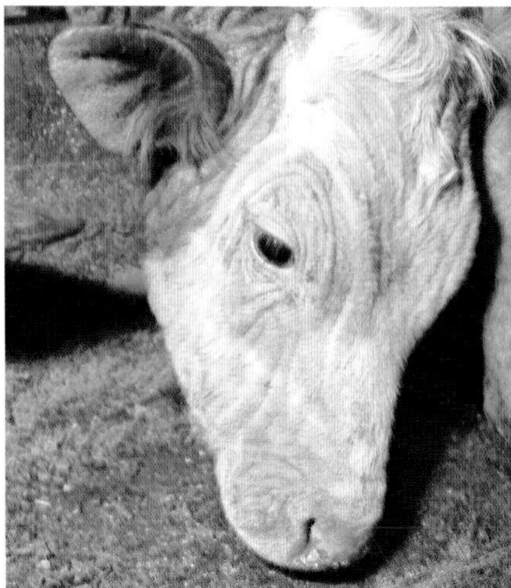

**Term**

Infestation with lice causes extensive changes of the skin and the coat of cattle. Lice are small (2–4 mm), blood-sucking insects living in the coat.

**Incidence**

Slight infestation with lice is common in cattle and does not cause any problems during the grazing period. However, after the cattle have been housed, the lice may multiply considerably.
Where cattle are housed throughout the year, especially with large cattle stocks, e. g. for calf fattening and rearing, bull fattening and keeping milk cattle in covered yards, we have increasingly seen lice infestation in recent years, with considerable impairment of the animals' condition.

**Pathogen**

In Europe, three types of louse predominate. They usually occur at the same time in cattle:

- Short-headed cattle louse (Haematopinus eurysternus)
- Long-headed cattle louse (Linognathus vituli)
- Small cattle louse (Solenopotes capillatus).

The lice attach their small tun-shaped eggs (nits), measuring 0.5–1.0 mm, individually to the hairs of cattle. After 1 or 2 weeks larvae are hatched which suck blood, shed their skins three times and develop to maturity within 25 to 30 days.

Fig. 406

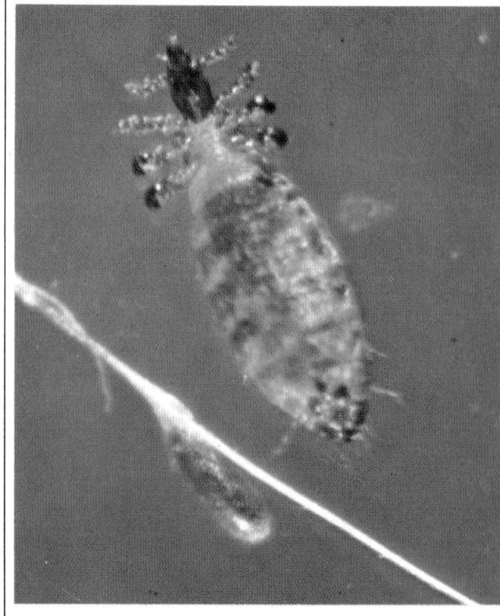

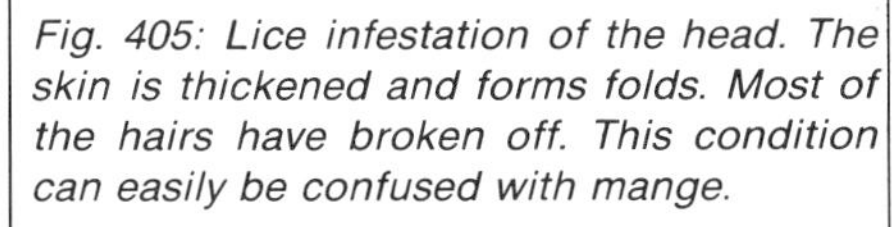

*Fig. 405: Lice infestation of the head. The skin is thickened and forms folds. Most of the hairs have broken off. This condition can easily be confused with mange.*

*Fig. 406: Long-headed cattle louse under the microscope. A nit is attached to the hair shown next to it.*

*Fig. 407: Severe lice infestation of the whole body with intense itching.*

*Fig. 408: Slight lice infestation is often seen in calves, leading to skin areas with thin hair cover. The development of the calves is impaired by itching and restlessness.*

*Fig. 407*

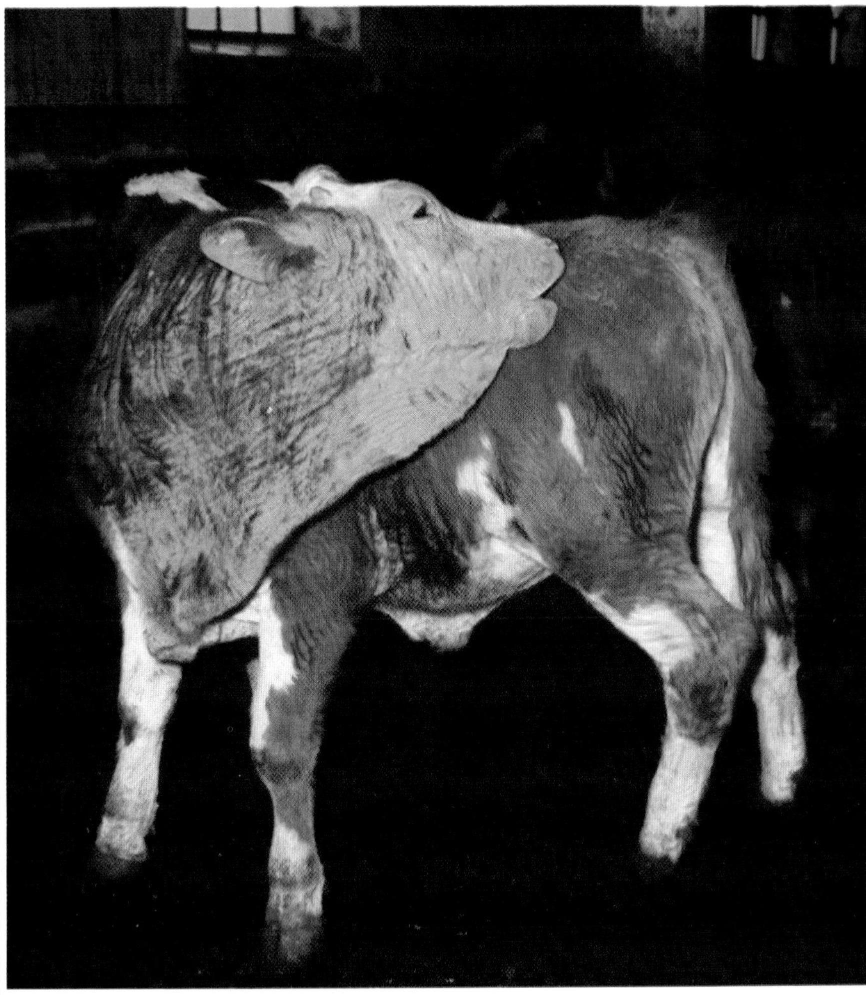

Cattle lice also transmit the pathogens of other diseases, e. g. ringworm.

*Fig. 408*

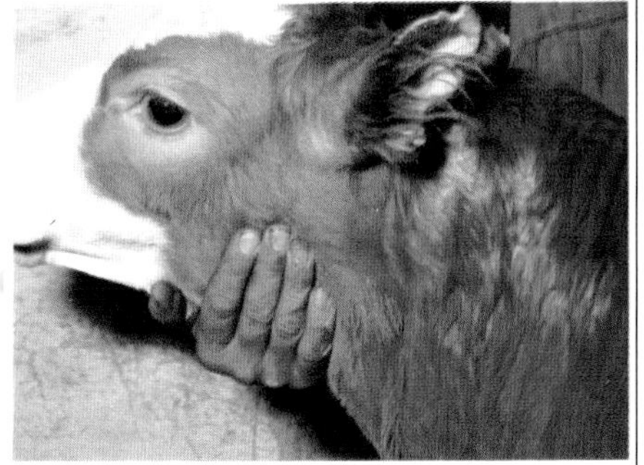

**Importation / Route of infection**

Lice are usually transmitted direct from one animal to another, less commonly indirectly via cleaning implements or infested cattle houses (walls of pens, places where cattle rub themselves). Away from the host animal, lice cannot survive for longer than one week. High-density housing favours transmission from animal to animal and promotes the multiplication of lice.

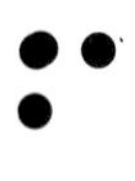

Symptoms

Slight infestation with lice hardly affects the animals. With more severe infestation the coat becomes rough and dull. The blood-sucking of the lice provokes a defence reaction of the skin with increased growth leading to scale formation. The migration and blood-sucking of the lice cause itching which manifests itself in increasing restlessness (licking, scratching, rubbing). If the itching persists for long periods, these mechanical "counter-measures" of the animals cause the hairs to break off and result in skin areas with sparse hair cover.

*Fig. 410*

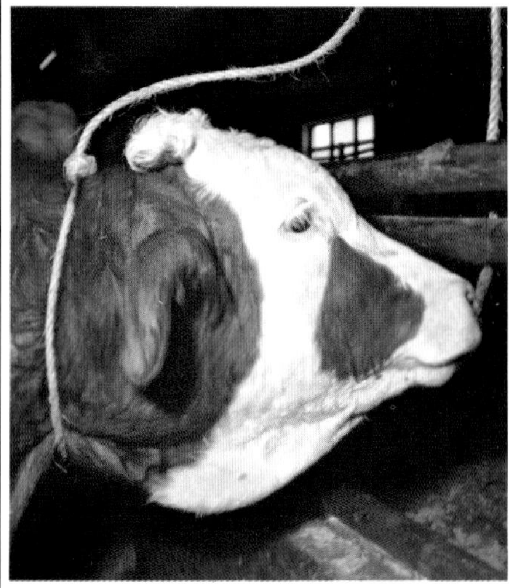

*Fig. 409*

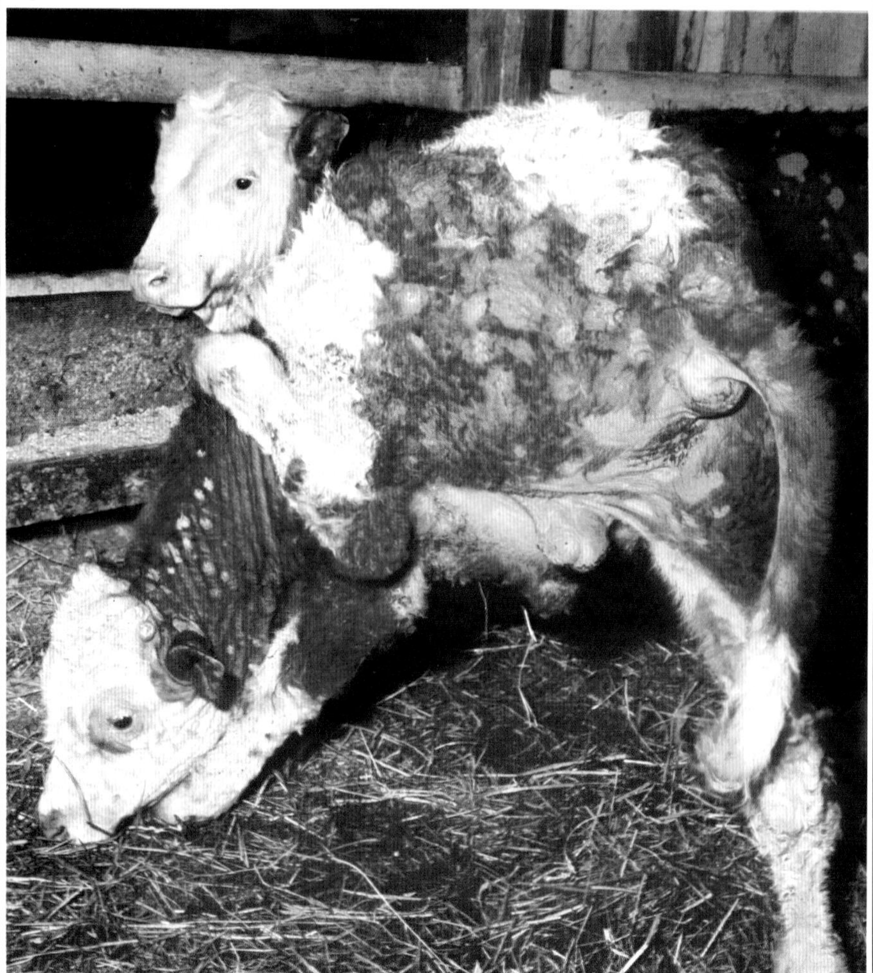

Fig. 411

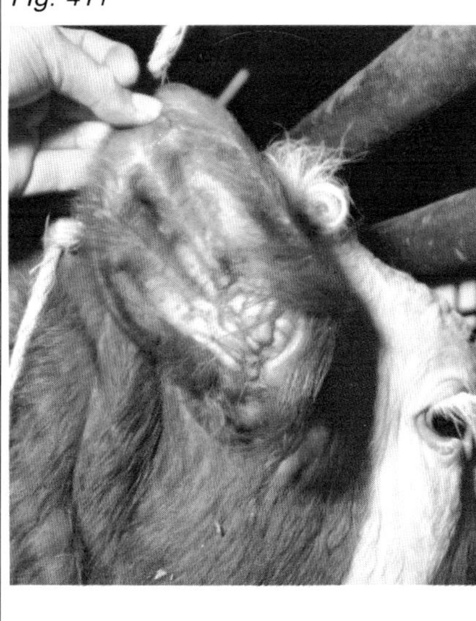

Massive infestation, particularly with the short-headed cattle louse, causes substantial loss of blood and leads to anaemia in undernourished cattle.

**Similar symptoms**

Mange is often confused with lice infestation, since the skin changes are similar. Both conditions very frequently occur simultaneously. In addition, there may also be trichophytosis.

**Diagnosis**

If lice infestation is suspected, the hair is parted at the affected sites. The lice and the nits which are attached to the hairs, may be seen as white specks with the naked eye. In order to confirm the diagnosis and to determine the type of louse involved, a tuft of hair is removed from a heavily infested site and examined under the microscope.

**Treatment**

Lice are combated by wash or spray treatment of the whole animal body, using insecticides like halogenated hydrocarbons or phosphoric acid esters. These products also kill mange mites. The treatment of lice infestation is therefore the same as for mange (see Fig. 400).
Concomitant trichophytosis needs to be treated with different products. The eggs of lice (nits) have very resistant shells which are not destroyed by the insecticides used. For this reason the treatment has to be repeated after the next generation of lice has been hatched.
The pour-on method with TIGUVON is a very convenient procedure. However, the dosage has to be adjusted very carefully to the body-weight, in order to avoid intoxication.

**Prevention**

On livestock farms with frequent purchase and change of animals the cattle should be regularly examined for lice.

*Fig. 409: Mixed infestation with lice and ringworm. The lice spread the spores of the fungi over the whole body.*

*Figs. 410 and 411: Drooping ears. Proliferating inflammation of the external auditory canal, caused by constant irritation in lice or mange infestation.*

## Phosphoric acid ester poisoning

Fig. 412

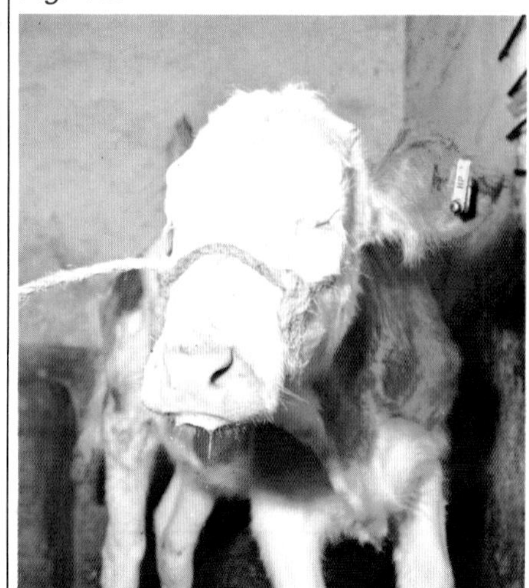

Fig. 413

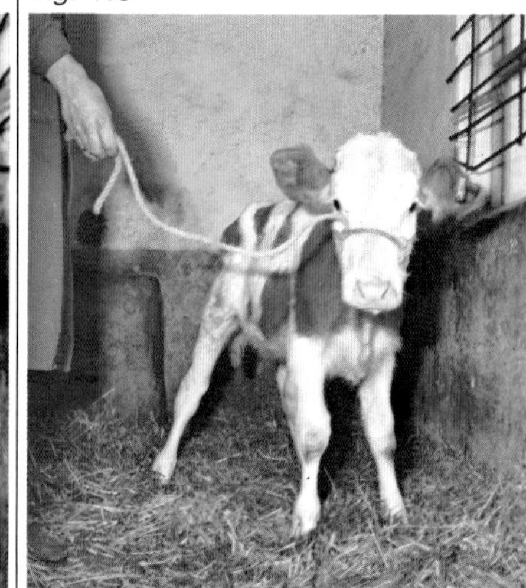

**Term**

Many products used today for the treatment of skin and intestinal parasites are based on phosphoric acid esters. These products offer the advantage of high efficacy and good biological degradability. Their disadvantage lies in their toxic effect on the animal, even with slight overdosage.

**Incidence**

Phosphoric acid esters are administered by mouth for anthelmintic treatment. For the treatment of lice, mange mites and warble-flies, they are applied to the skin (pour-on or washing).
The active ingredients are introduced into the body through the intestine or the skin. If they are given in overdosage, signs of intoxication may appear in individual animals or in entire herds. Young animals are more sensitive to phosphoric acid esters than adult cattle. We mainly use the following phosphoric acid ester products for antiparasitic treatment: ASUNTOL, DIAZINON, NEGUVON and TIGUVON.

**Cause**

If these products are given in excessive concentration or at too short an interval, toxic effects result. At the motor nerve endings acetylcholine is released as transmitting substance. If phosphoric acid esters are given in overdosage, the enzyme acetylcholinesterase which breaks down acetylcholine, is inhibited. A shortage of acetylcholinesterase leads to an excess of acetylcholine. This excess causes a disturbance of stimulus conduction in the central nervous system.

*Figs. 412 and 413: Phosphoric acid ester poisoning in a calf. Hypersalivation; shunning light. Fig. 413 shows the unsteady posture (central nervous dysfunction) and increased timidity of the animal.*

*Figs. 414 and 415: The greatly increased bowel action caused by phosphoric acid ester poisoning, leads to diarrhoea and straining. At a later stage, blood admixtures in the faeces are observed.*

*Fig. 414*

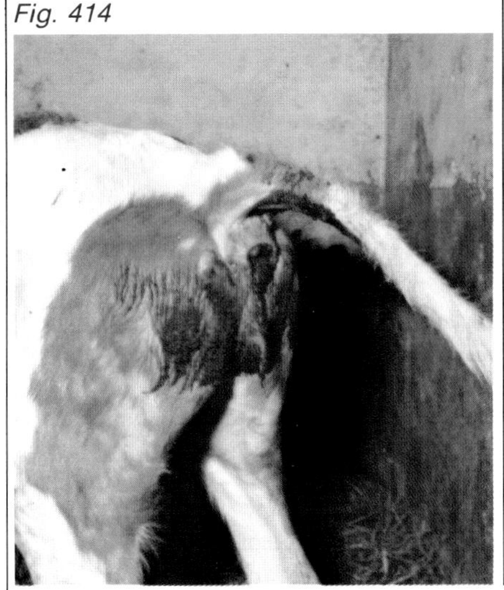

*Fig. 415*

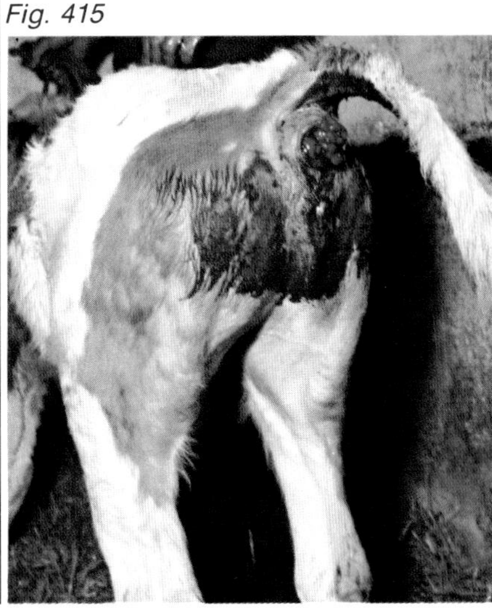

**Symptoms**

These disorders manifest themselves in muscular tremor, staggering gait, difficulty in breathing with stretched-out tongue and audible groaning. These symptoms are accompanied by hypersalivation, diarrhoea, frequent urination and colic. The contraction of the pupils is particularly striking.
These signs of intoxication appear within 2 to 24 hours of inappropriate use of phosphoric acid esters.

**Diagnosis**

The typical symptoms point to phosphoric acid ester poisoning. The diagnosis is established by ascertaining preceding antiparasitic treatment. It can be confirmed by determining the cholinesterase level in the laboratory.

**Similar symptoms**

All diseases associated with central nervous disorders show a similar clinical picture to that of phosphoric acid ester poisoning. This applies particularly to hypersomnia (ISTME) and vitamin $B_1$ deficiency. However, in neither of these conditions are blood admixtures in the faeces, hypersalivation or contraction of the pupils observed.

**Treatment**

Atropine is used as an antidote in the treatment of phosphoric acid ester poisoning. 50 to 200 mg atropine sulphate is injected, half the dose being given intravenously, the other half intramuscularly. The intravenous injection is given very slowly, while monitoring the heart rate and the diameter of the pupils. When the pupils become dilated, the quantity of atropine required as an antidote has been reached, and the intravenous injection is terminated.

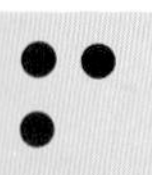

# Tail-tip inflammation in beef bulls

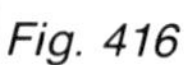

*Fig. 416*

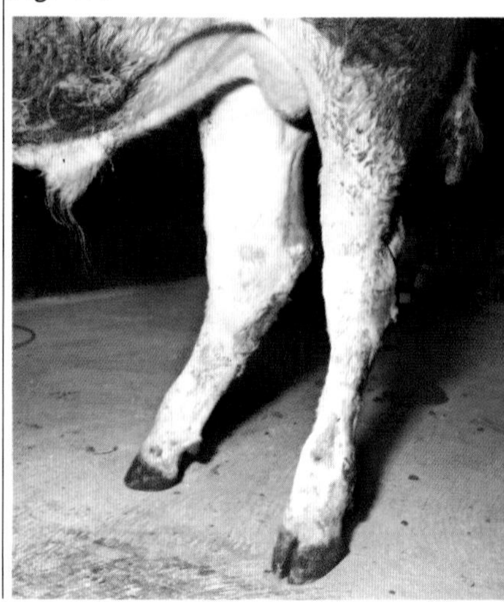

*Fig. 417*

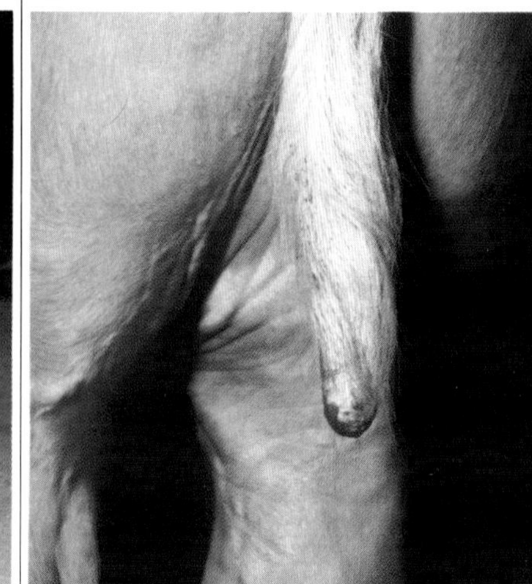

**Term**

Tail-tip inflammation, formerly also called "tail necrosis", is an inflammatory change of the tip of the tail, which is aggravated by pyogenic organisms. The infection with pyogenic bacteria is initially localised, but usually develops into a severe general condition.

**Incidence**

The condition occurs particularly on livestock farms where intensive beef bull fattening is carried out. Up to now, inflammation of the tail tip has mainly been observed in stocks kept on slatted floors. We have rarely seen tail-tip inflammation in deep litter houses. The condition even occurs in calves weaned on slatted floors, but it does not become a problem until the animals weigh 200 kg or more. The frequency of the affection increases with increasing body-weight. During the final fattening period, as many as 50 to 60% of bulls may suffer from inflammation of the tail-tip.

**Cause**

The cause of the condition is as yet unknown. Neither pathogenic organisms (bacteria, fungi) nor errors in feeding have been clearly established as the cause. However, it is certain that housing the animals on slatted floors significantly contributes to the appearance of tail-tip inflammation. We have found that calves weaned on slatted floors showed inflammation of the tail tip at an early stage. After rehousing the calves on deep litter, the changes disappeared within a short time, whereas rehousing such calves on slatted floors aggravated the condition.

*Fig. 418*

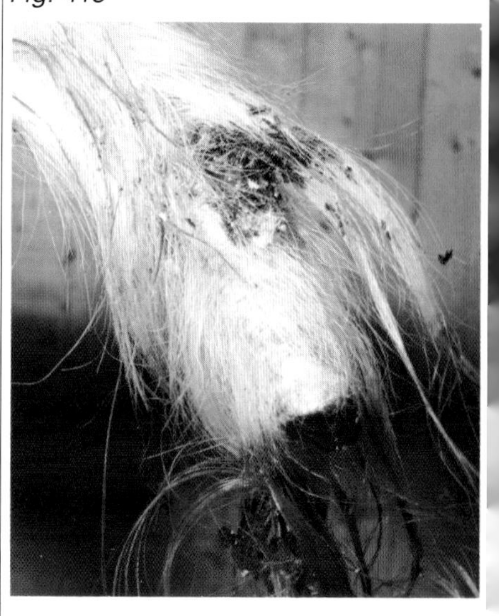

*Fig. 419*

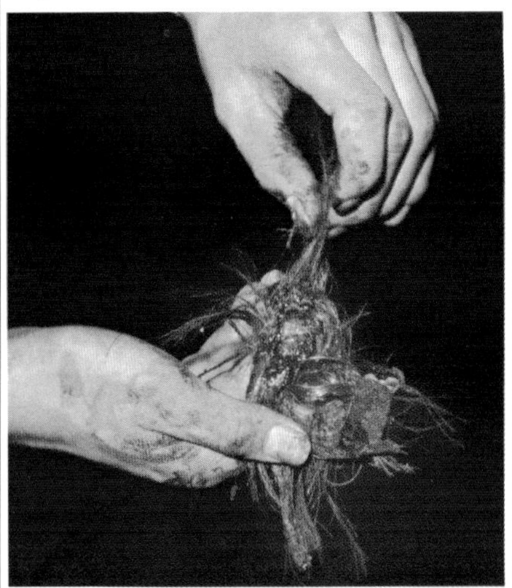

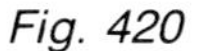

*Fig. 420*

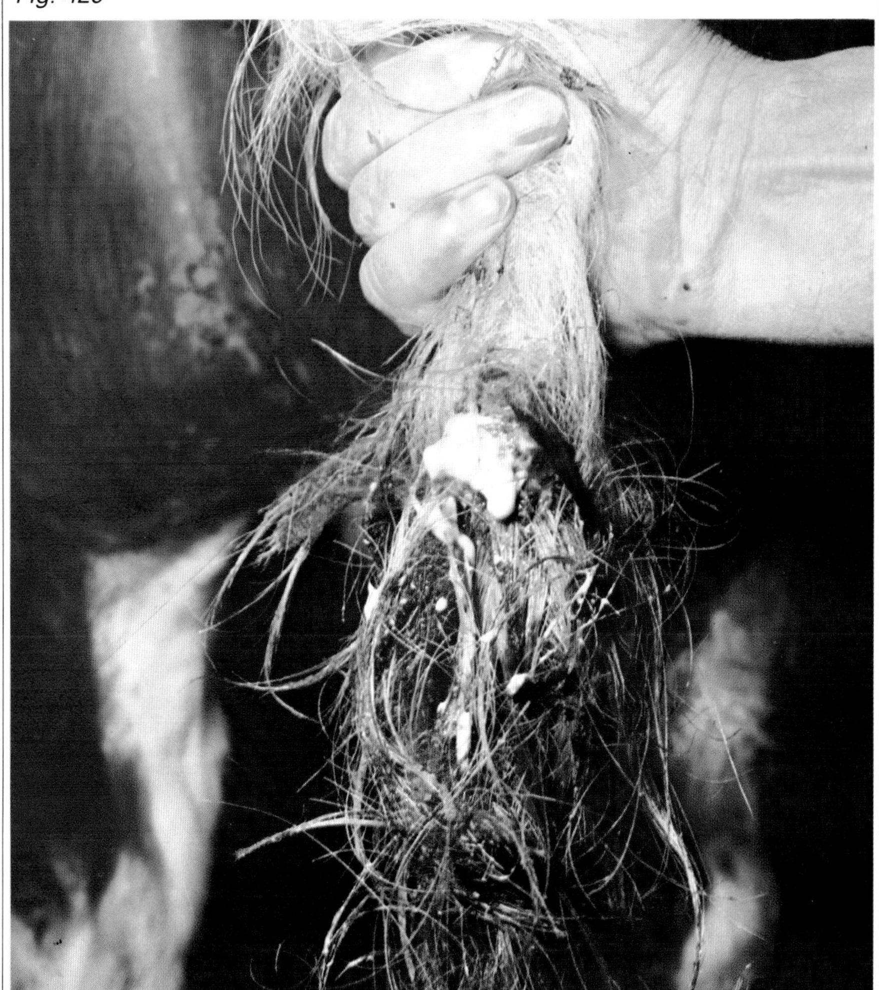

*Fig. 416: Inflammation of the ankle joint, starting from an inflammation of the tail tip.*

*Fig. 417: Hairless tail tip with necrotic skin.*

*Fig. 418: Tail tip inflammation where the necrotic, numb tip of the tail was severed by the animal treading on it on the slatted floor.*

*Fig. 419: Inflamed tail tip. After spreading the soiled moist hairs of the switch, the inflamed tip of the tail can be seen.*

*Fig. 420: Suppurative inflammation of the entire tail, starting from an inflammation of the tail tip. When the tail is squeezed, thick pus oozes out.*

**Cause**

The permanently moist switch leads to the first signs of inflammation. In high-density housing with high air humidity, the concrete planks remain constantly wet. The ammonia content of the cattle house air is particularly high above the dung passage, irritating the skin and promoting inflammation.

*Fig. 421*

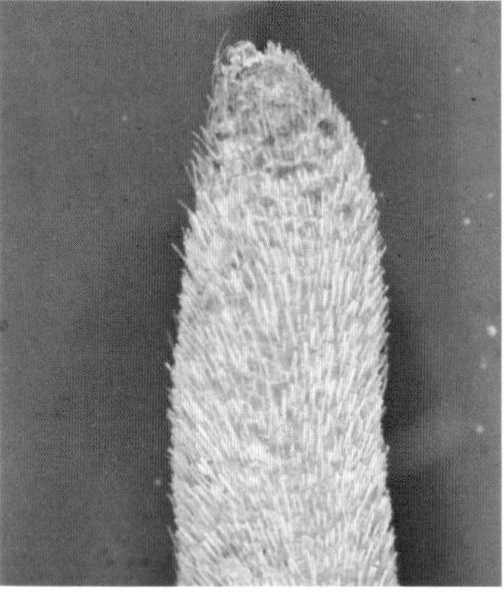

*Fig. 422*

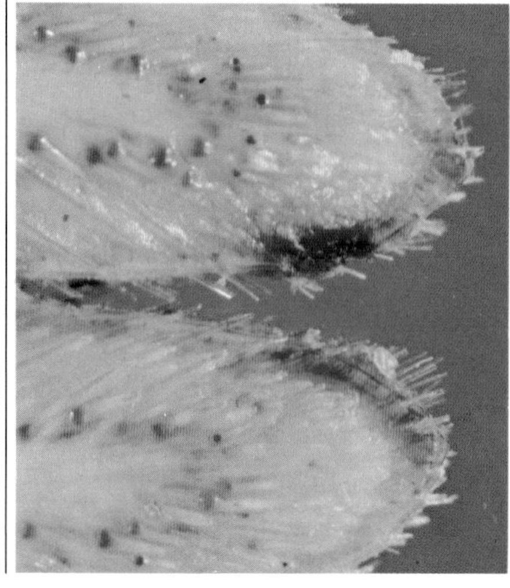

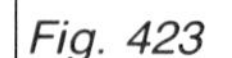

*Fig. 423*

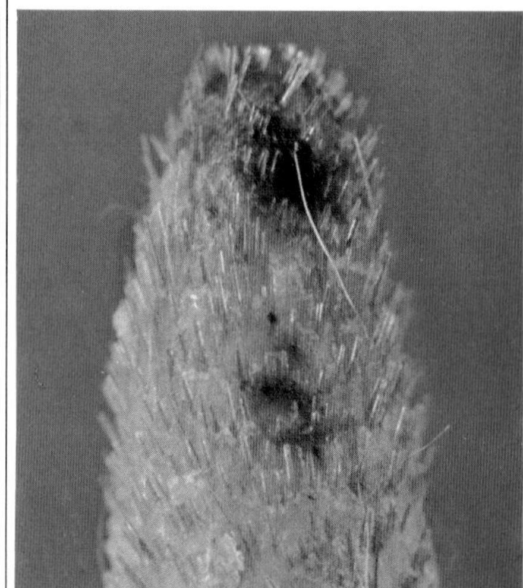

**Symptoms**

According to our observations, the inflammation starts with a small weeping eczema at the tail tip. The eczema usually develops on the upper side of the tail. The initial stage, which can even be seen in calves housed on slatted floors, is often overlooked. The livestock farmer notices the condition when it has become chronic after several weeks or months. The skin at the inflamed site is thickened and chapped and tends to lacerate because of the reduced blood supply. Cracks or rhagades are formed which often break open and bleed easily. The hair at the tail tip becomes matted with blood, serous fluid and moisture. This creates ideal conditions for the multiplication of pyogenic bacteria which invade the wounds and penetrate into the subcutaneous tissue where they cause extensive suppurative inflammations (phlegmon).

The inflammatory process spreads in the direction of the root of the tail. The spinal canal ends at the first vertebrae of the tail. The bacteria can thus reach the spinal cord and can cause ascending infections. This results in impaired mobility with a stiff gait, unilateral or bilateral lameness and permanent lying-down of the animals. These symptoms appear quite suddenly, but the animals affected may first show an arched back, reduced appetite, dull coat and poor weight gain.

*Fig. 424*

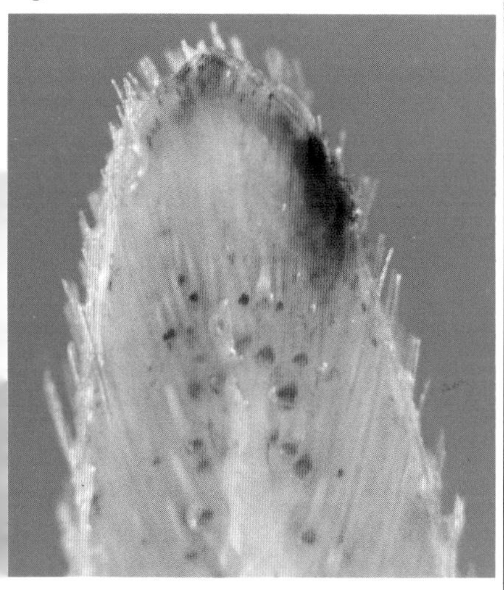

*Fig. 425*

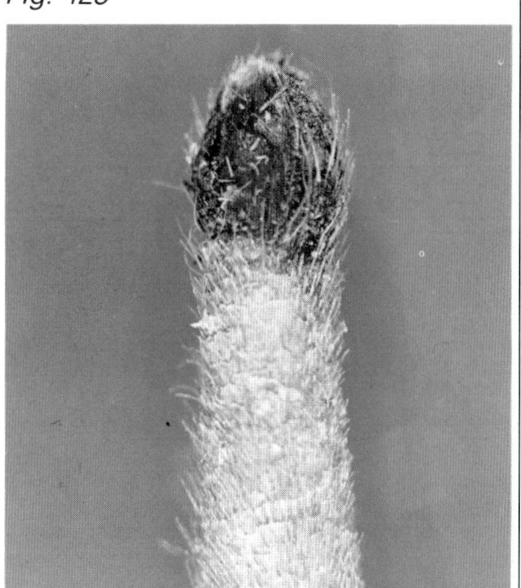

*Fig. 426*

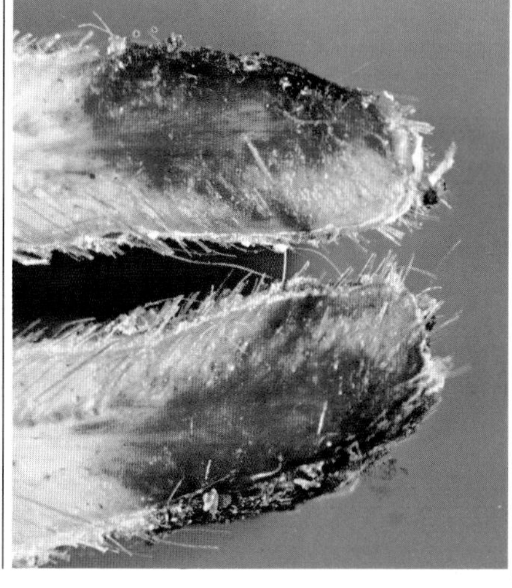

*ig. 421: Initial stage of tail tip inflammation. Weeping eczema on the upper side of he tail, reddened with inflammation.*

*ig. 422: Cracks or rhagades are formed which are invaded by pyogenic organisms.*

*igs. 423 and 424: Incipient tail tip inflammation. In Fig. 424 the tail tip has been cut open. Since the upper side of the tail is in close contact with the moist slatted floor when the animal lies down, it is here that the inflammation usually begins.*

*igs. 425 and 426: Deep-seated inflammation with superficial histolysis (necrosis).*

**Symptoms**

If lameness, reduced weight gain or swelling of the joints is observed, the tail tip should be carefully examined for changes.

With regular thorough examinations, the early stage of tail tip inflammation can be recognised. Weighing of the animals offers a good opportunity for such examinations.

**Diagnosis**

If the bacteria reach the blood stream or lymphatic channels, they are carried to all organs of the body, resulting in abscesses in the liver, the lungs, the muscles and the testes. Articular inflammations are often seen at the hindlegs where inflammations of the ankle, fetlock and claw joints occur.

**Similar symptoms**

Fig. 427

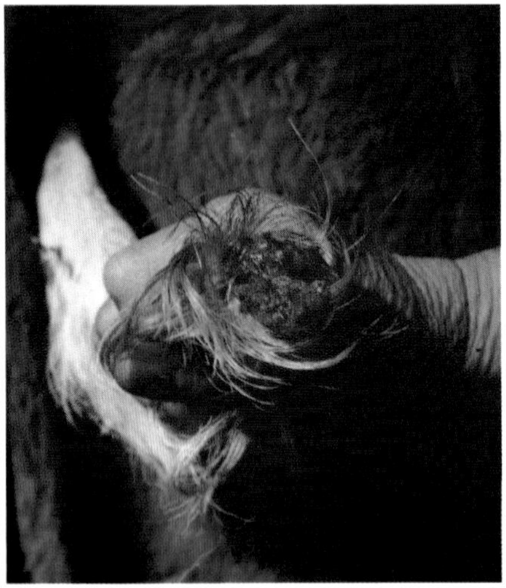

Fig. 428

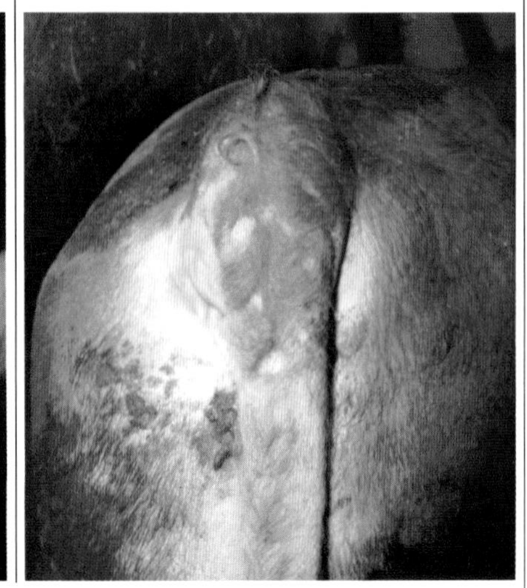

Fig. 429

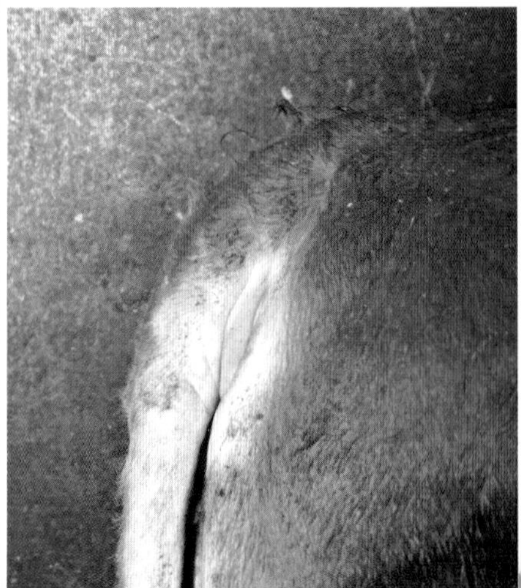

Similar manifestions on the tail are observed in the following conditions:

- **Tail mange:** Mainly at the root of the tail, but also at the tip; caused by mites. Secondary infection with pyogenic bacteria produces a similar picture to that of tail tip inflammation.
- **Bites:** Sucking and biting the tails of other calves (cannibalism) results in injuries which often suppurate. Crude fibre deficiency may promote cannibalism.
- **Tail worm:** Pus nodes (acne) which may reach the size of hazelnuts, distributed over the entire tail. There is local alopecia and itching.

*Fig. 427: Cannibalism. Bitten-off tail tip. Secondary infection with pyogenic bacteria produces a similar clinical picture to that of tail tip inflammation.*

*Figs. 428 and 429: Tail worm: Pus nodes up to hazelnut size in the region of the base of the tail, with circumscribed alopecia.*

*Fig. 433: In older animals and in those where the inflammation is already present, amputation should not be carried out by means of the rubber ring.*

Fig. 430

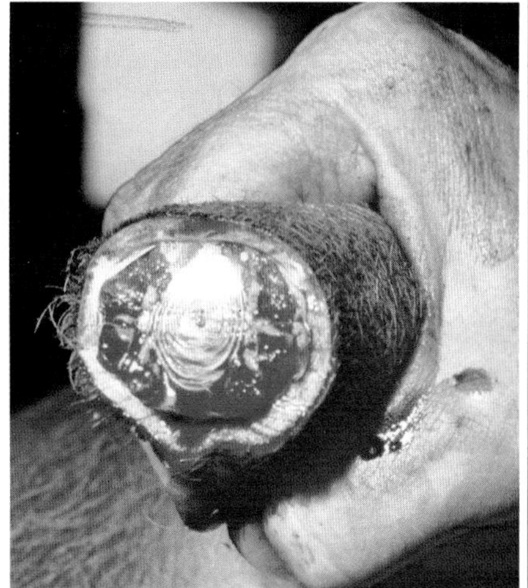

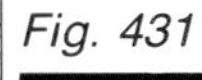

Fig. 431

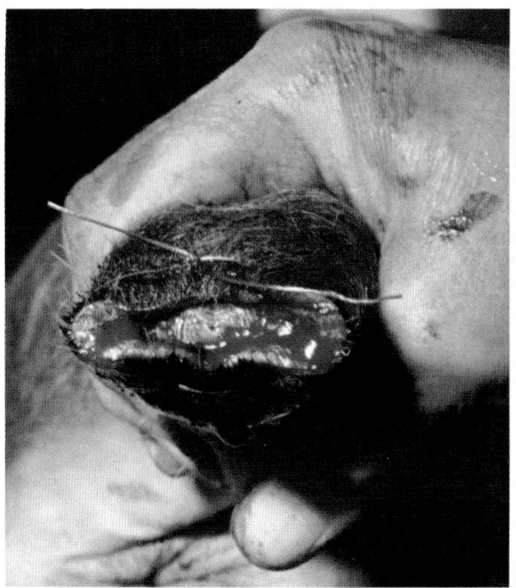

Fig. 432

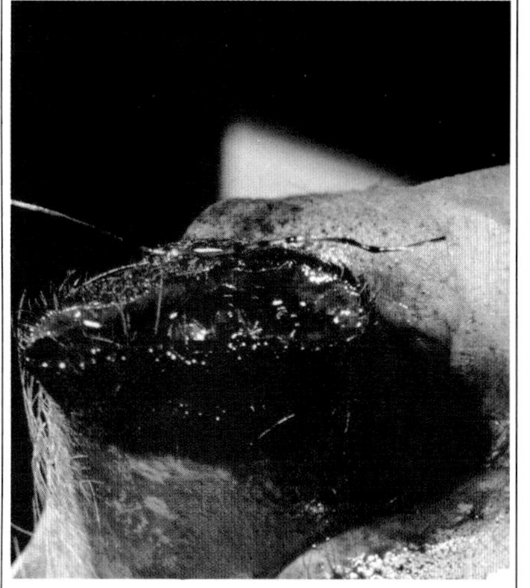

*Figs. 430 to 432: Surgical amputation in advanced inflammation. The tail is severed between the vertebrae under local anaesthesia.*

*By means of a U-shaped suture the skin is tightly pulled together over the edge of the vertebra.*

*The stump is thoroughly sprayed with BLAUHOLZTINKTUR.*

Fig. 433

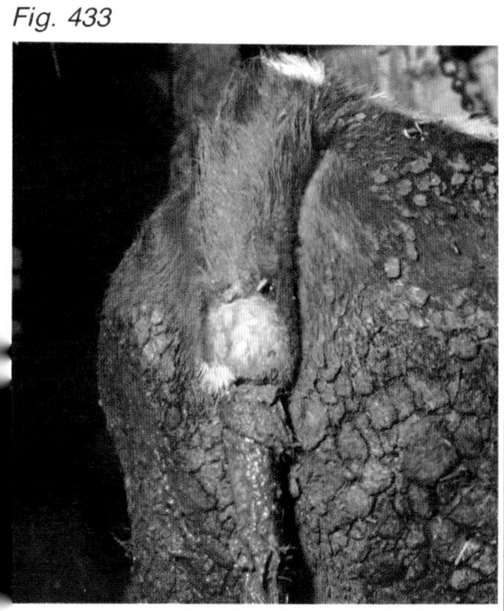

If the tail tip inflammation is recognised at an early stage, the inflammatory process can be arrested by housing the bulls on deep litter. In addition, the tail is shorn and the affected sites are treated with antibiotic and disinfectant ointments (BOVOFLAVIN) or tinctures (BLAUHOLZTINKTUR).

The safest method of treatment is the amputation of the tail, which has good prospects of success if the inflammatory process is confined to the lower part of the tail. Under no circumstances should the amputation be carried out with a rubber ring in the advanced stage of the condition.

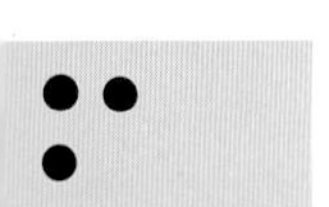



*Fig. 434*

*Shearing the amputation site in the region of the 7th and 8th vertebrae of the tail.*

*Fig. 435*

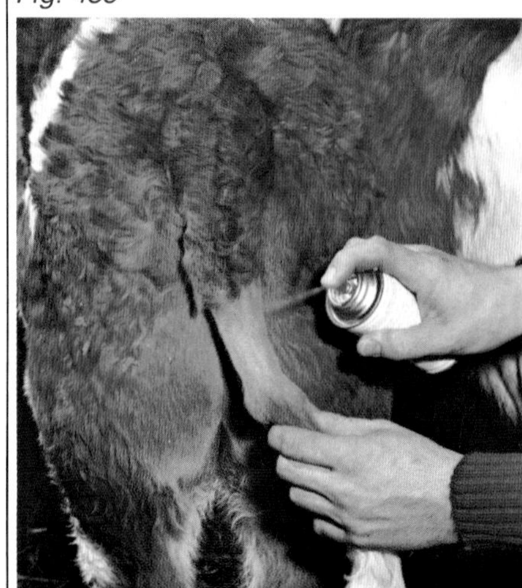

*Disinfection of the skin.*

*Fig. 436*

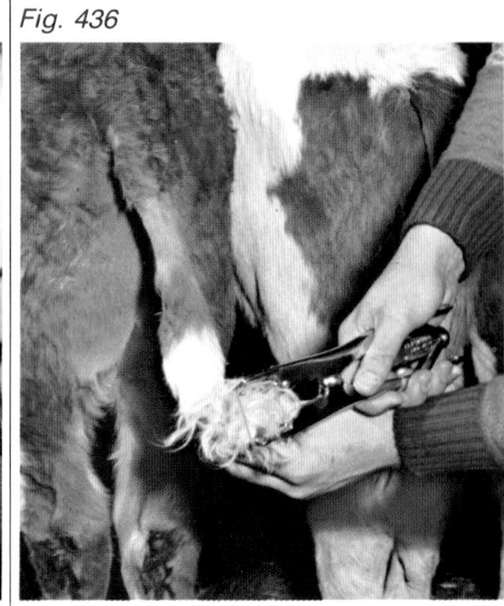

*Applying the rubber ring by means of an elastrator.*

The docking of the tail by means of rubber rings is a safe method of overcoming this problem.

The docking rings must not be applied later than at the age of three months. The rubber ring is applied with specially designed tongs (elastrator) approx. 2 or 3 hand-breadths (preferably between the 7th and 8th vertebrae of the tail) below the base of the tail (see Figs. 434 to 442).

*Figs. 434 to 442: Docking the tails of calves by means of a rubber ring.*

Fig. 437

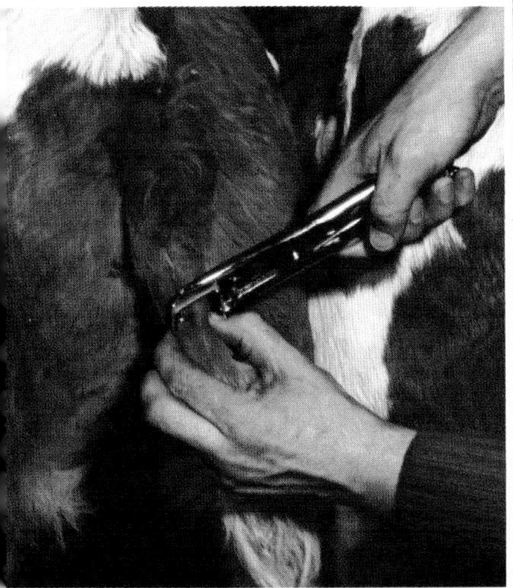

Feeling the amputation site between the vertebrae. It lies in a small pit on the raised section between the two vertebrae.

Fig. 438

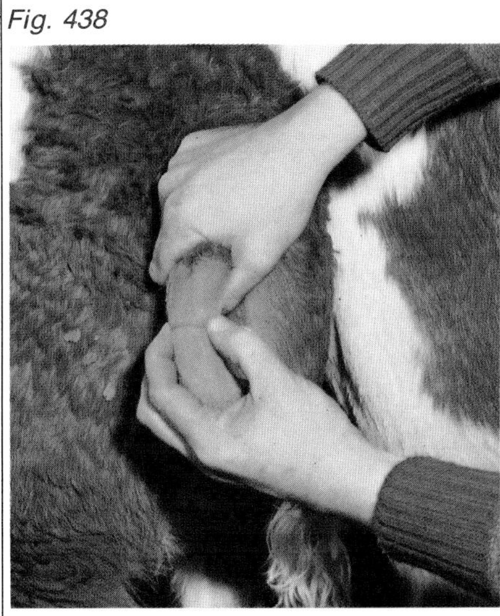

Checking that the rubber ring is correctly positioned.

Fig. 439

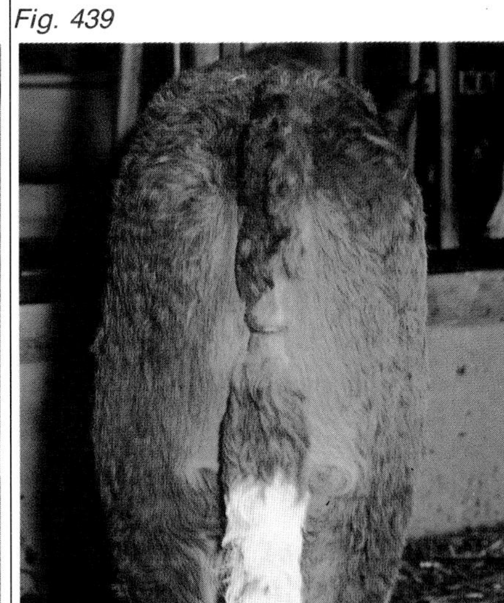

Within a few minutes, the rubber ring forms a constriction. The calves show no sign of pain.



Approx. 14 days after amputation the tail has dried out.

Fig. 440

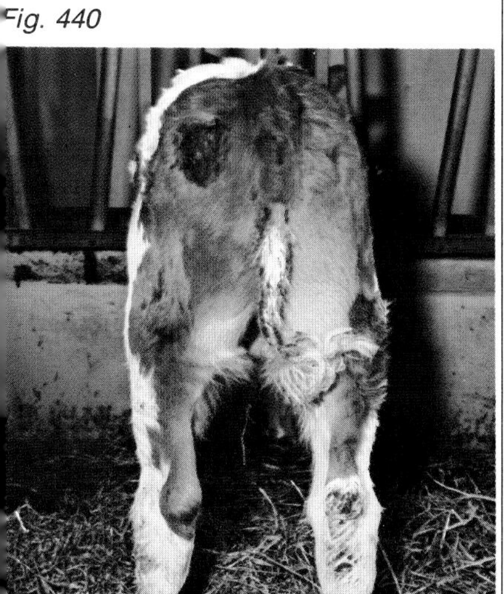

The tail falls off in the third week.

Fig. 441

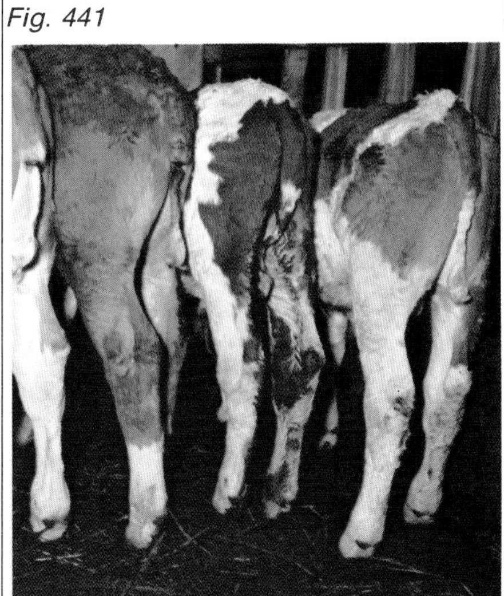

An examination of the amputation site and the application of wound tincture are indicated.

Fig. 442

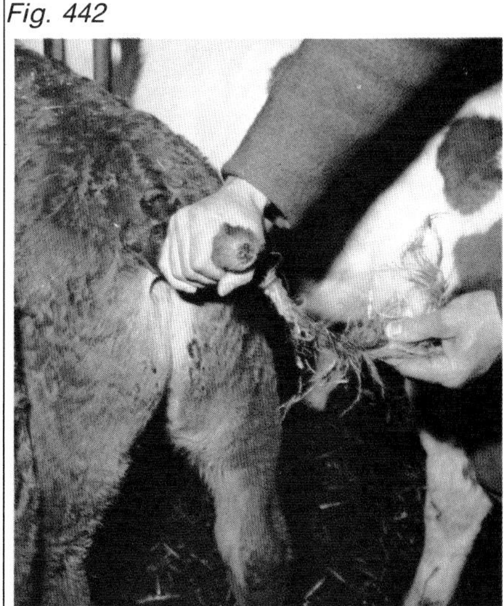

# Abscess formation

Fig. 443

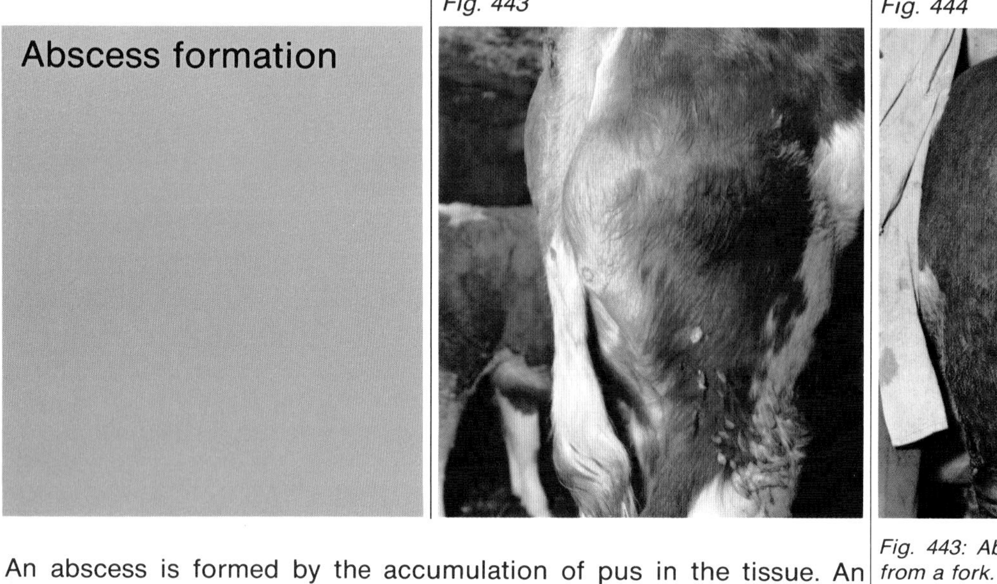

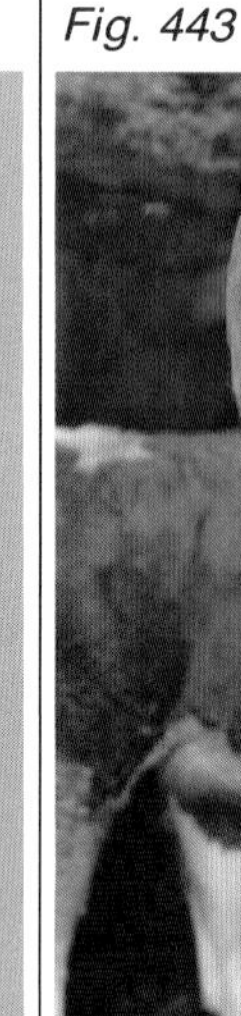

Fig. 444

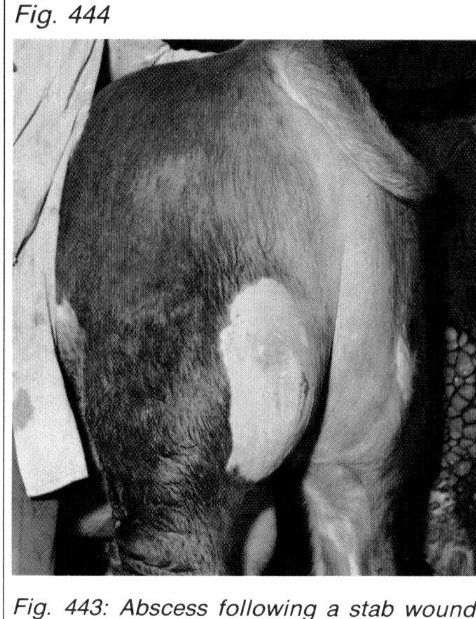

*Fig. 443: Abscess following a stab wound from a fork.*

*Fig. 444 to 451: Abscess treatment.*

**Term**

An abscess is formed by the accumulation of pus in the tissue. An abscess cavity develops which is demarcated from the remaining tissue by the pyogenic membrane which encapsulates the abscess.

**Incidence**

Abscesses occur in all organs. If they form in the skin, the subcutis or the muscles, boil-like distensions can be seen.

**Cause**

Abscesses are formed when pyogenic organisms get into the skin or the muscles. This can happen in the case of injuries, e.g. stab wounds from forks, butting with the horns or incorrect injection (for correct injection procedure, see page 242).

**Symptoms**

The inflamed, usually swollen site is initially hot, reddened and painful. Increased body temperature in conjunction with loss of appetite may be observed. The inflammation then becomes localised. The abscess comes to a head. The gathered abscess becomes soft and can be indented. The accumulation of pus "wobbles" on palpation.

**Treatment**

When the abscess has come to a head, it often bursts on its own accord. If it does not, it should be lanced at its lowest point to allow the pus to flow out freely.

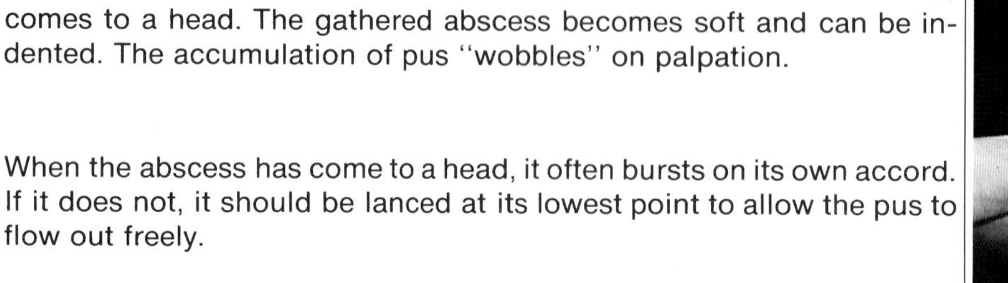

*Palpating the abscess cavity and opening up any associated abscess chambers.*

Fig. 448

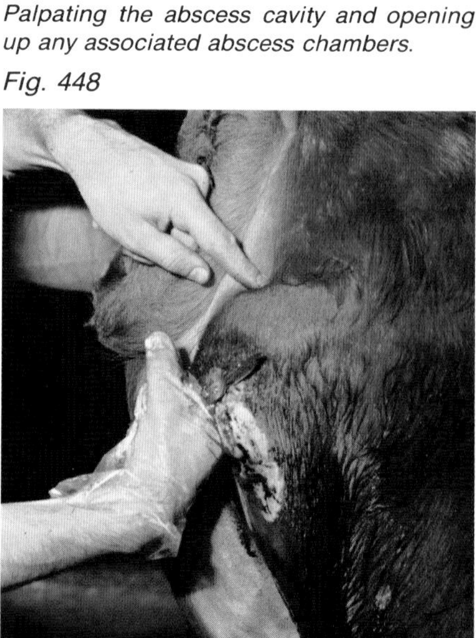

Fig. 445

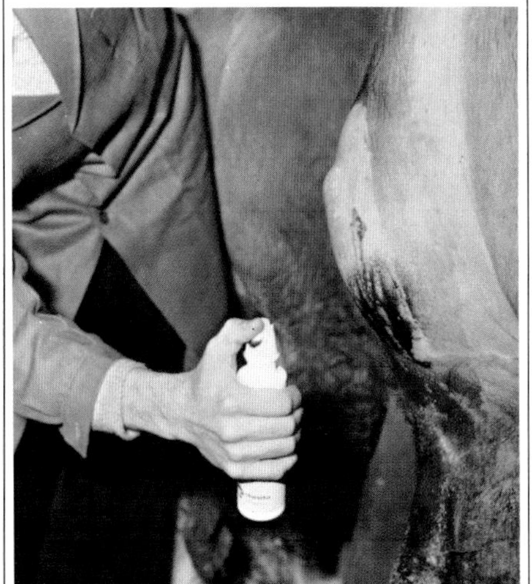

*Disinfecting the skin*

Fig. 446

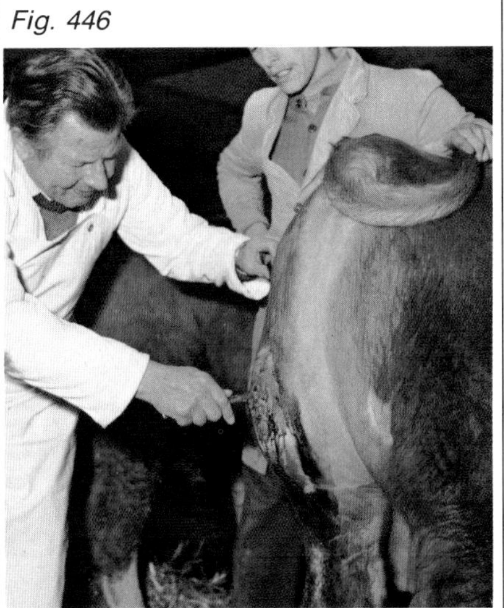

*Lancing the gathered abscess*

Fig. 447

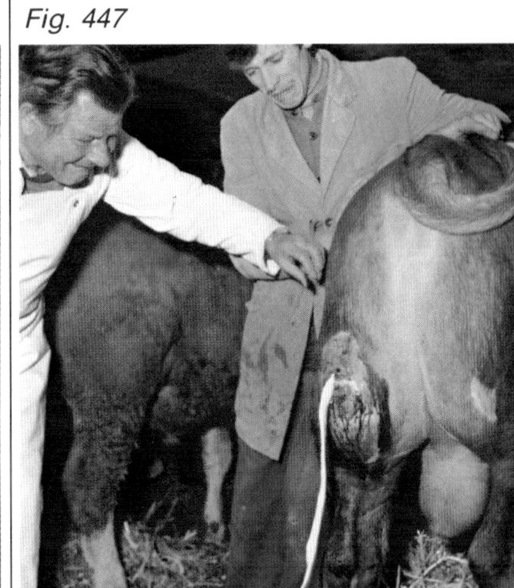

*Ample incision down to the lowest point.*

*Repeated spraying with BLAUHOLZTINKTUR will prevent licking by other animals and granulations.*

Fig. 449

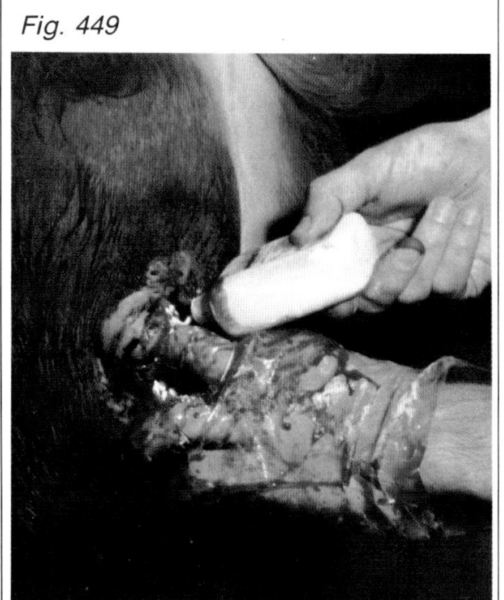

*Wound 12 days after lancing of abscess.*

Fig. 450

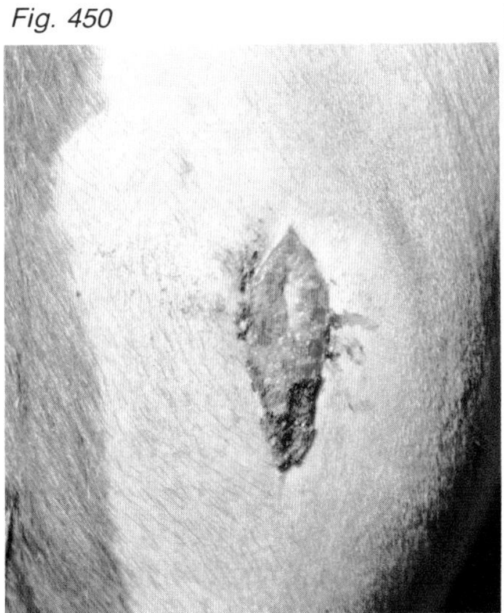

*Separating the edges of the wound and generous application of P/S powder.*

Fig. 451

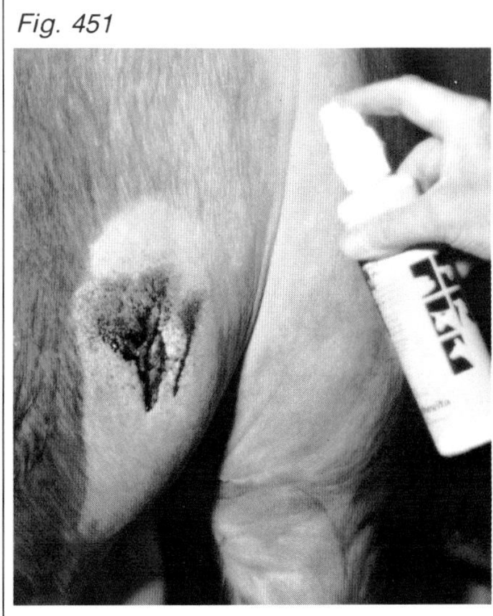

# Diseases of the claws

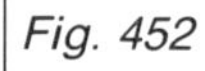

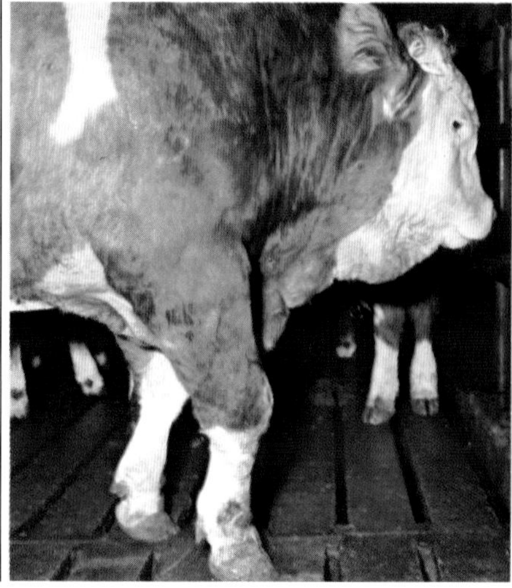

*Fig. 452*

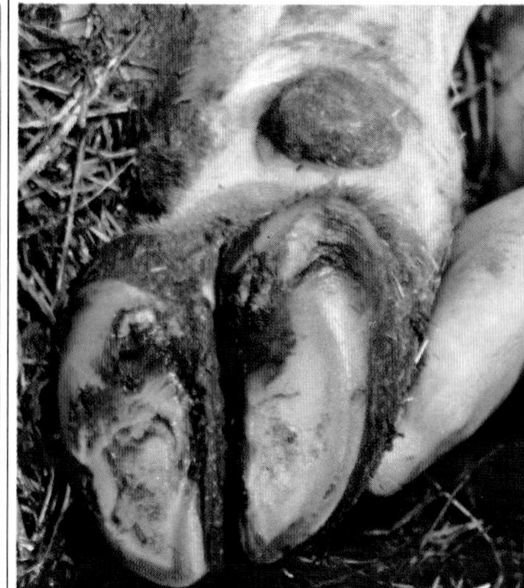

*Fig. 453*

**Term**

The increasing importance of economic considerations and rationalisation has brought about a change in the housing systems for cattle. Today, a small number of attendants have to look after as many animals as possible. For this reason the **stanchion stable** was initially replaced by the **deep litter house** in cattle rearing and fattening. In recent years, the **slatted floor house** has been given almost exclusive preference whenever new cattle housing has been built.

Diseases of the limbs and claws occur with all three forms of housing, the distribution – according to the type of cattle house – being as follows:

- Deep litter house: Dislocation, sprain, contortion, foul-in-the-foot, haematoma, abscess.
- Slatted floor house: Cuts from rough or badly fixed planks; sores and callosities from lying down; ulcers of soles and balls; worn claws; laceration of horn and claw bone fractures if the gap between the planks is too wide; articular changes, postural anomalies.
- Stanchion stable: Articular changes and postural anomalies, particularly in the forelegs; inflammation of the ankle joint; callosities from lying down; carpal boils.

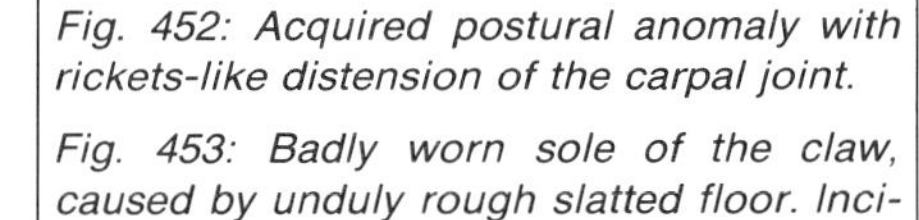

Fig. 452: Acquired postural anomaly with rickets-like distension of the carpal joint.

Fig. 453: Badly worn sole of the claw, caused by unduly rough slatted floor. Incipient ball rot.

Fig. 454: Pronounced articular changes in both forelegs. This bull was kept in a stanchion stable for a long period, where the feeding trough was too low.

Fig. 454

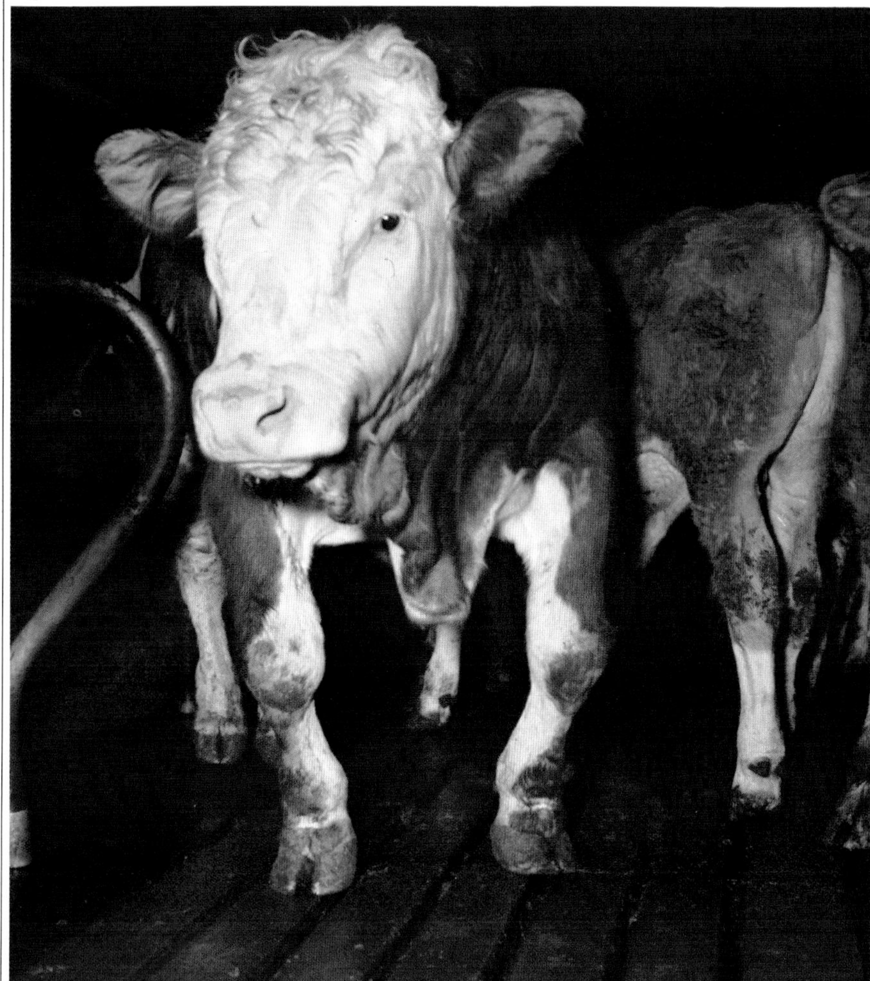

Term

From the large number of diseases of the limbs and claws that may occur, we have selected injuries to the claws and foul-in-the-foot for consideration here. We have found that these conditions are of frequent occurrence and can cause problems in entire stocks.

Fig. 455

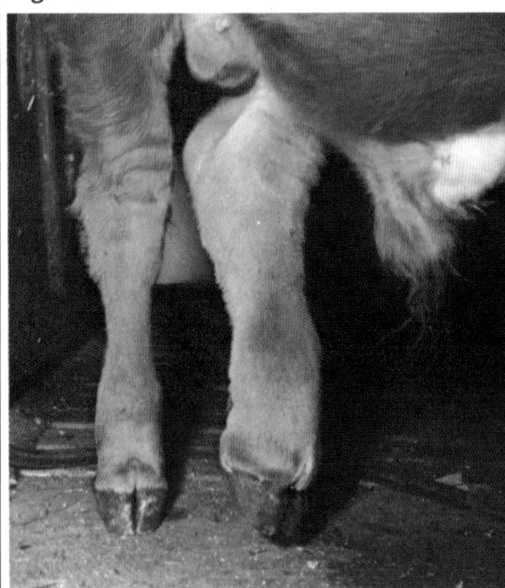

Fig. 456

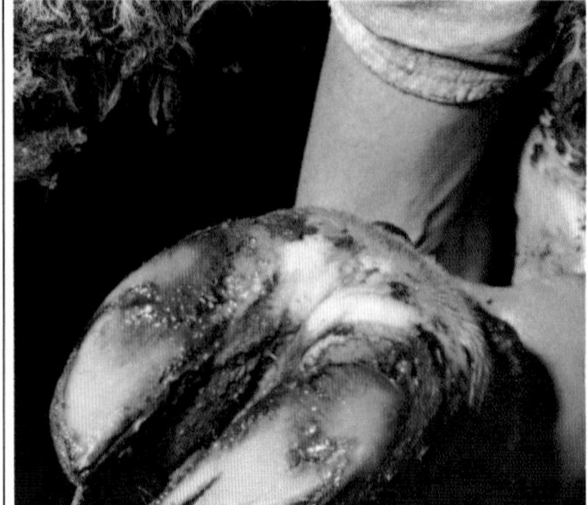

Fig. 457

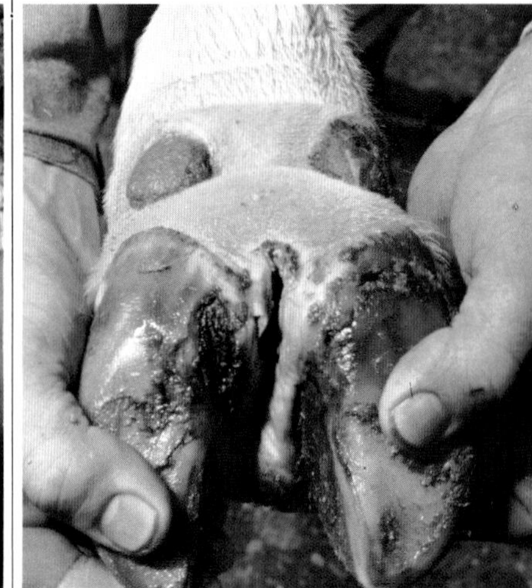

## Injuries to the claws

**Incidence**

When bulls are housed on slatted floors, injuries to the claws are increasingly observed, if the following points are disregarded:

- Form and size of the pens, and the number of animals housed in them (optimum: 8 to 10 bulls per pen) must be in the right proportion. This will provide a calmer atmosphere in the cattle house. Do not house the animals too densely; otherwise injuries from kicking and, in the summer months, heat accumulation (heat stroke) may occur.
- The slatted floor must have a non-slip surface, so that the animals do not lose their footing even if the planks are temporarily moist (high air humidity, sudden change in the weather). Uneven concrete planks with sharp, ragged or projecting edges cause cuts on the claws and balls. The width of the gap should be 3 to 3.5 cm, the width of the plank 10 to 13 cm.
- With an appropriate ration and fodder of constant quality, the bulls remain calm even with intensive feeding. Strict adherence to the feeding times is especially important. If the animals are fed irregularly, restlessness in the pens – and thus the risk of injuries – increases.

Fig. 458

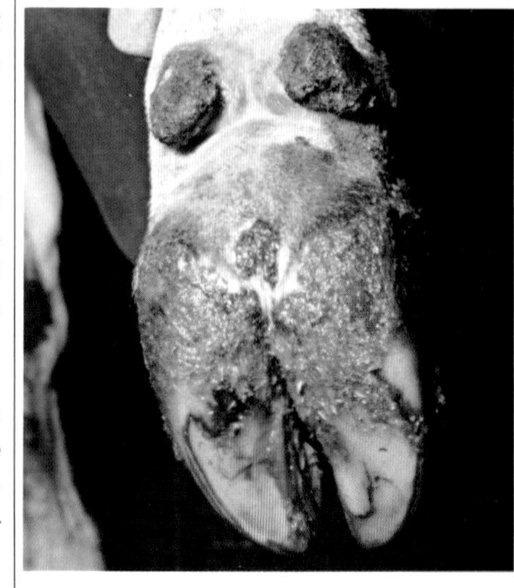

*Figs. 455 and 456: Deep cut in a claw followed by infection from dirt. The extremity is painful; swelling reaching up to the ankle joint.*

*Fig. 457: Separation in the interdigital area. Severe swelling and inflammation at the back of the fetlock joint.*

*Fig. 458: Partial rupture of the tip of the claw and deep-reaching separation of the sole. Severe inflammation of the ball of the foot.*

*Fig. 459: Badly worn sole with fissured horn in the area of the ball of the foot.*

*Fig. 459*

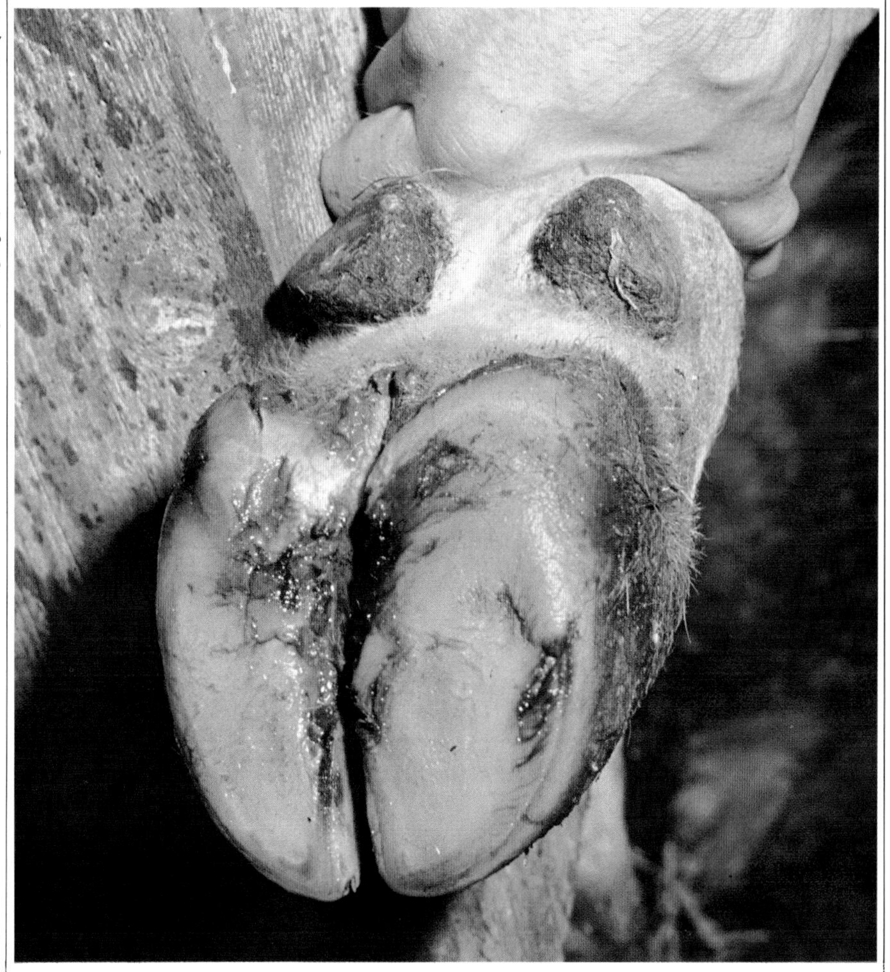

**Symptoms**

We see an increasing number of cuts and tears in the claws of the hind feet. Differing degrees of lameness of the affected limbs draw attention to these injuries. Raising the affected foot and cleaning the claw and ball with brush and water will reveal the extent of the injury. If the separation of the horn of the claw reaches down into deeper layers, invading pyogenic organisms can cause inflammation. In such cases the back of the fetlock joint and the interdigital space are often hot, swollen and painful. Suppuration of the sole and of the hollow wall of the claw and inflammation of the claw joint are not usually noticed until the claws are trimmed.

Treatment

Injuries to the claws and inflammation always involve badly soiled wounds.

Thorough cleaning and appropriate preparation of the claws are necessary. This is followed by local treatment of the injury with disinfectant sprays or antibiotic ointments and powders. In deep-seated inflammation with suppuration, the claws should be thoroughly trimmed to enable adequate drainage. The application of a bandage and housing in a separate shed with straw litter are essential for the healing process.

*Fig. 460: Treatment schedule for injuries to the claws.*

*Figs. 461 to 466: Treatment of a suppurative cut on the ball of the foot.*

*Fig. 460*

| | | |
|---|---|---|
| Environment | Housing in **"sick pen" with straw litter** for at least 3 weeks. Claws to be cleaned with soap and water. Brush thoroughly. | Immediately |
| Local treatment | If necessary, sedation with COMBELEN. Trim gaps in horn, spray in tincture of haematoxylon. Apply claw bandage and renew on 4th, 8th and 12th day. | Immediately + 4th, 8th, 12th day |
| Injection | Subcutaneous injection of 15 ml THERANEKRON per animal. Repeat after 1 week in persistent cases. | 1st and 8th day |
| Oral Administration | Give 1 BOVIBOL/150 kg body-weight. Repeat on 5th day in persistent cases. | 1st and 5th day |

Fig. 461

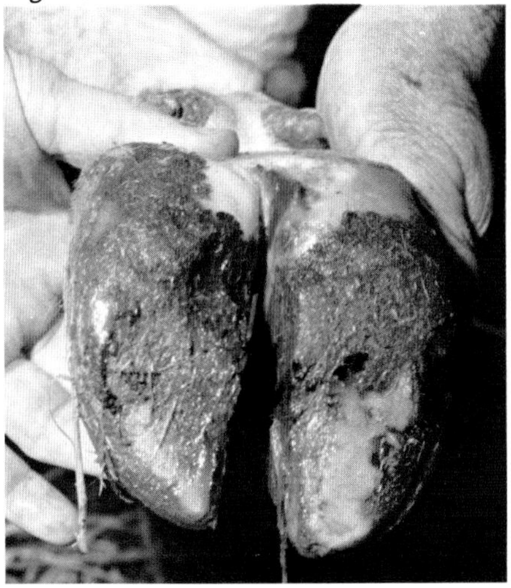

Cleaning and exposing the wound.

Fig. 462

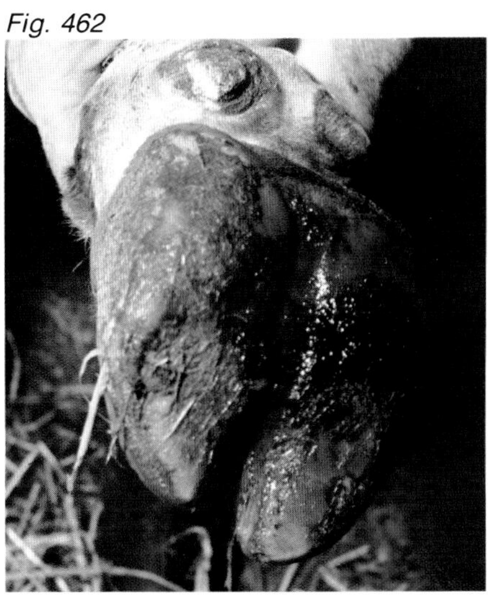

Spraying with wound tincture.

Fig. 463

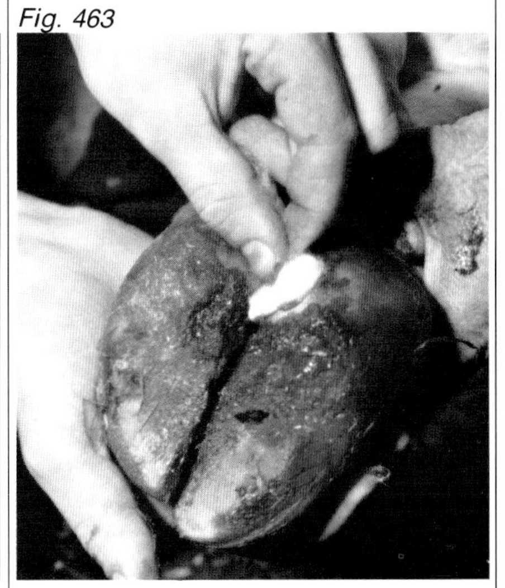

The suppurating wound is extended with a knife to enable better drainage.

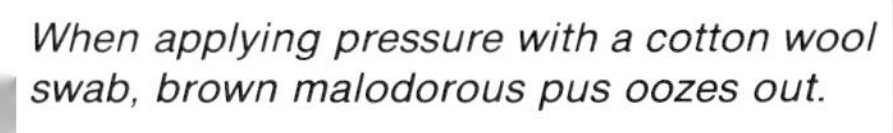

When applying pressure with a cotton wool swab, brown malodorous pus oozes out.

Fig. 464

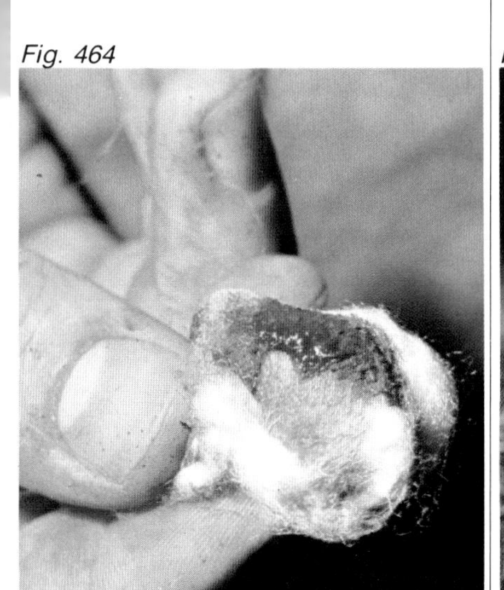

After further disinfection, a padded claw dressing is applied.

Fig. 465

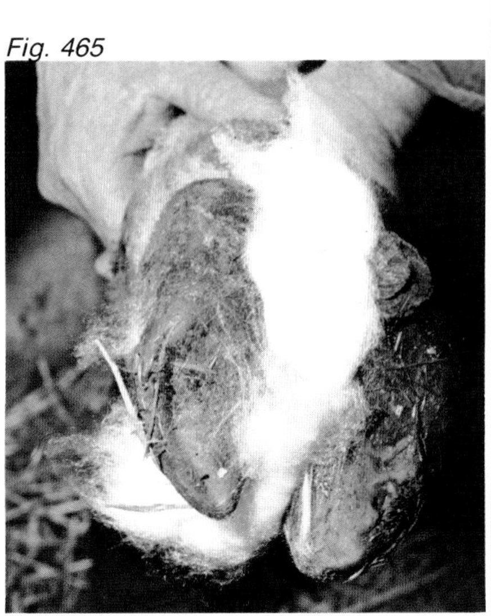

Internal dressing. The outer dressing consists of several layers of firm elastic bandages or sack-cloth.

Fig. 466

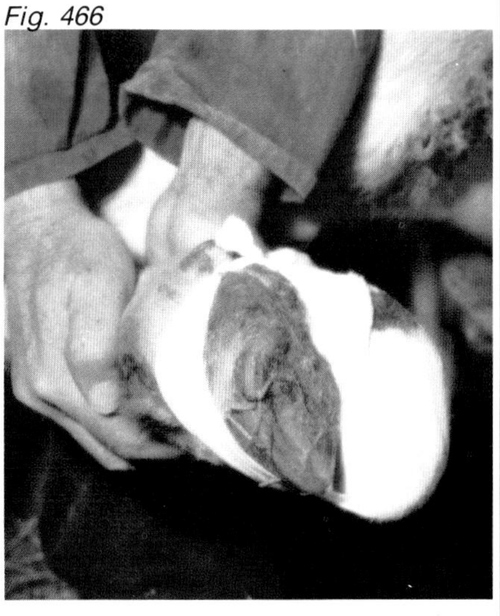

## Foul-in-the-foot (panaritium)

This term covers all inflammatory changes in the region of the claws, but refers in particular to interdigital panaritium and to inflammation of the coronal edge and the ball of the foot (phlegmon).

**Term**

Errors in housing and feeding lead to skin changes in the region of the claws which, if bacterial infection supervenes, cause "panaritium".

Fig. 467

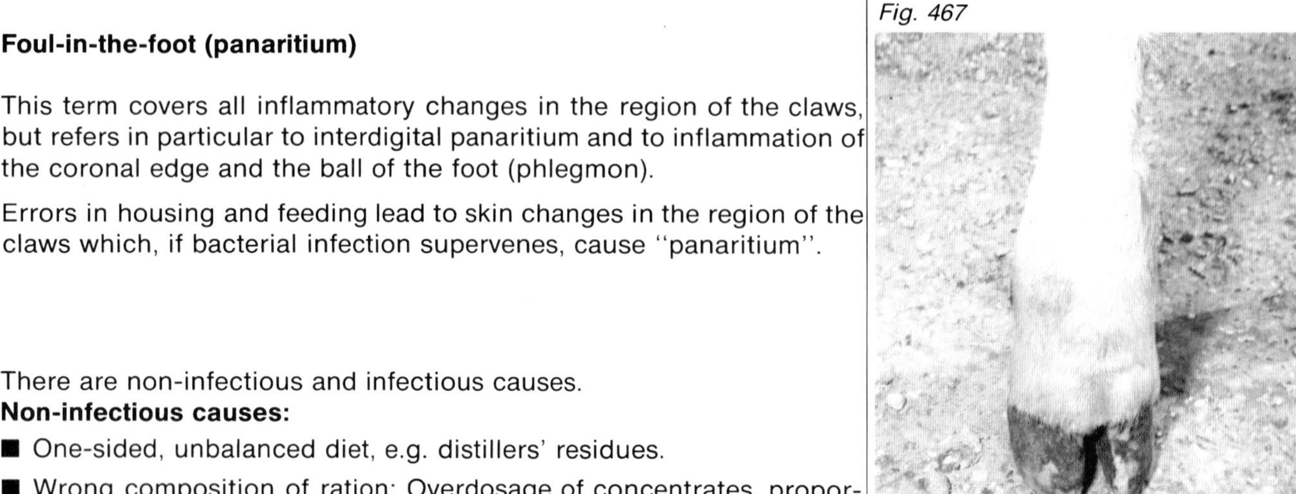

**Cause**

There are non-infectious and infectious causes.

**Non-infectious causes:**

- One-sided, unbalanced diet, e.g. distillers' residues.
- Wrong composition of ration: Overdosage of concentrates, proportion of roughage too small. With a high volume of concentrates, the ration must contain a certain amount of roughage, and the concentrates should be distributed over several feeds, in order to prevent hyperacidity of the rumen contents (acidosis of the rumen). Otherwise, breakdown products (histamines) are formed in the rumen which, after passing into the blood stream, cause inflammation of the skin of the claws and impairment of horn growth.
- Deteriorated fodder; large amounts of green forage without sufficient roughage. This causes diarrhoea which, due to the excretion of body salts, leads to electrolyte deficiency which in turn reduces the elasticity of the skin and of the claw horn.
- Inadequate intake of vitamins, particularly vitamin A (which protects the epithelium).
- Shortage or excessive quantity of minerals in the diet (see feeding, page 275).
- Poor controlled environment. Unduly moist lying areas involve the danger of slipping and of injury.

**Infectious causes:**

As a result of the above-mentioned, non-infectious causes, the resistance of the skin, particularly in the region of the claws, is reduced. The skin becomes cracked and fissured leading to very small superficial injuries which are then invaded by bacteria, especially Spherophorus necrophorus, Fusiformis nodosus and Corynebacterium pyogenes.

Fig. 468

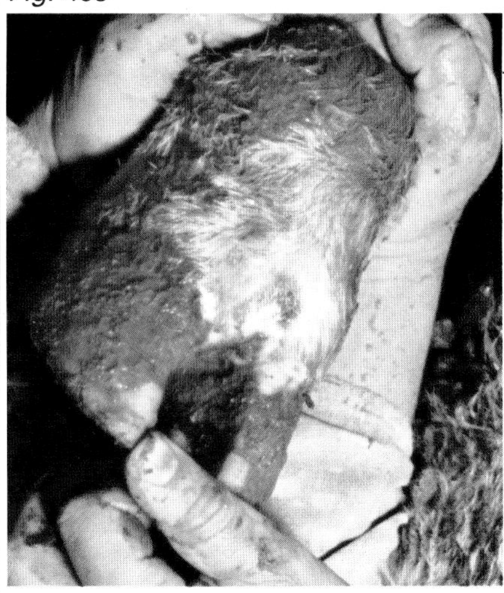

Fig. 469

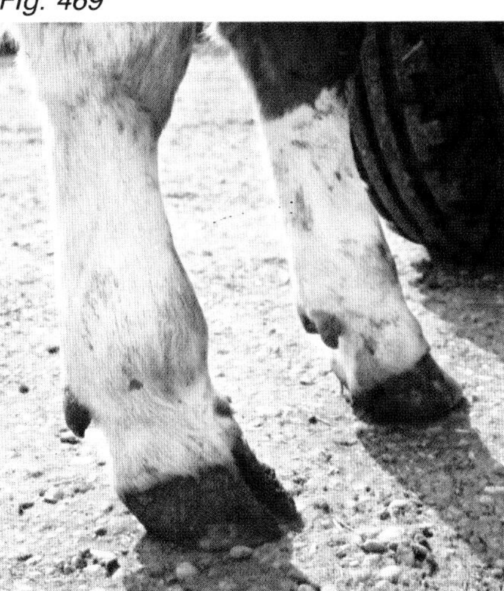

Fig. 470

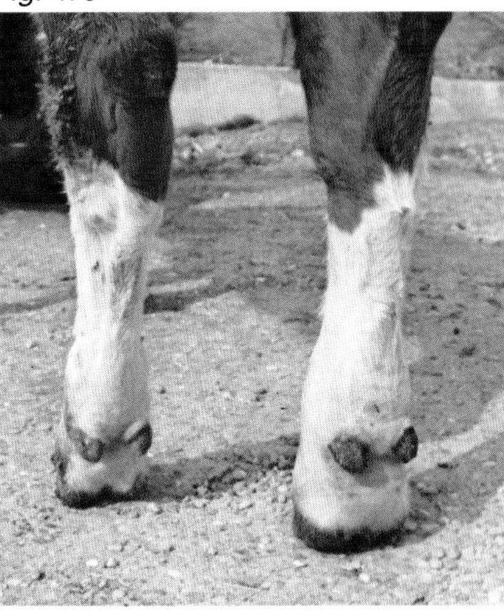

Symptoms

In **interdigital panaritium** the skin is initially reddened, hot and tight. Later on it becomes chapped and fissured, secreting a dirty and greasy fluid which has an unpleasant stale, sweetish odour. The animals are reluctant to walk, and when they do, they move very carefully putting their weight alternately on the affected limbs. In the advanced stage, a bulge can be seen between the claws as well as pronounced swelling and reddening of the adjacent skin areas.

In **panaritium of the coronal edge and the ball of the foot** (phlegmon) the hairs at the line of transition from the claw horn to the haired skin initially stand on end. The coronal edge and the ball of the foot are increasingly hot to the touch and show a bluish red, painful and hard swelling which may involve one or both claws. The animals are very cautious in putting their weight on the claws.

In interdigital panaritium and in phlegmon of the coronal edge and the ball of the foot, the inflammation may reach deep-lying tissue, like tendon sheaths, tendons and joints. Pronounced swelling reaching beyond the fetlock joint, severe lameness and suppuration in the region of the claws are the result.

*Fig. 467: Incipient interdigital panaritium. Reddening of the skin between the claws. Swelling of the coronal edge.*

*Fig. 468: Advanced stage of interdigital panaritium. Secretion of dirty and greasy fluid which has an unpleasant stale, sweetish odour.*

*Fig. 469: Inflammation of fetlock joint as a result of chronic ball phlegmon.*

*Fig. 470: Incipient panaritium of the coronal edge and the ball of the foot. Hard, bluish red, painful swelling.*

If panaritium occurs frequently, feeding and the controlled environment should be checked.

**Treatment**

In the initial stage, injections of sulphonamides result in rapid improvement and healing. In order to obtain a long-lasting sulphonamide blood level and to avoid disturbing the animals by further injections, BOVIBOL is given after the sulphonamide injection. The BOVIBOL bolus is given by mouth with the aid of an applicator and passes into the dorsal sac where it releases sulphamethazine for a period of 4 to 5 days. In addition, we inject THERANEKRON which contains spider venom and helps to confine the inflammation.

With deep-lying inflammatory processes and suppuration, ICHTHYOL ointment dressing or surgical intervention to open up the abscess, is required. Subsequent bandaging of the claw and housing on straw are necessary.

The prognosis is poor for severely affected animals with impairment of their general condition, increased body temperature and refusal to feed.

*Fig. 471*

| | | |
|---|---|---|
| Injection | Intramuscular injection of 1 ml THERACANZAN per 10 kg body-weight. 10 ml THERANEKRON per animal, subcutaneously. | 1st day |
| Oral Administration | In addition to the injection give 1 BOVIBOL/150 kg body-weight | 1st day |
| Fodder | **Follow-up treatment:** 10 g RP. RINDER I/ animal per day, independent of body-weight, for 2 or 3 weeks. | 1st to 21st day |
| Environment | Make sure the slatted floors are dry. If necessary, spray floor with superphosphate. Keep litter dry in deep-litter house. | |

*Fig. 471: Treatment schedule for panaritium.*

Fig. 472

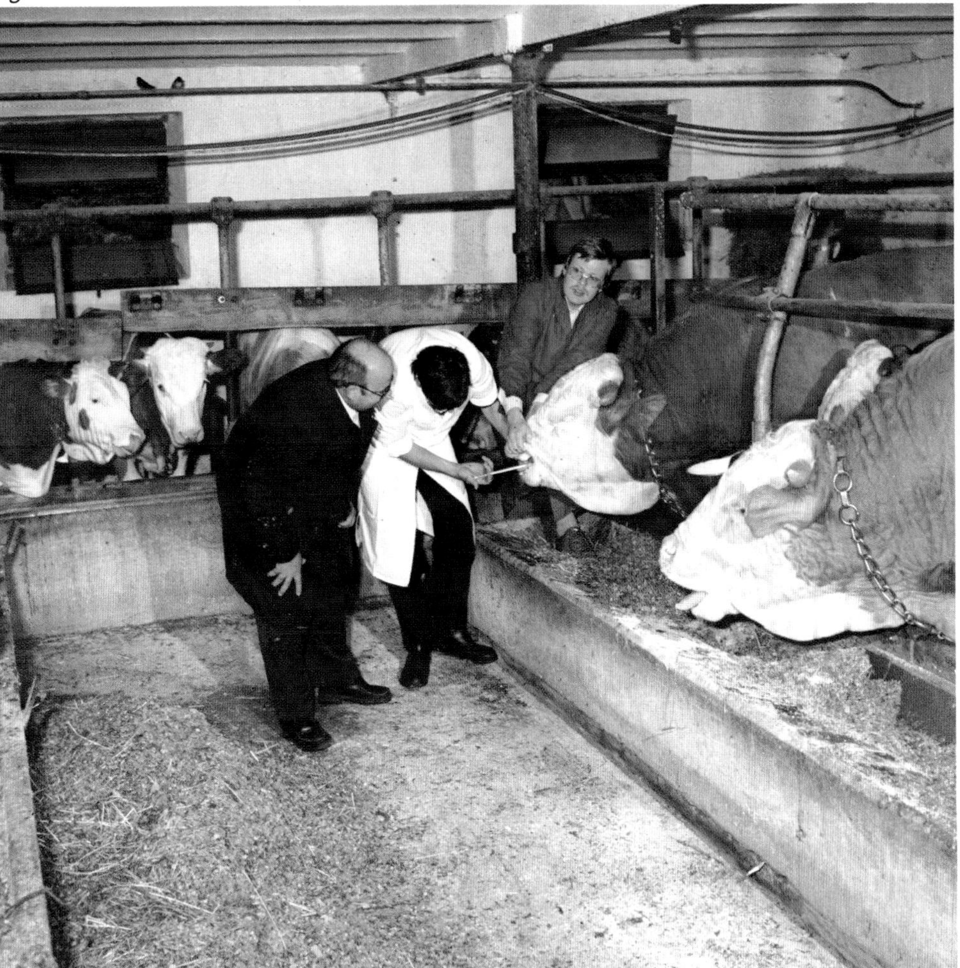

*Administration of a long-acting sulphonamide bolus: The success of treatment depends on the selection of the right active substance, the dosage and adequate duration of application.*

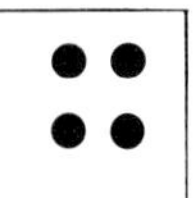

# Part 4

## Guidelines for treatment

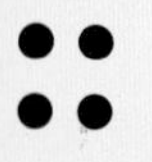

# Guidelines for treatment

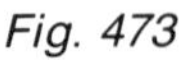

Fig. 473

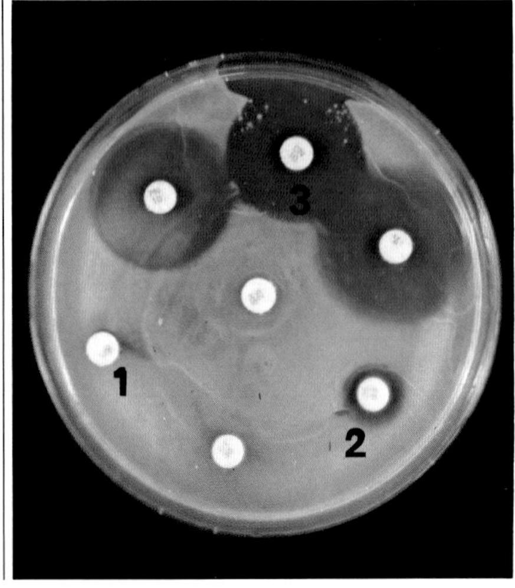


*Figs. 473 and 474: Action spectra of drugs. The circular diagram shows the action spectra of various drugs. Blank or only partly filled sections indicate no effect or insufficient action against the pathogen. For active substances with a narrow spectrum, but good effect against specific pathogens (e. g. furane derivatives against intestinal bacteria, like salmonella and E. coli), the diagnosis needs to be confirmed. In many cases these substances are then the drug of choice for the specific condition concerned.*

*In selecting a drug for causal treatment of a disease, a resistance test of the pathogen demonstrated is helpful. In Fig. 473 a sensitivity test for a known pathogen (salmonella) has been carried out on an agar plate (see also page 44). Test disc 1 – impregnated with an antibiotic – has not effected any inhibition of bacterial growth. The antibiotic is not effective. A small "zone of inhibition" has formed around test disc 2. This antibiotic is likely to have only a slight effect. The antibiotic of test disc 3 shows good effect.*

For the treatment of sick animals, fundamental guidelines should be observed. Adherence to these therapeutic principles will determine success or failure.

The treatment of infectious diseases aims to combat presumed or actually demonstrated pathogens. In addition, the defence mechanisms of the animal body can be reinforced by supportive treatment (symptomatic treatment) and vital functions can be maintained (e. g. by support of the circulatory system). In some diseases, for instance in virus infections, this is the only possible form of treatment.

Metabolic disorders and diseases induced by housing conditions must be combated by changing the housing conditions and by giving supportive treatment.

**Causal treatment**

## Combating the cause

In bacterial infections, fungal infections and the presence of ecto- and endoparasites, causal treatment is carried out. Success in combating the pathogens mainly depends on three conditions:

- Selection of the right active substance
- Dosage
- Adequate duration of application

*Fig. 474*

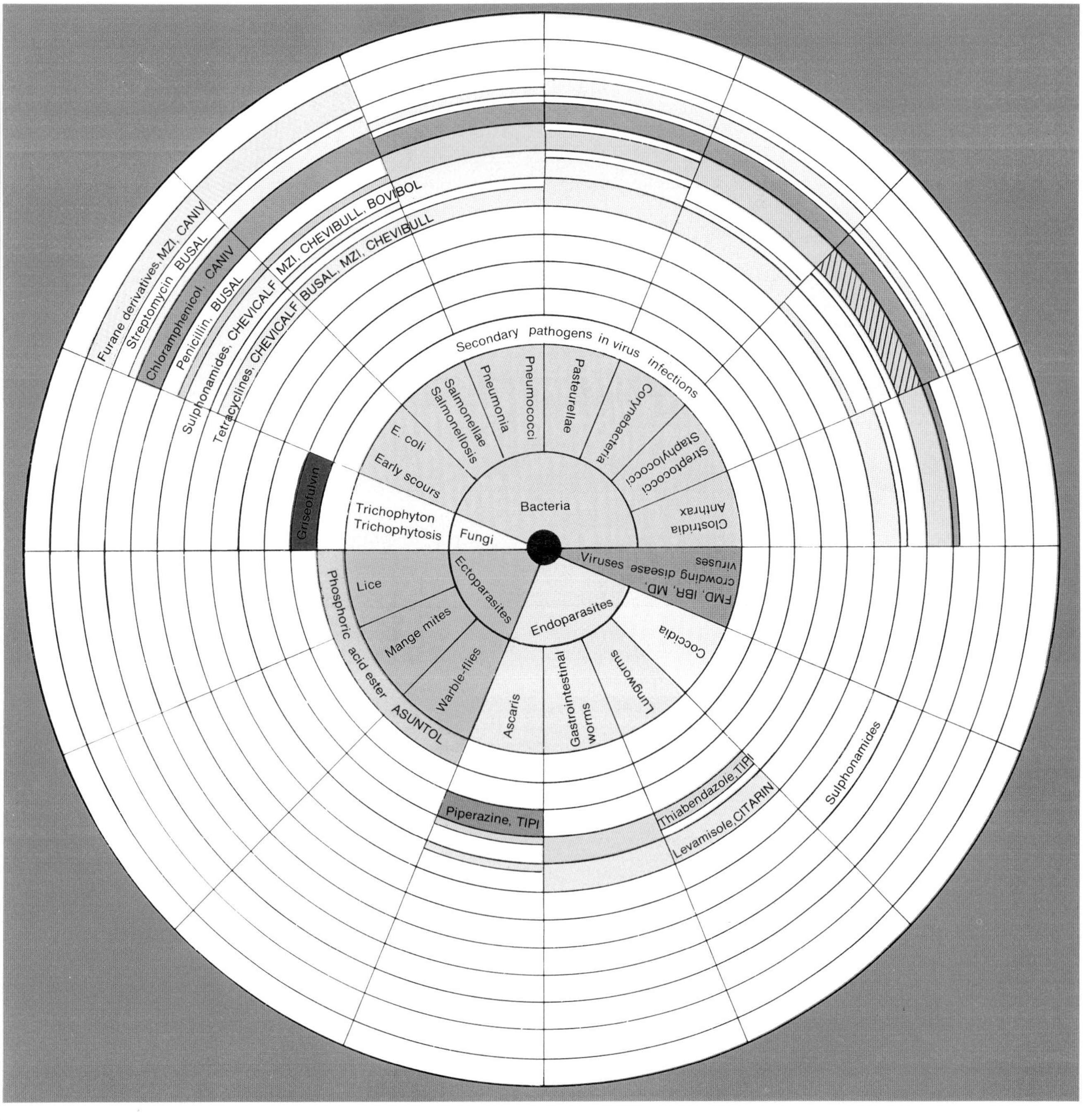

Bacteria
Secondary pathogens in virus infections
Pneumococci
Pasteurellae
Corynebacteria
Staphylococci
Streptococci
Anthrax
Clostridia
Pneumonia
Salmonellae
Salmonellosis
E. coli
Early scours
Fungi
Trichophyton
Trichophytosis
Griseofulvin
Viruses
FMD, IBR, MD, crowding disease viruses
Endoparasites
Coccidia
Lungworms
Gastrointestinal worms
Ascaris
Ectoparasites
Lice
Mange mites
Warble-flies
Phosphoric acid ester ASUNTOL
Furane derivatives, MZI, CANIV
Streptomycin BUSAL
Chloramphenicol, CANIV
Penicillin, BUSAL
Sulphonamides, CHEVICALF MZI, CHEVIBULL, BOVIBOL
Tetracyclines, CHEVICALF BUSAL, MZI, CHEVIBULL
Piperazine, TIPI
Thiabendazole, TIPI
Levamisole, CITARIN
Sulphonamides

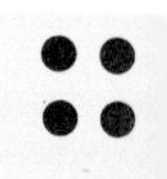

**Causal treatment**

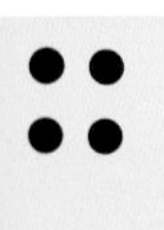

Correct treatment

Fig. 475

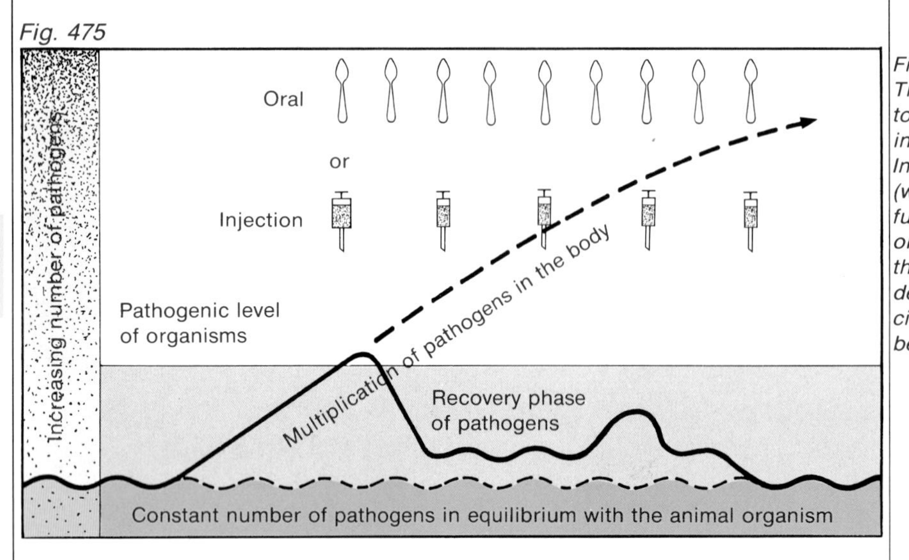


*Fig. 475: Diagram of correct treatment. Timely treatment starts when the first symptoms of the disease appear (outbreak). This inhibits the multiplication of the pathogens. In the recovery phase of the pathogens (when the disease seems to have abated), further treatment needs to be carried out, in order to prevent renewed multiplication of the pathogens and a relapse. The intrinsic defence mechanisms of the body and sufficiently long medication restore the balance between the body and the pathogens.*

Infective pathogens are either in the blood and body fluids or in organs (liver, lungs, muscles, skin). The level of the active substance, e. g. an antibiotic, at the site of the pathogen is therefore of decisive importance. If the blood or tissue level of the drug is inadequate, the disease may take an insidious (chronic) course, giving rise to periodic relapses, stunting and the constant excretion of pathogens.

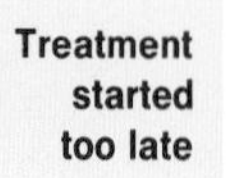

Treatment started too late

Fig. 476

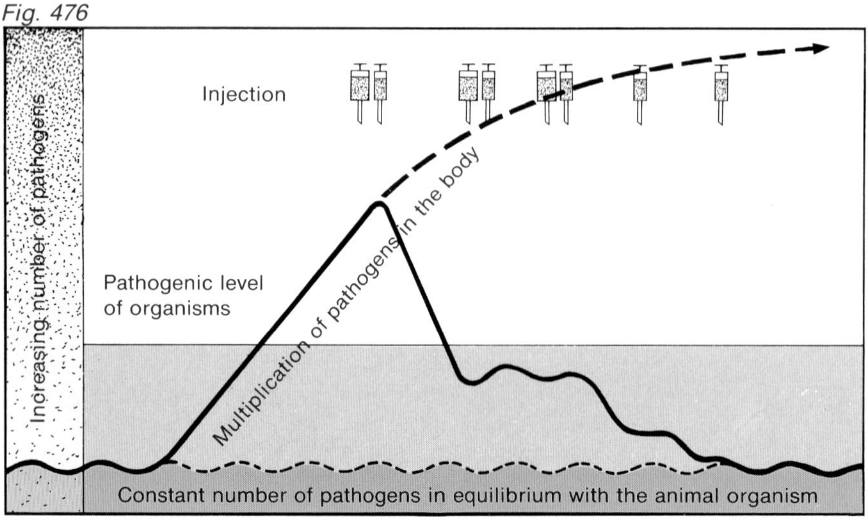


*Fig. 476: Diagram of treatment started too late.*
*Since the animal body is already extensively invaded by pathogens, additional symptomatic treatment (support of circulation, antipyretic therapy) is required in order to maintain vital functions (Symbol: small syringe). With further damage to the body, a longer period of follow-up treatment is likely (pneumonia, crowding disease).*

*Fig. 477: Diagram of treatment given for too short a period. If treatment is given in time, but for an insufficient period, the pathogens recover during the recovery phase. If the dosage is too low or the duration of treatment too short, the pathogens remaining become more resistant and multiply even more quickly than before, leading to a relapse.*

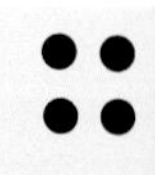

*Fig. 477*

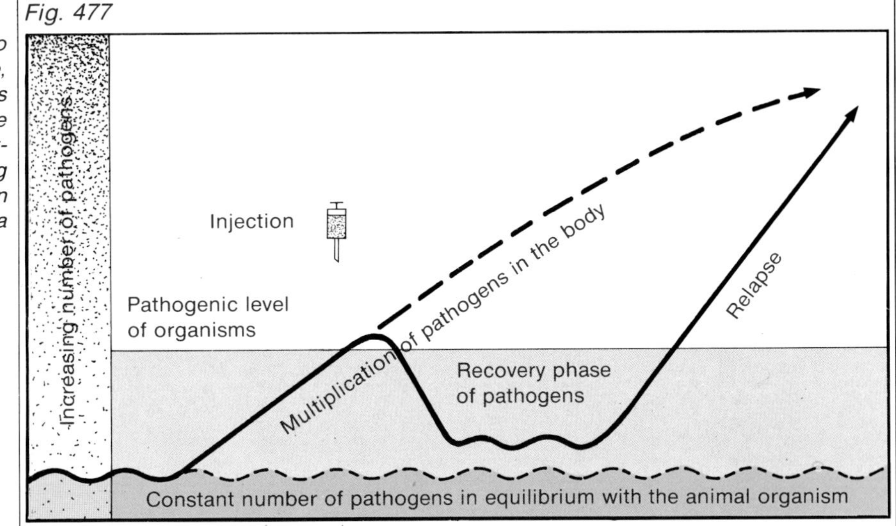


**Inadequate duration of treatment**

If these three therapeutic principles are disregarded, the pathogens are not sufficiently damaged. After a brief period of recovery, they multiply again and cause a relapse. The pathogens remaining after an inadequate dosage has been given, are usually the most refractory organisms and are most likely to become resistant.

**Modes of administration**

The success of the causal treatment of pathogens – apart from the timely start of therapy – essentially depends on the concentration of the drug in the blood and the tissue. Several modes of administration are available to achieve these blood and tissue levels. Whilst an injection will produce rapidly rising blood levels, oral administration is likely to achieve a slowly rising, but longer lasting level. Several injections will also provide an adequate long-term effect, but have the disadvantage of disturbing the animals on several occasions. Economy is also an important factor in selecting the form of administration. In many cases, combined treatment – e.g. injection plus oral application – is indicated.

The diagrams shown overleaf illustrate the rise and maintenance of blood and tissue levels with the most important types of administration.

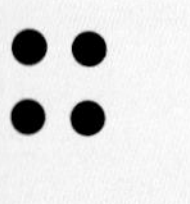

Modes of administration

*Figs. 478/480/482*

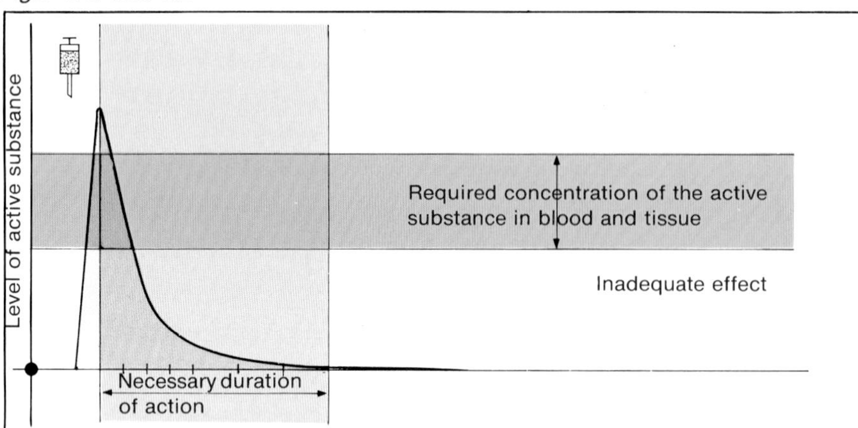


*Fig. 478: Single injection. After a short period, the drug quickly reaches the required level in the blood and tissue. Excretion depends on the drug used, but is usually quick. The curve shows that the necessary active substance level is not maintained for a sufficiently long period.*

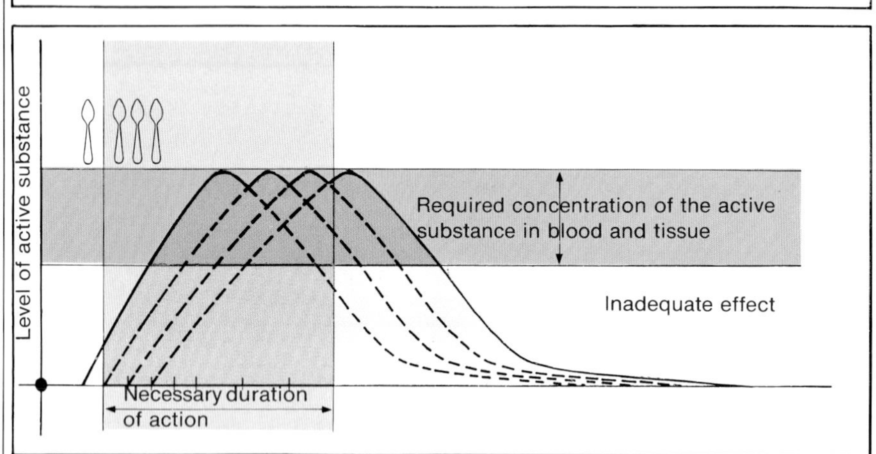


*Fig. 480: Oral administration in the fodder or via the drinking-fluid.*
*Ingestion by mouth, the passage through the body into the intestine and the time required for absorption delay the onset of action.*
*Continual administration with the feed results in a virtually even active substance level in the blood and tissue.*

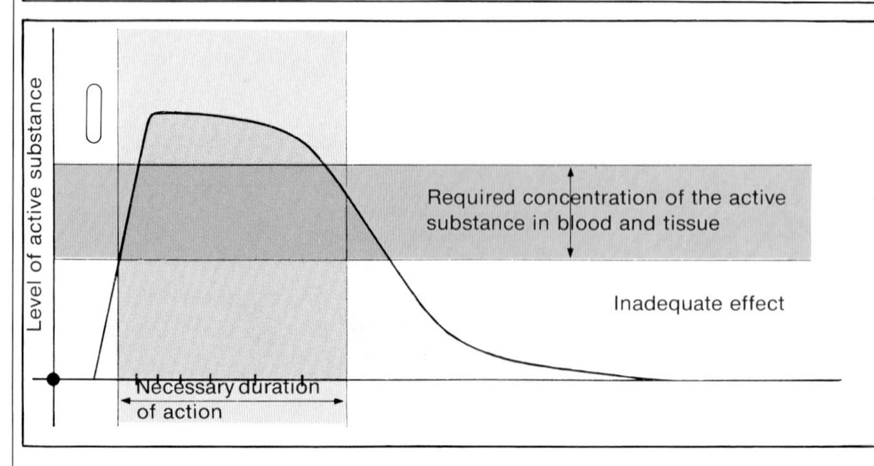


*Fig. 482: Administration of a long-acting sulphonamide bolus (BOVIBOL). This special form of oral treatment is only possible in cattle with a fully developed compartmental stomach system. Following administration by means of an applicator, the bolus passes into the dorsal sac where it slowly dissolves over a period of 4 to 5 days.*

Figs. 479/481/483

*Fig. 479: Several, repeated injections provide a sufficiently long duration of action. If the disease takes a highly acute course and if absorption from the intestine is impaired, several injections must be given. This method has the disadvantage of having to disturb the animals repeatedly. Giving the injections may also be a problem.*

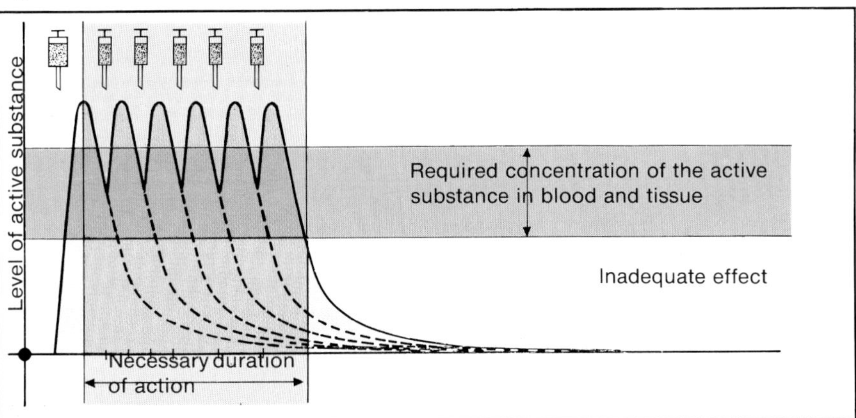


*Fig. 481: Combination of injection and oral administration. With this method, the drawback of the slow onset of action is overcome by giving an injection at the start of treatment.*

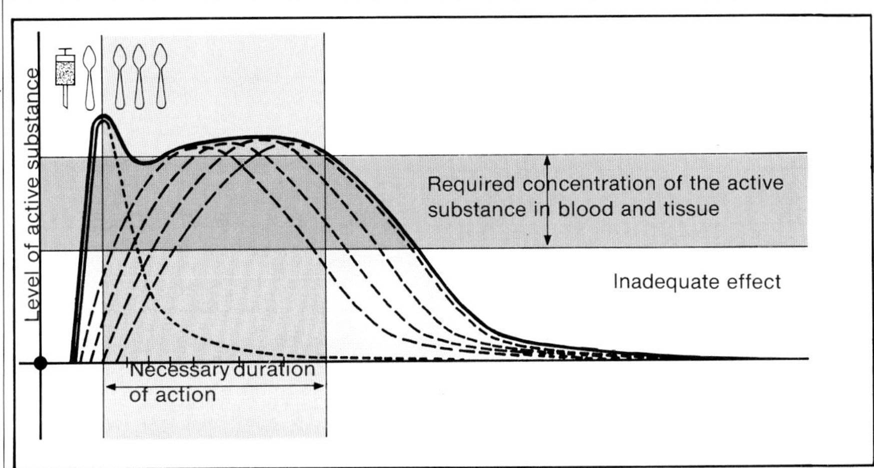


*Fig. 483: Combination of injection and bolus.*
*The injection given at the start of treatment ensures a very rapid onset of action.*

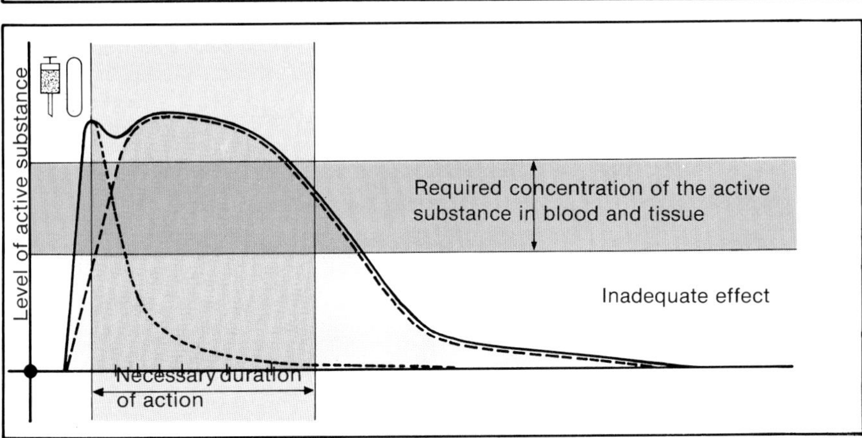

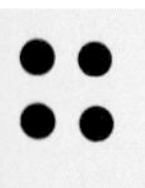

## Supportive (symptomatic) treatment

**Supportive treatment**

If causal therapy of the pathogen is not possible, we need to fall back on treatment that limits or alleviates the extent and severity of the disease. In this way, life-threatening manifestations can be contained and the animal organism can form antibodies to overcome the cause of the disease.

For instance, in the respiratory condition IBR, causal treatment of the pathogen, a herpes virus, is not possible. It is the animal body itself that has to overcome the viral infection by forming antibodies. Alleviating symptomatic treatment mainly aims to prevent an obstruction of the airways with mucus. Anti-inflammatory mucolytic drugs have the effect of decongesting the mucosae and of facilitating the removal of mucus from the airways. In conjunction with the administration of circulatory agents, symptomatic treatment has a life-saving effect.

Since the virus infection IBR always involves a secondary bacterial infection, antibacterial treatment with antibiotics is carried out at the same time. The administration of antibiotics will not have any effect on the progress of the viral infection. The high body temperature which is a defence reaction of the body to suppress the multiplication of viruses, is not directly influenced by antibiotics. In the initial stage of a viral infection, the existing fever must be regarded as a defensive measure of the animal organism to increase the metabolic processes and to stimulate the development of immunity. The use of antipyretics (e. g. cortisone) is only indicated if the fever persists for long periods and if the animal's general condition is poor.

*Fig. 484*

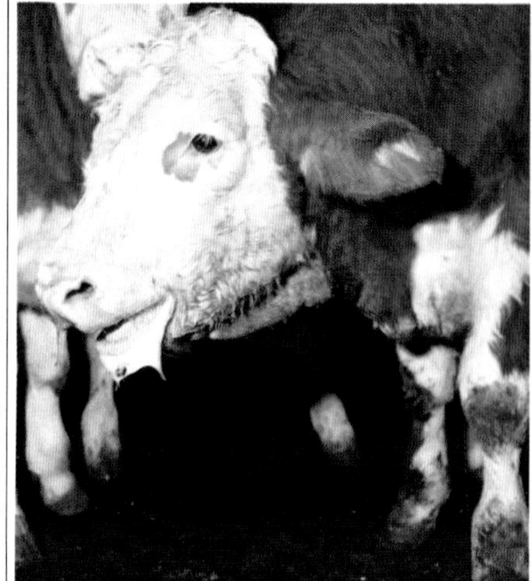

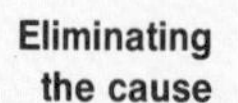

## Elimination of causally involved errors in housing and feeding

**Eliminating the cause**

Errors in feeding and housing, i. e. stress factors that lead to infectious diseases, have to be remedied (see page 252). Supportive symptomatic treatment is necessary in the majority of cases. Since such diseases usually develop slowly, prolonged periods of treatment up to the complete recovery of the animals, should be anticipated. The cause should be eliminated permanently.

*Fig. 484: Young bull with symptoms of severe respiratory distress in IBR.*
*The actual pathogen of IBR, a herpes virus, cannot be combated specifically in this case. Treatment is concentrated on support of the circulation, reduction of body temperature and administration of mucolytic drugs. Antibiotics will only prevent a secondary bacterial infection.*

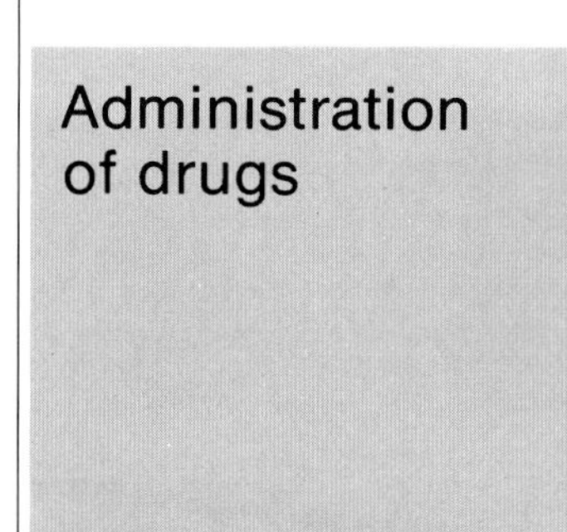

# Administration of drugs

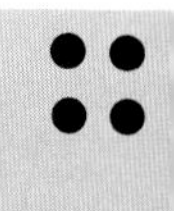

Drugs are administered to animals in various ways. In selecting the type of administration to be used, the following questions need to be answered:

- Which organ is affected?

  Gastrointestinal infections, for instance, are best treated by giving the drug in the fodder or by mouth, because in this way the active substance passes direct to the site of the disease process.

- Is it a local condition (e. g. an abscess) or a disease involving the entire body (generalised disease)?

  With an abscess, local treatment such as lancing the gathered abscess, will be most successful. With a generalised condition (e. g. blood poisoning – septicaemia) the pathogens or their toxins have to be combated throughout the animal body by inducing high blood and tissue levels of the drugs used.

- Has the animal suddenly fallen ill, or has the condition developed slowly, without immediate danger to life?

  In order to ensure rapid distribution of the drug in the body of severely ill animals, injections often need to be given. If the disease takes an insidious, chronic course, prolonged treatment will be necessary for which the oral administration of drugs is indicated.

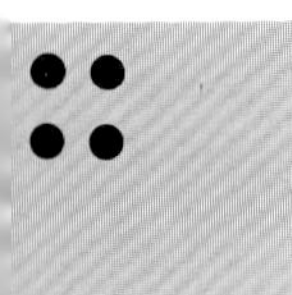

Fig. 485

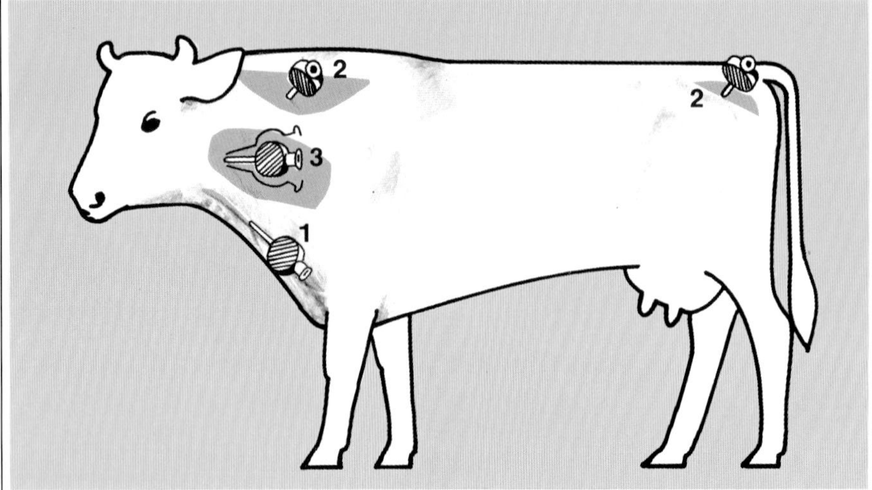


The mode of administration also depends on the nature and formulation of the active ingredients contained in the medicinal product. Here it should be considered that some active substances are tolerated by the animal only in one specific formulation which may call for a certain type of administration. Thus some solutions of calcium and magnesium can only be given intravenously. Conversely, commonly used penicillin suspensions cannot be administered intravenously.
Some drugs can only be injected up to a certain maximum volume at any one site. If this maximum dose per injection site is exceeded, incompatibility with the tissue and poor assimilation result.

Injection

## Administration by injection

**Intravenous injection** is best carried out into the jugular vein. Blood flow in the vein is blocked and the needle is inserted rapidly. Intravenous injection offers the advantage of a very quick onset of action. The intravenous injection of drugs usually has to be carried out slowly. With some drugs, the circulation, respiration and pulse rate need to be monitored during the injection.

*Fig. 485: Common injection sites in cattle.*
*1 Intravenous injection into the jugular vein.*
*2 Intramuscular injection into the muscles of the neck or croup.*
*3 Subcutaneous injection into the neck.*

*Figs. 486 to 488: Subcutaneous injection into the neck.*

*Fig. 486: Using thumb and forefinger, the needle is firmly pressed against the barrel of the syringe before it is inserted.*

*Fig. 487: A skin fold is raised with the left hand and the needle is inserted into its base. The needle is freely movable under the skin.*

*Fig. 488: During the injection the needle is held with the left hand and the plunger is pressed forward with the right hand. The injected fluid causes the formation of a small protrusion under the skin.*

*Fig. 489*
*1 Injection syringes and cannulae: Glass syringes with metal plungers can be sterilised by boiling. Today, plastic disposable syringes are widely used, which are supplied in sterile packs.*
*2 Injection gun and cannulae with screw-on fittings. By means of a dosing device, the fluid volume to be injected per injection, can be adjusted.*
*3 Vaccinating gun for vaccinations. After each injection, the next vaccine dose is automatically sucked up from the vaccine bottle.*

*Fig. 486*

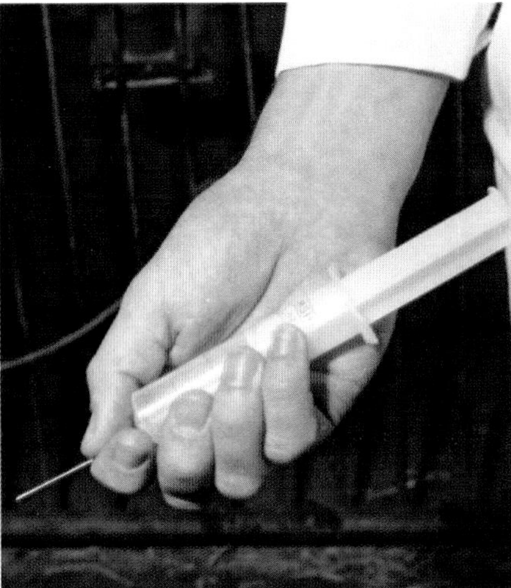

*Fig. 487*

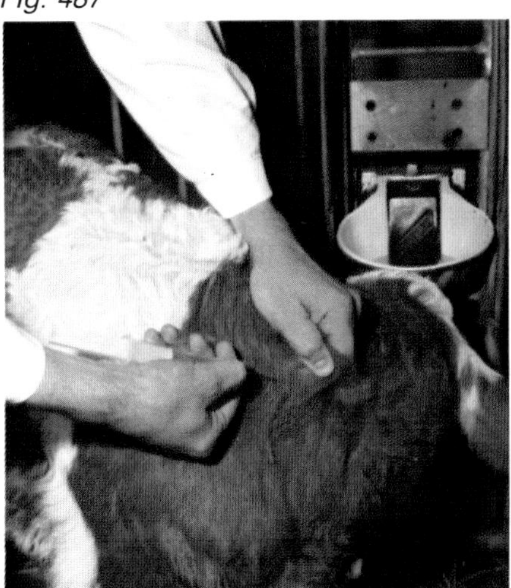

*Fig. 488*

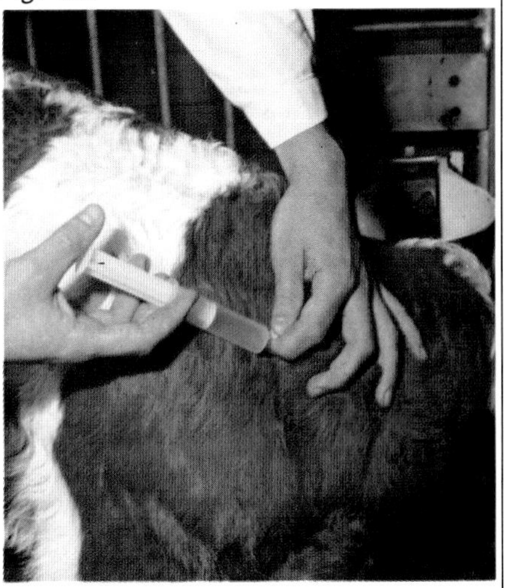

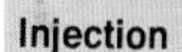



The **intramuscular injection** is the most widely practised type of injection. Muscular body sites like the croup, shoulder and neck are suitable for intramuscular injections. The croup muscles are particularly suitable. Here the needle is inserted in the centre of a triangle formed by the tuberosity of the hip, the base of the tail and the ischial tuberosity.

The **subcutaneous injection** is given into the loose subcutis on the neck, whereby a skin fold is raised with one hand and the needle is inserted with the other hand at the base of the skin fold. The needle must be freely movable below the skin. The fluid injected forms a protrusion under the skin.

*Fig. 489*

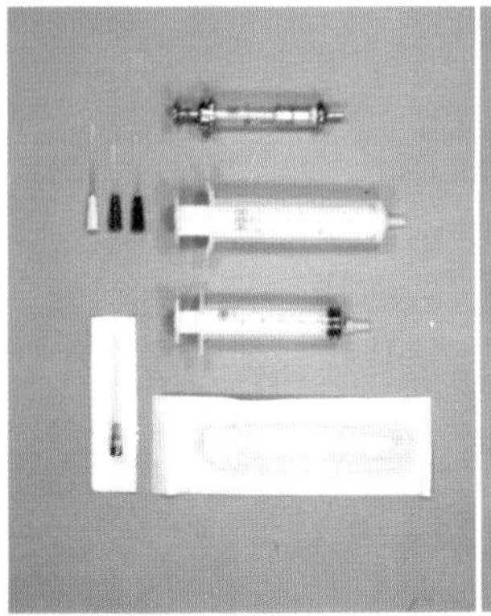

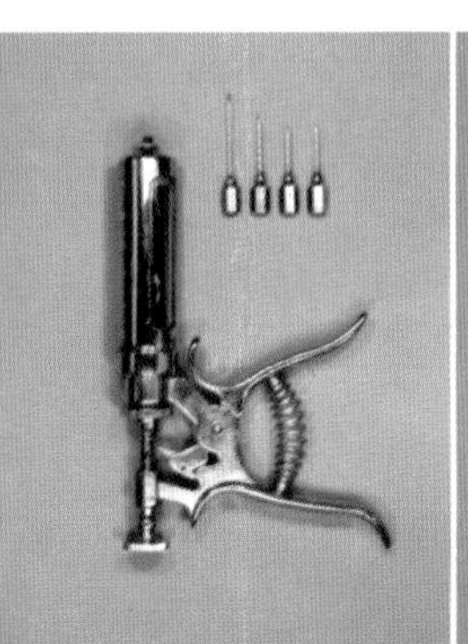

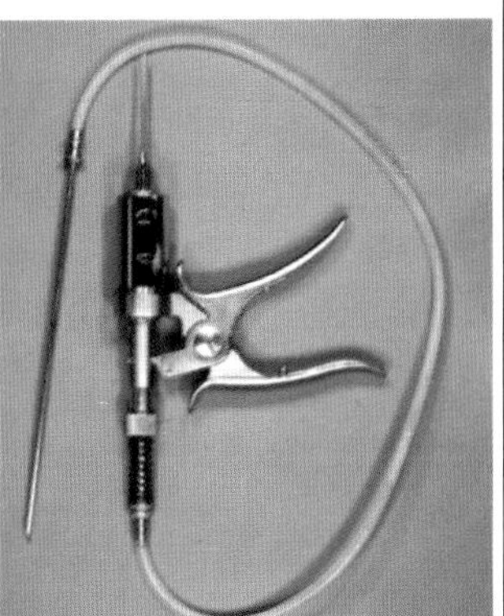

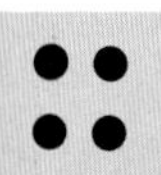

## Oral administration

The treatment of individual animals or groups of animals can be carried out with drugs in powdered form, given in the fodder. Here special attention should be paid to even distribution of the drug in a fodder (concentrate) which the animals like to eat.

**Medicated feeds**

For individual animals, the medicated pre-mix should be well mixed with the appropriate quantity of concentrate and then offered to the animal. If drug and fodder are mixed in the trough, the distribution of the drug is usually inadequate. Also, mixing in the feeding trough leads to the formation of dust from the fine drug particles, and drugs with a somewhat unpleasant taste are then taken up only reluctantly by the animal.

For the treatment of groups, the drug is best distributed in the concentrate by means of a mixer. Even a concrete mixer can be used for this purpose. Adding individual active substances to the fodder without previously preparing a premix, is not without danger. For instance, the formation of clumps with moist fodder can lead to a high drug dosage that is not tolerated, or to a low, ineffective dosage.

In bull fattening in deep litter houses where 2 or 3 animals share one feeding place, the quantity of drug required first needs to be mixed into the concentrate and then into the total ration.

Calves fed on milk are best given the drug via the drinking fluid. Only water-soluble drugs can be used for this purpose. If treatment is carried out via automatic drinkers, the drug must be introduced during the preparation of the milk substitute.

*Fig. 490*

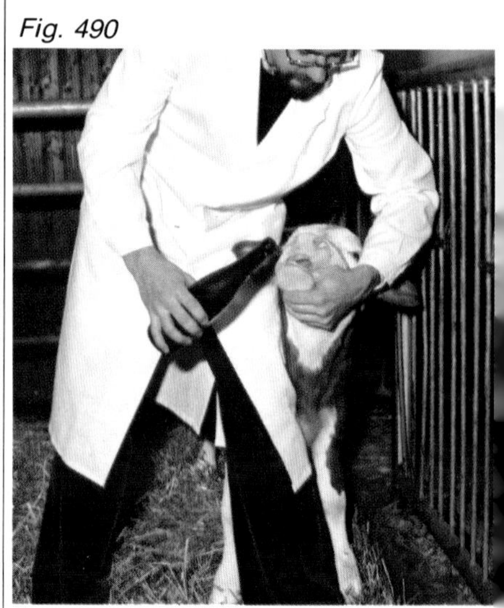

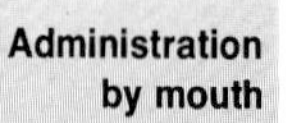

**Administration by mouth**

Drugs which the animals do not take up themselves, are dissolved or mixed with water and poured into the cheek pouch using a long-necked bottle, whereby the animal's head is slightly raised so as to ensure that the contents of the bottle are gradually emptied into the cheek pouch and swallowed. If large volumes of fluid are administered in this way, the bottle should be removed from the mouth for brief intervals (after $^1/_8$ to $^1/_4$ of a litre has been swallowed).

Pills are administered by means of an applicator or are placed by hand on the back of the tongue. They are swallowed by reflex deglutition and remain in the ventral sac where they dissolve.

*Fig. 490: Administration of liquid drugs with a long-necked bottle:*
*The mouth of the calf is opened by inserting the thumb whereby the mandible is firmly held between the thumb and the fingers. The liquid is poured in portions into the cheek pouch, raising the head slightly.*

*Fig. 491: Administration of a bolus by means of an applicator. The plunger of the applicator is not pushed forward until the end of the applicator has reached the back of the tongue.*

*Fig. 492: Correct position of the applicator with the bolus in the throat. Once the bolus is at the back of the tongue, it is swallowed by reflex deglutition.*

*Fig. 493: How the waiting time is arrived at. Illustration of the elimination time of active substances. Following the administration of the last dose, the blood and tissue levels of the active substance decrease relatively quickly. At 1 the level falls below the effective concentration. The elimination rate then slows down considerably. At 2 the level has decreased to below the limit of demonstration. At 3 the active substance has been completely eliminated or metabolised. The time span between 3 and 4 serves as a safety margin, since elimination may be delayed by unforeseen biological processes.*

*Fig. 494: Waiting times of the drugs mentioned in this book (pages 246 and 247).*

Fig. 491

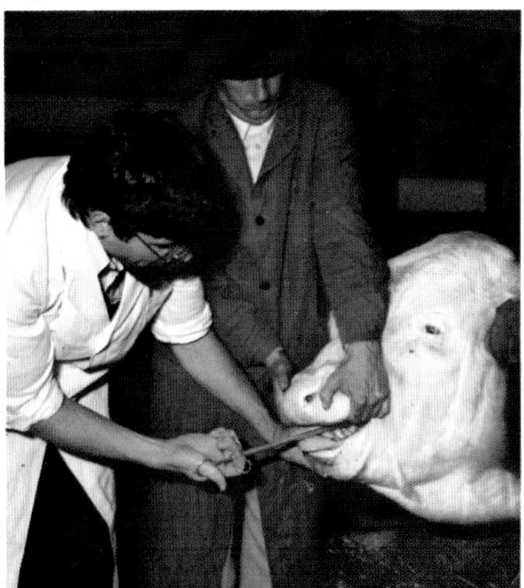

Fig. 492

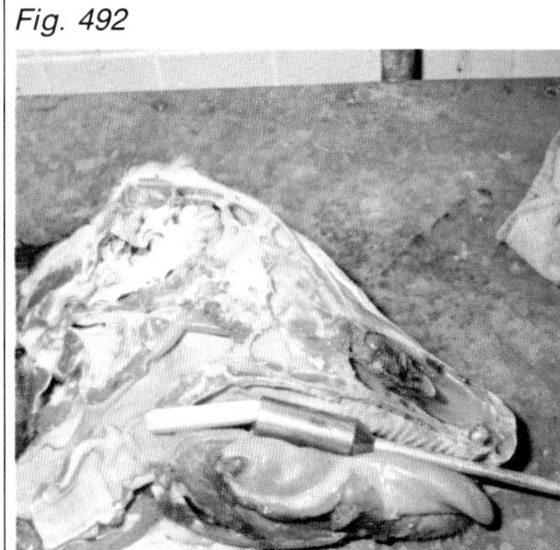

Waiting time

## Waiting times

Drugs form residues in the body. These residues are retained for a certain time and are then excreted in the urine and the faeces. After the last dose has been administered, the waiting time shown on the pack or stated in the directions for use circular, should be observed before the animal is slaughtered.
The waiting times of the drugs mentioned in this book are listed on pages 246 and 247.

Fig. 493

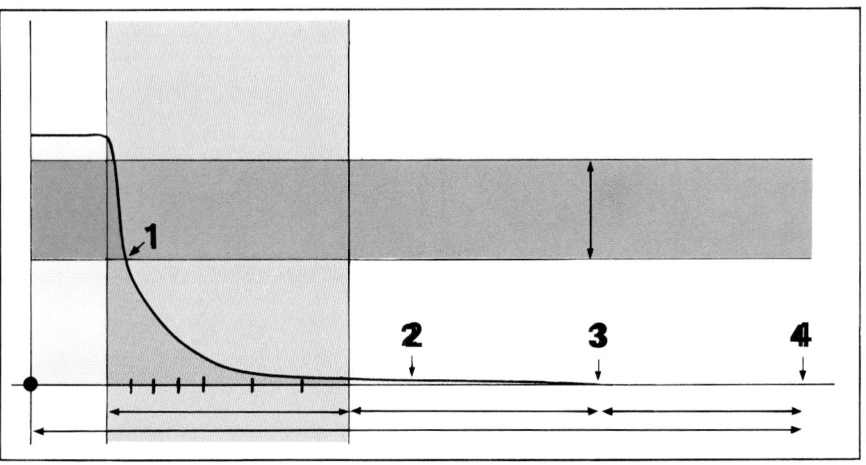

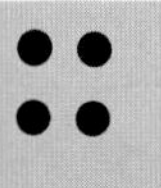



*Fig. 494*

| Trade name | Active ingredient | Manufacturer | Mode of administration |
|---|---|---|---|
| **A**suntol | Coumaphos | Bayer | external |
| **B**ayferon | Interferon inducer | Bayer | vaccination |
| Bisolvon | Bisolvon | Boehringer | injection |
| Blauholztinktur | Aqueous haematoxylon extract, phenol | Chevita | local |
| Bovibol | Sulphamethazine | Chevita | oral |
| Bovigrip | Vaccine with PI III, adeno 1, 3, 5, reo 1, 3 viruses | Behringwerke | vaccination |
| Bovoflavin | Acridine, quinaldine | Hoechst | ointment |
| Busal | Chlortetracycline, streptomycin, penicillin, vitamins A, $D_3$, E, C, B-complex | Chevita | oral |
| Buscopan compositum | Hyoscine butylbromide, aminophenazone | Boehringer | injection |
| BVD-MD vaccine | Vaccine with BVD viruses | Vemie | vaccination |
| **C**aniv | Nifurprazine, chloramphenicol, arsanilic acid, vitamin complex | Chevita | oral |
| Catosal | Organophosphorus compound and vitamin $B_{12}$ | Bayer | injection |
| Chevi 45 | Aldehydes, quaternary ammonium compounds, alcohol | Chevita | disinfection |
| Chevi 75 | Phenol, perchloroethylene, alcohol | Chevita | disinfection |
| Chevibull | Chlortetracycline, sulfadimidine, vitamins A and $B_1$ | Chevita | oral |
| Chevicalf | Chlortetracycline, sulfadimidine, vitamin A, citric acid | Chevita | oral |
| Citarin-L 10% | Levamisole | Bayer | injection |
| Citarin-L Spot-on | Levamisole | Bayer | external |
| Caffeine-sodium 50% | Caffeine-sodium salicylate | Atarost | injection |
| Combelen | Phenothiazine derivative | Bayer | injection |
| **D**efungit | Benzylcarboxymethyltetrahydro-thiadiazone-thiosodium | Hoechst | external |
| Derma-Trichex Concentrate | Thymol, propionic acid | Friesoythe | external |
| Diazinone 25% | Phosphoric acid ester | Aesculaap | external |
| Dovenix | Nitroxynile | Vemie | injection |
| **E**kparol | Hexachlorocyclohexane | Chevita | local |
| Elrisal | Electrolyte salts | Chevita | oral |
| **F**oracol | Chloramphenicol | Forachemie | injection |
| Forapen | Penicillin, streptomycin | Forachemie | injection |
| **G**ambul | Bovine gammaglobulin | Chevita | oral; injection |
| Glykofusal | Invertose in isotonic saline solution | Asid | infusion; injection |
| Griseofulvin Supplement | Griseofulvin | Praemix | oral |
| **H**epamugol | Glucose, calcium lactate, asparaginate, methionine | Mucos | infusion |

| Trade name | Active ingredient | Manufacturer | Mode of administration |
|---|---|---|---|
| Hepaston | Vitamin B complex | Chevita | injection |
| Hostacain | Butylaminoacetanilide | Hoechst | injection; local |
| **I**chthyol ointment 40% | Ammonium Sulfoichthyolicum | Friesoythe | local |
| **K**elfizin | Sulphamethoxypyrazine | WdT | injection |
| **M**ultivitamin R 12 | Vitamins A, $D_3$, E, C, B-complex | Chevita | oral |
| MZ I | Tylosine tartrate, furazolidone, chlortetracycline, sulfadimidine, citric acid, salicylic acid | Chevita | oral |
| MZ II | Chlortetracycline, sulfadimidine, sodium salicylate, methylene blue | Chevita | oral |
| **N**eguvon | Phosphoric acid ester | Bayer | external |
| Novalgin | Aminophenazone derivative | Hoechst | injection |
| **P**enbrock | Ampicillin | Beecham | injection |
| Perlacar | Extract from bovine foetal skin, procaine hydrochloride | Asid | injection |
| Phenylarthrit Forte | Phenylbutazone, dexamethasone | Selectavet | injection |
| Phlegmalon Ointment | Camphor, ichthyol, iodine, chloroform | Albrecht | ointment |
| PI III Vaccine | Vaccine and interferon inducer | Mérieux-Rentschler | vaccination |
| Pneumovac Plus | Vaccine with PI III, adeno 3, reo 1, IBR/IPV, BVD-MD | Hydrochemie | vaccination |
| Prednisolone | Prednisolone acetate | Forachemie | injection |
| Procaine | Procaine hydrochloride, adrenaline | Aesculaap | injection |
| **R**aniden 2.5% suspension | Rafoxanide | Therapogen | oral |
| Rompun | Xylacine | Bayer | injection |
| **S**icaden | Polymeric organo-silicium compound | Byk Gulden | oral |
| Spectam | Spectinomycin | Abbott | injection |
| **T**ardomyocel comp. III | Penicillin, streptomycin | Bayer | injection |
| Theracanzan | Sulphadimethoxine | Therapogen | injection |
| Theranekron | Spider venom from Tarantula cubensis | Therapogen | injection |
| Tiguvon | Phosphoric acid ester | Bayer | external |
| Tipi | Thiabendazole, piperazine citrate | Chevita | oral |
| Tympanol | Thymol, chlorocresol | Aesculaap | oral |
| **V**etoprim 24 | Trimethoprim, sulfadimidine, sulphathiazole | Friesoythe | injection |
| Vitamin-AD$_3$EC-100 | Vitamins A, $D_3$, E and C | Chevita | injection/oral |
| Vitamin E + Selenium | Vitamin E, sodium selenite | Vemie | injection |
| Vitin | Vitamins A, $D_3$, E, B-complex | Chevita | injection |
| Voren | Dexamethasone | Boehringer | injection |

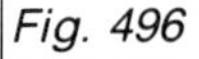

Fig. 495

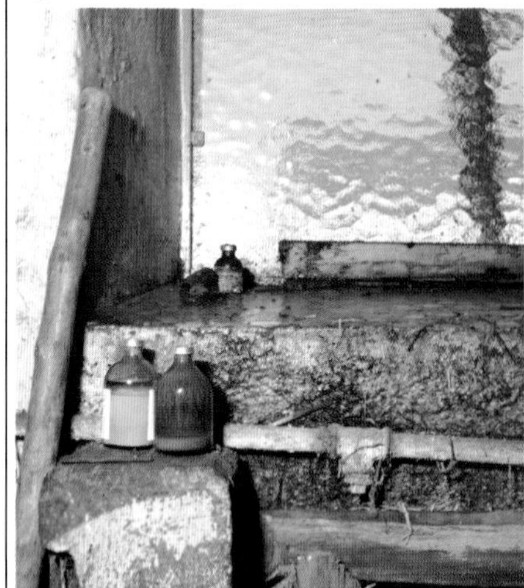

Fig. 496

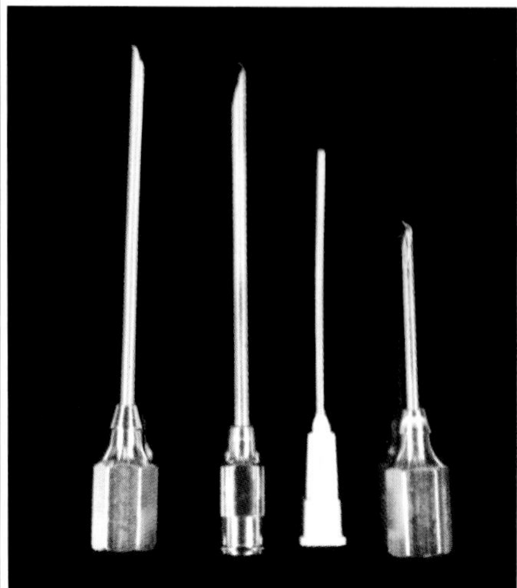



# Most common errors in the administration of drugs

- Dirty instruments, syringes and cannulae
  After an injection, the syringe and the cannula must be thoroughly rinsed with water. Residues of blood and drugs should be removed. Blunt cannulae and cannulae with bent tips make injection difficult and punch out small pieces of skin which are thus introduced into the tissue when the cannula is inserted. This often causes an abscess.

- Mixing of drugs
  Mixing different injectable products simultaneously in a syringe often produces precipitations which make the effect of the drug uncertain.

- Correct storage of drugs
  Drugs should be stored in a cool, dry place out of the reach of children. Some drugs need to be kept in a refrigerator, others must be protected from light during storage. Cooled drugs should not be administered until they have been warmed to room temperature.

*Fig. 495: Wrong storage of drugs. Drugs should be stored in a cool, dry place out of the reach of children.*

*Fig. 496: Blunt cannulae and cannulae with bent tips make injection difficult and punch out small pieces of skin on insertion of the cannula. This often causes an abscess.*

*Fig. 497*

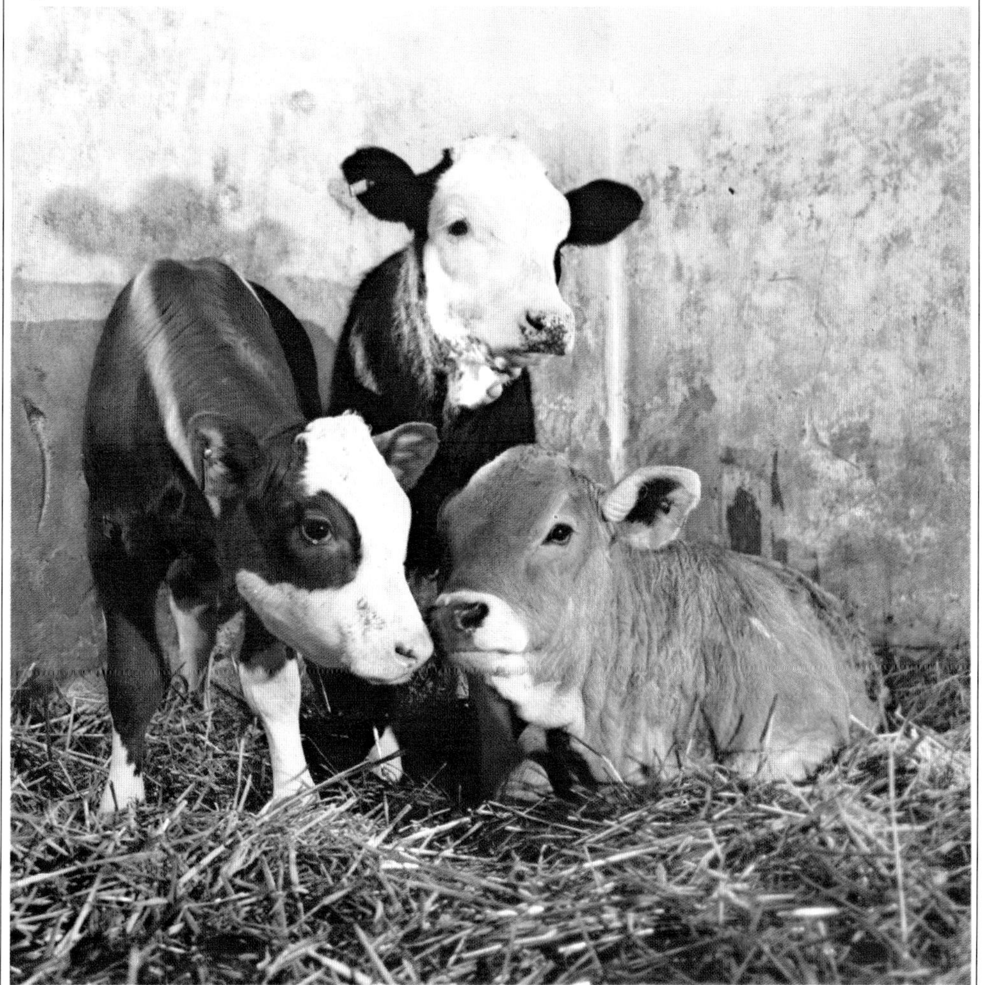

*Preserving the health of large stocks and preventing the outbreak of disease are economic requirements. Purposeful prevention and preventive treatment during periods of unforeseeable stress contribute to meeting these requirements. The necessary preventive measures are taken during periods of life in which the utilisation of the animals for human consumption does not arise (e. g. prophylaxis on housing after purchase). An animal kept healthy during the entire period of rearing and fattening yields high-quality meat that is free from residues.*

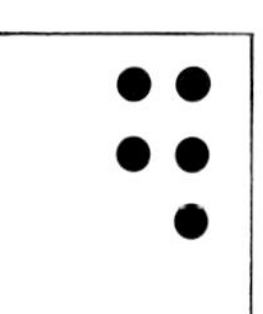

# Part 5

## Prevention and preventive treatment

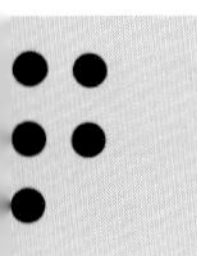

# Prevention and preventive treatment

Fig. 498

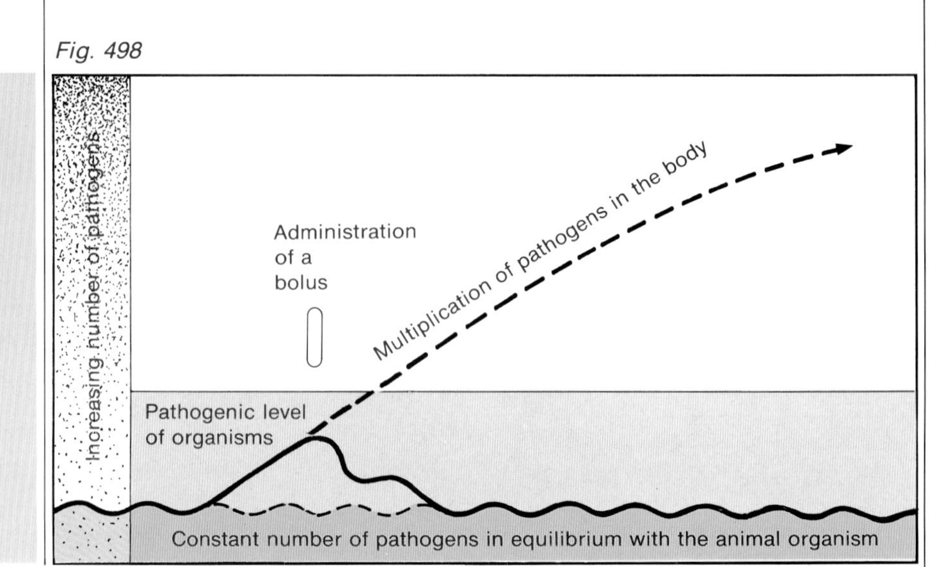


A large number of rearing diseases in cattle belong to the group of **infectious diseases.** They are caused by viruses, bacteria and fungi. Among the so-called **invasive diseases** we include those that are caused by ectoparasites and endoparasites.

In addition to these two groups of diseases caused by infective pathogens and parasites, there are **nutrition-induced and housing-induced diseases.** These occur as a result of intensive production where an environment appropriate to the animal is often neglected. Errors in housing and feeding are recognised too late or are disregarded. If they are not counteracted in time, these diseases will appear.

There is no clear line of demarcation between infectious and invasive diseases on the one hand and nutrition-induced and housing-induced conditions on the other. Thus errors in nutrition and housing (inadequate provision of vitamin A, high degree of air humidity in the cattle house) promote an outbreak of infectious crowding disease. On the other hand, infectious diseases and, in particular, invasive diseases (worm infestation) may cause deficiency states despite adequate feeding.

An appreciation of these multiple interactions has led to the introduction of new methods in the care of animal stocks. The recognition of disturbance factors and attempts at their elimination have given **prevention (prophylaxis)** and **preventive treatment (metaphylaxis)** an increasingly prominent place in animal husbandry.

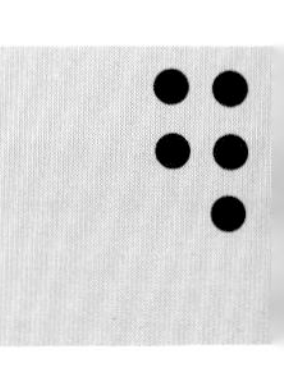



# Prevention (Prophylaxis)

*Fig. 498: Principle of preventive treatment: Experience shows that there is an increased incidence of disease after stress, which is due to a reduction in the intrinsic defence mechanisms of the animal body resulting in increased propagation of pathogens. Preventive treatment arrests the development of the disease process and restores the balance between pathogen and animal organism (Example: rehousing on slatted floors; see page 272). Low-dosed medication is usually sufficient for this purpose.*

*Fig. 499: Overcoming stress factors by prevention and preventive treatment, in order to avoid disease (pages 252 and 253).*

Starting points of specific prevention in cattle management:

- Adapting the housing conditions to the animal's needs
- Feeding appropriate to requirements
- Setting up a programme of hygiene and disinfection
- Carrying out vaccinations

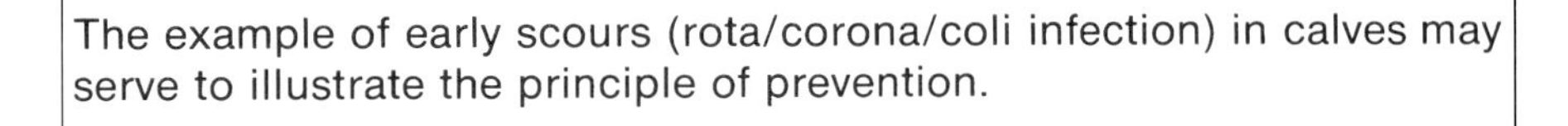

The example of early scours (rota/corona/coli infection) in calves may serve to illustrate the principle of prevention.

Since early scours is a virus infection against which the calf has no or only inadequate protection from maternal antibodies, we try, first of all, to avoid any infection with rota and corona viruses after birth. We remove the mucus from the mouth of the calf by expressing it, with clean hands, from the outside to prevent any pathogens being introduced by the hands into the oral cavity (hygiene). Immediately after birth we place the calf in a cleaned and disinfected calf pen (housing, hygiene and disinfection). The environment of the calf thus has a low pathogen content. Ingestion of virus-containing faeces, as occurs when the calves are tied up behind the cows in the dung passage, is avoided in this way. During the first few hours of life we administer bovine gammaglobulin before colostral milk is given. This in fact amounts to **passive immunisation.** We then administer vitamin A in high dosage which reinforces non-specific protection against infection (feeding appropriate to requirements).

Cleanly milked colostrum (if possible, 2 litres during the first four hours) further increases protection against infection.

As preventive treatment of early scours in calves, a medicated feed (CHEVICALF) consisting of chlortetracycline, sulphamethazine, citric acid, vitamin A and glucose is given daily, in order to eliminate any bacterial pathogens during the first few days of life.

This example shows that disease can be prevented by the combined effect of several preventive measures.

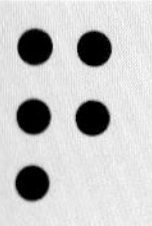

*Fig. 499*

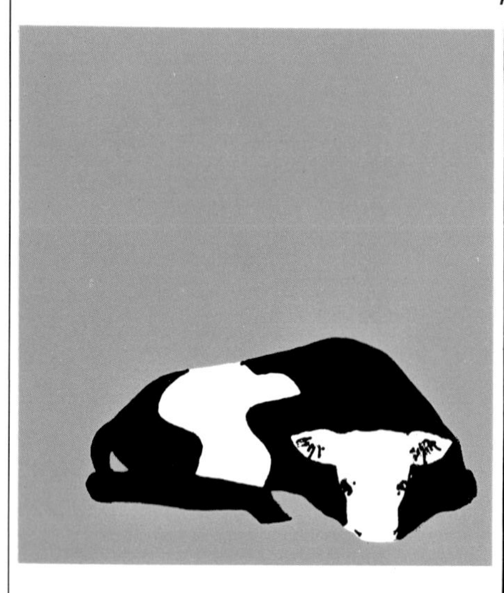

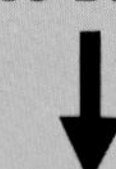

**Stress-Disease**

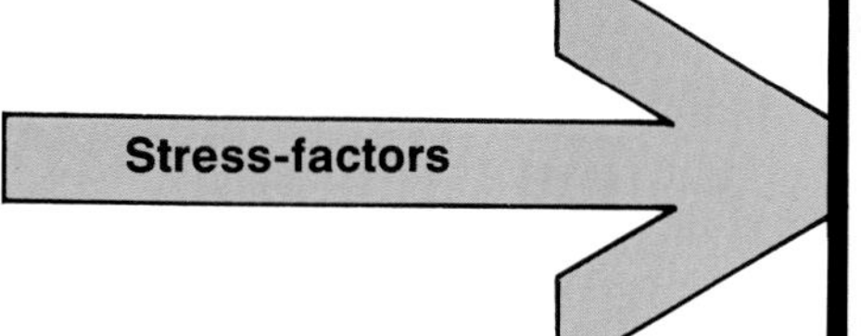



**Factors that can be eliminated**

- Controlled environment:
  air humidity too high,
  movement of air too great,
  ammonia concentration too high,
  change in temperature too sudden.
- Feeding:
  unbalanced supply of nutritive substances,
  crude fibre and structural deficiencies,
  supply of minerals, vitamins and trace elements not adapted to the basic ration,
  irregular feeding.
- Housing:
  inappropriate housing of calves,
  purchase without provision of reception house,
  animal groups too large,
  density of housing too high or too low.

**Factors that cannot be eliminated**

- Purchase:
  market, transport, dealer's cattle houses, change of cattle house,
  possible infection from purchased calves,
  change in feeding and attending personnel.
- Weaning:
  change to roughage.
- Necessary measures that cause stress:
  dehorning, docking of tail,
  vaccinations,
  re-grouping,
  rehousing on slatted floor.

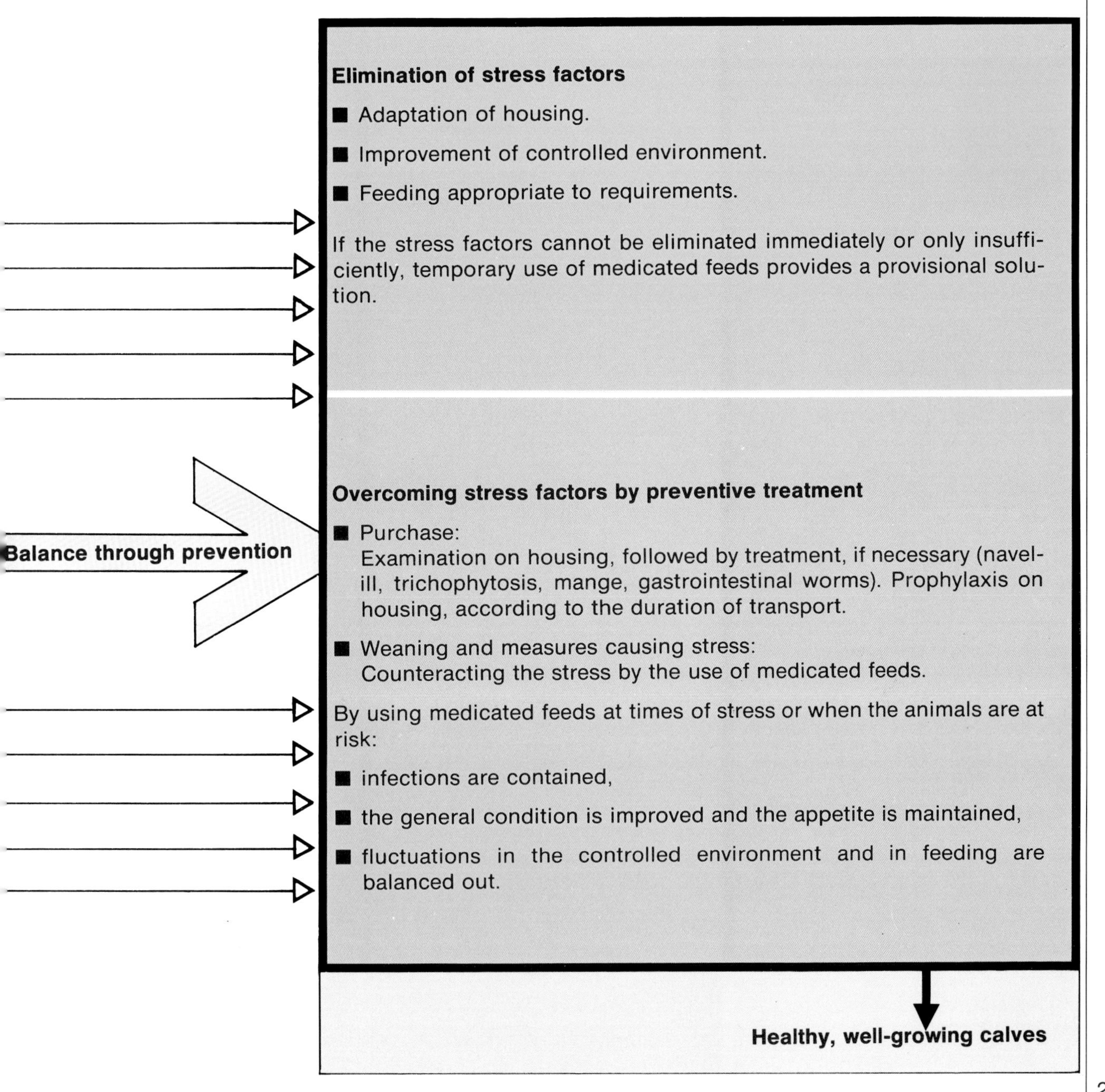


**Elimination of stress factors**

- Adaptation of housing.
- Improvement of controlled environment.
- Feeding appropriate to requirements.

If the stress factors cannot be eliminated immediately or only insufficiently, temporary use of medicated feeds provides a provisional solution.

**Overcoming stress factors by preventive treatment**

- Purchase:
  Examination on housing, followed by treatment, if necessary (navel-ill, trichophytosis, mange, gastrointestinal worms). Prophylaxis on housing, according to the duration of transport.
- Weaning and measures causing stress:
  Counteracting the stress by the use of medicated feeds.

By using medicated feeds at times of stress or when the animals are at risk:

- infections are contained,
- the general condition is improved and the appetite is maintained,
- fluctuations in the controlled environment and in feeding are balanced out.

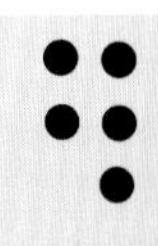

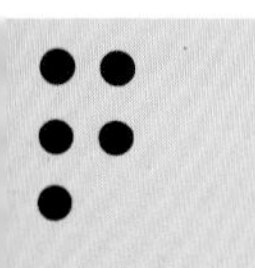

Preventive treatment

# Preventive treatment (metaphylaxis)

At times of foreseeable stress, unavoidable stress factors can be counteracted by preventive treatment. The example of the purchase of calves may serve to illustrate the principle of preventive treatment.

Despite the careful selection of healthy and vital calves, health problems may occur during the first few weeks following purchase.

Transport to the market and from the market to the fattening farm, or the transport from the breeding farm to the dealer's cattle house and from there to the fattening house, is a most severe stress for the calves. Changes in the controlled environment and in feeding also constitute stress factors which give rise to colds and scours, particularly during the first fortnight following housing. In addition, all calves have a different immune status, that is they have been exposed and have adapted to the pathogens present on their farm of origin, but have no immunity to pathogens present in other stocks.

In its new environment, the purchased calf comes into contact with pathogens from other stocks which have been introduced by calves of different origin. It has to build up its own active immunity against these pathogens.

When calves are purchased, we add CHEVICALF, BUSAL or MZ I to the drinking fluid as preventive treatment. The duration of use and the selection of the drug are adapted to individual requirements (cf. pages 262 and 270). Additional preventive measures (reception house, programme of hygiene and disinfection) should be carried out at the same time.

In selecting suitable products for such preventive treatment, the following should be considered:

- Side-effects should be slight, even with prolonged use. In the newborn calf, the liver and the kidneys are especially sensitive and should not be exposed to full stress. Damage to the sites of blood formation, such as the bone-marrow, has a detrimental effect on further growth. In sucking calves, for instance, chlortetracycline or furazolidone should only be used if there is a compelling reason for doing so (resistance test).

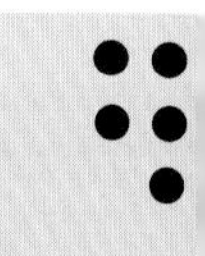

Preventive treatment

- Preventive treatment is carried out orally with medicated feeds. In this way it can be given over a long period. Since an adequate and prolonged effect is achieved with a relatively low dosage, there is little stress in the animal organism. If preventive treatment were carried out with injections, the animals would have to be rounded up on each occasion, involving a considerable amount of extra work for the stockholder and repeated disturbance of the animals.

- Damage to the gastrointestinal flora should be avoided by selecting suitable formulations.
  Calves in which the compartmental stomach system has not yet developed, require drugs in water-soluble, easily absorbed form. Although cattle with a fully functioning compartmental stomach system can utilise undissolved drugs, they do react sensitively to overdosage with antibiotics. Chlortetracycline, for example, is best absorbed by sucking calves in water-soluble form as hydrochloride. Fattening calves can utilise chlortetracycline in less prepared form.
  Prolonged administration in unduly high dosage has a detrimental effect on the flora of the first three stomachs in ruminants.

- Combinations of different substances of complementary action will alleviate the stress caused by drugs. In sucking calves we prefer a combination comprising chlortetracycline, sulphamethazine, vitamin A, citric acid and glucose in water-soluble form (CHEVICALF) for preventive treatment. The antibiotic chlortetracycline has a selective effect on the intestinal flora, that is it inhibits the growth of pathogens without affecting the bacteria required for the digestion. It is well absorbed from the intestine and produces high blood and tissue levels. The sulphonamide sulphamethazine is effective both in intestinal and in respiratory infections. Citric acid stabilises the degree of acidity in the intestine. In this way, the multiplication of E. coli pathogens which are known to cause diarrhoea and severe generalised conditions in calves, is suppressed. The glucose provides energy. Vitamin A protects the epithelium and thus supports the general defence mechanisms.

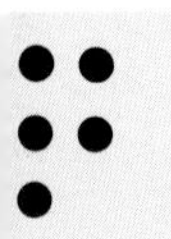

# Summary of preventive measures

## 1st to 4th week of life

Fig. 500

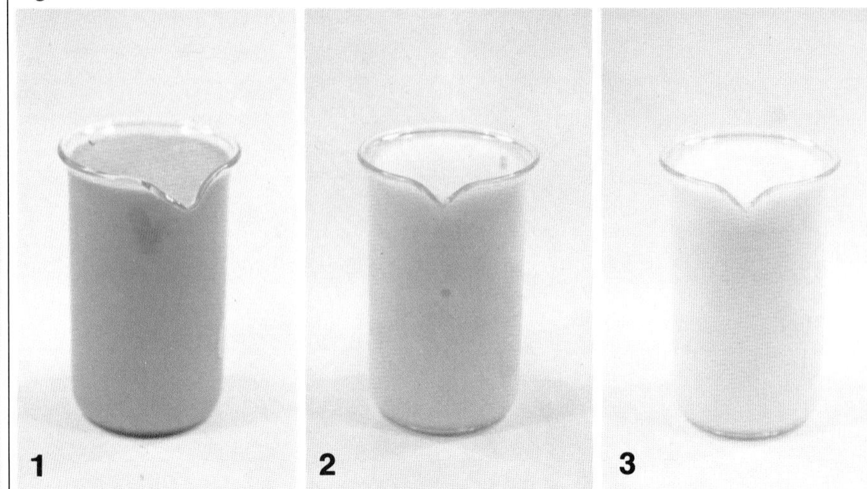


Birth

## Care of the calf after birth

- Removing amniotic fluid and mucus from the oral and nasal cavities: Hold mouth and nose with both hands and squeeze out mucus.
- Touch navel only with clean and disinfected hands. If necessary, tear off umbilical cord one hand-breadth below its point of exit. Squeeze out residual blood and spray with BLAUHOLZ-TINKTUR both inside and outside.
- Rub calf dry with straw.
- Place in calf box or separate calf house immediately, if possible.

Early diarrhoea

## Calves with early diarrhoea

This is usually an infection with rota, corona and coli bacteria. Before the first colostral milk is given, we administer:

- 25 ml bovine gammaglobulin (GAMBUL) and 10 ml Vitamin-$AD_3EC$-100 by mouth.
- Subcutaneous injection of 25 ml bovine gammaglobulin (GAMBUL) and 10 ml Vitamin-$AD_3EC$-100.
- 10 g CHEVICALF per calf/day in the drinking fluid, starting on the first day and continuing for at least 14 days.

*Fig. 500: Milk after birth:*
*1 Colostral milk on the 1st day. Cocoa-like colour. Its viscosity is due to the high content of protein (gammaglobulin) and solid substances.*
*2 Colostral milk on the 3rd day. The decreasing cell content may be seen from the lighter colour.*
*3 Normal milk on the 14th day after birth.*

*Figs. 501 to 505: Navel care after birth*

*Fig. 501*

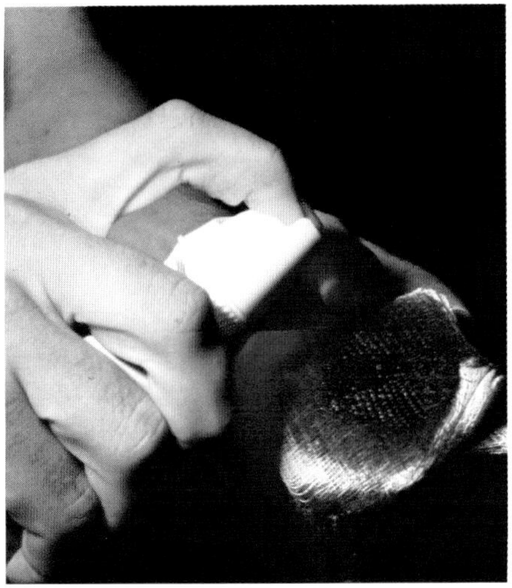

*Gauze swab soaked in BLAUHOLZTINKTUR*

*Fig. 502*

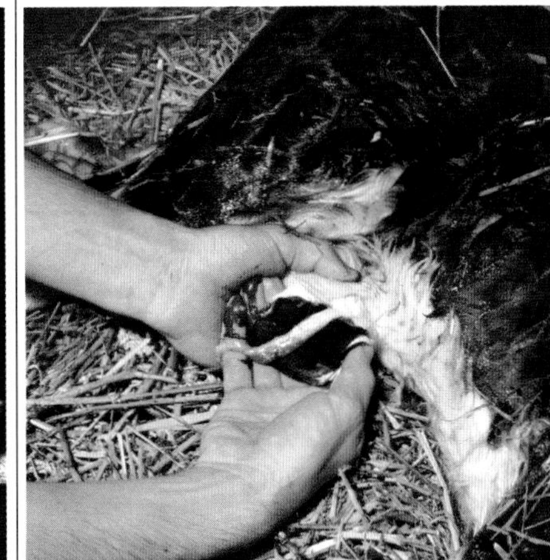

*Umbilical cord on the swab*

*Fig. 503*

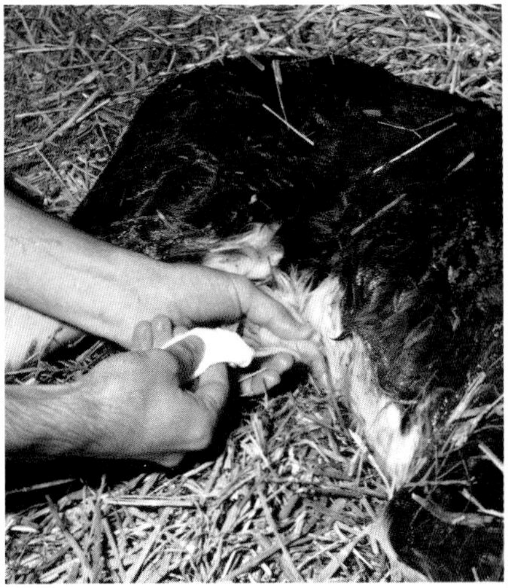

*Squeezing out residual blood with the swab*

*Fig. 504*

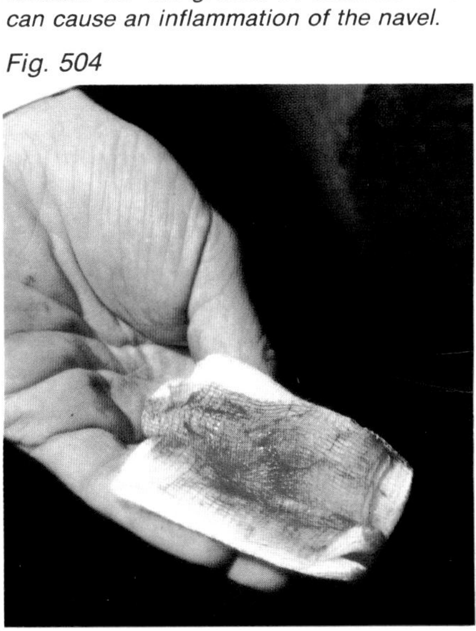

*Residual blood on the swab. This is an ideal medium for the growth of bacteria which can cause an inflammation of the navel.*

*Fig. 505*

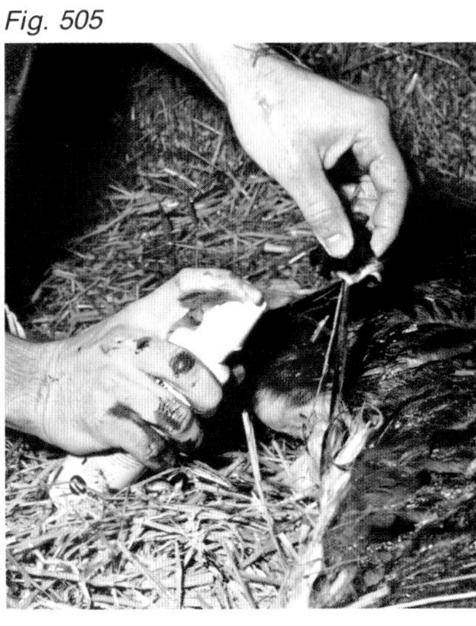

*Spraying the navel inside and outside*

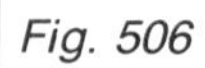

Fig. 506

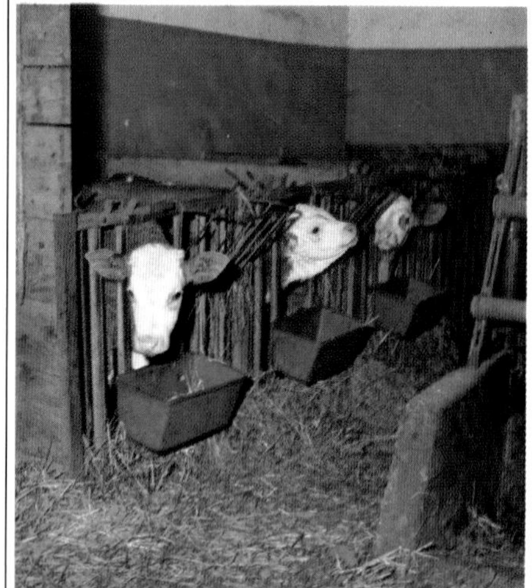

Fig. 507

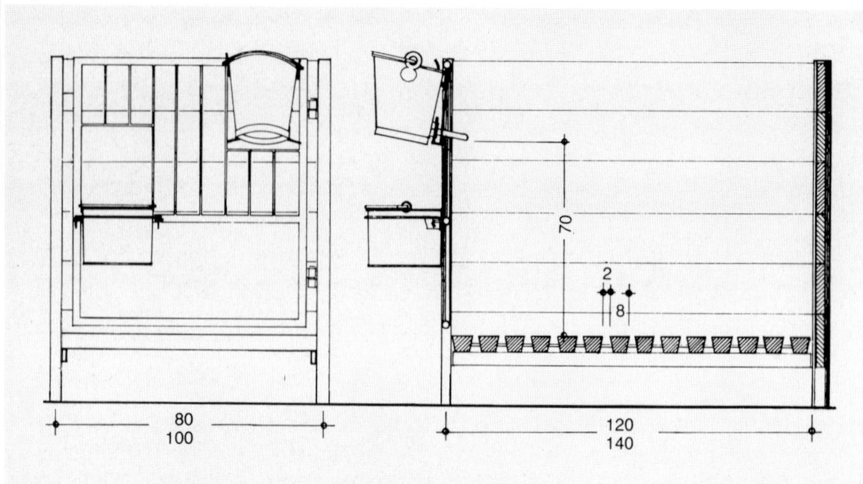


Calf box

## Requirements for a calf box

- Measurements: width 80 cm, length 120 cm, height 120 cm; floor grid, width of gaps 2 cm; width of battens 8 cm; clearance of floor grid from the ground: 25 cm.
- After clearing out calf box: thorough cleaning and disinfection (CHEVI 45 2%); allow to stand empty for approx. 1 week, preferably outside the cattle house, in the open air (drying out in the sun) if the weather is good. Use good quality straw litter.
- Calf box in the cow shed: heating lamp in the first week. Optimum temperature 18 to 20° C, minimum 16° C.

Calf house

## Requirements for a calf house

- Controlled environment: Minimum temperature 16° C, optimum temperature: 18 to 20° C. Maximum movement of air: 0.2 m/sec. Concentration of noxious gases: carbon dioxide 0.35% by volume, ammonia 0.003% by volume, hydrogen sulphide 0.001% by volume.
- Space required: individual animals up to 14 days old: 80 × 120 cm. If kept in groups on litter: 1 square metre per calf, 5 to 10 calves per group. Width of feeding place: 35 cm. Feeding rack required.

Air space per calf: 6 to 7 m$^3$ with a ceiling height of 270 cm.

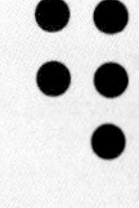

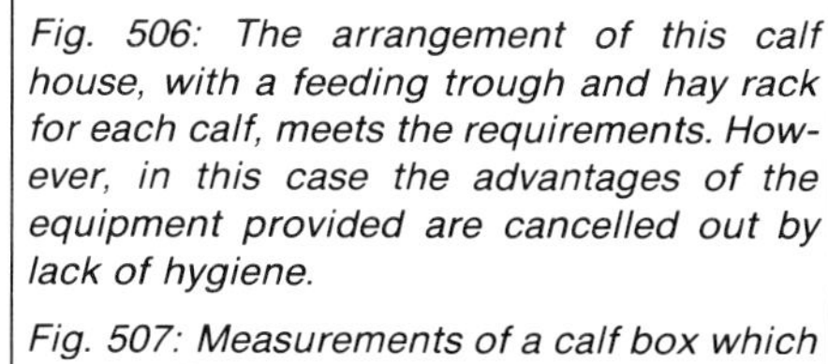

*Fig. 506: The arrangement of this calf house, with a feeding trough and hay rack for each calf, meets the requirements. However, in this case the advantages of the equipment provided are cancelled out by lack of hygiene.*

*Fig. 507: Measurements of a calf box which can easily be constructed from wood without expert help. If the box is enlarged to a width of 100 cm and a length of 140 cm, the calf can be housed in it up to the 10th week of life (Measurements quoted from: Koller, "Cattle Housing").*

*Fig. 508: Even if space is limited, an appropriate controlled environment can be created for the newborn calf by the construction of a calf box which ensures the necessary separation from the remaining animals. The crate shown on the left in the picture constitutes a short-term emergency solution.*

*Fig. 508*

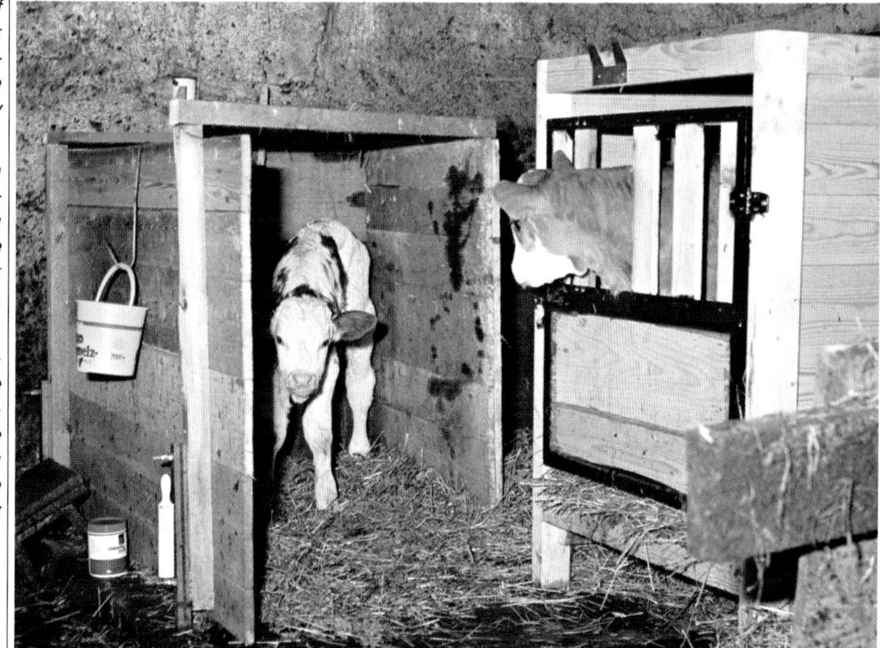



## Feeding requirements

- Colostral milk: If possible, 2 litres during the first 4 hours of life, from a bucket.
- Feeding plan: 1st day: 0.75 to 1 litre three times daily; 2nd and 3rd day: up to 1.5 litres three times daily; 4th to 7th day: up to 3 litres twice daily; from the 8th day gradual change-over from full-cream milk to milk substitute.
- Drinking temperature: 38 to 40° C, cow's milk in pre-warmed bucket; stir milk substitute at 50 to 60° C, depending on make. Check drinking temperature regularly. Give sour milk at 20 to 25° C.
- Calf growing ration: Prepare each feed freshly; store outside the cattle house.
- Total consumption of feed during the 1st to 4th week of life: 30 litres colostral milk, 100 litres milk substitute (corresponds to 12.5 kg milk substitute powder), 144 litres water (corresponds to 122 litres from the milk plus 22 litres given in addition).

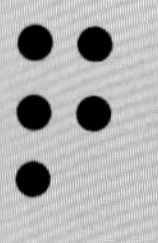

## Summary of preventive measures

## 5th to 12th week of life Rearing and weaning

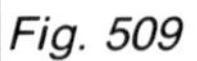

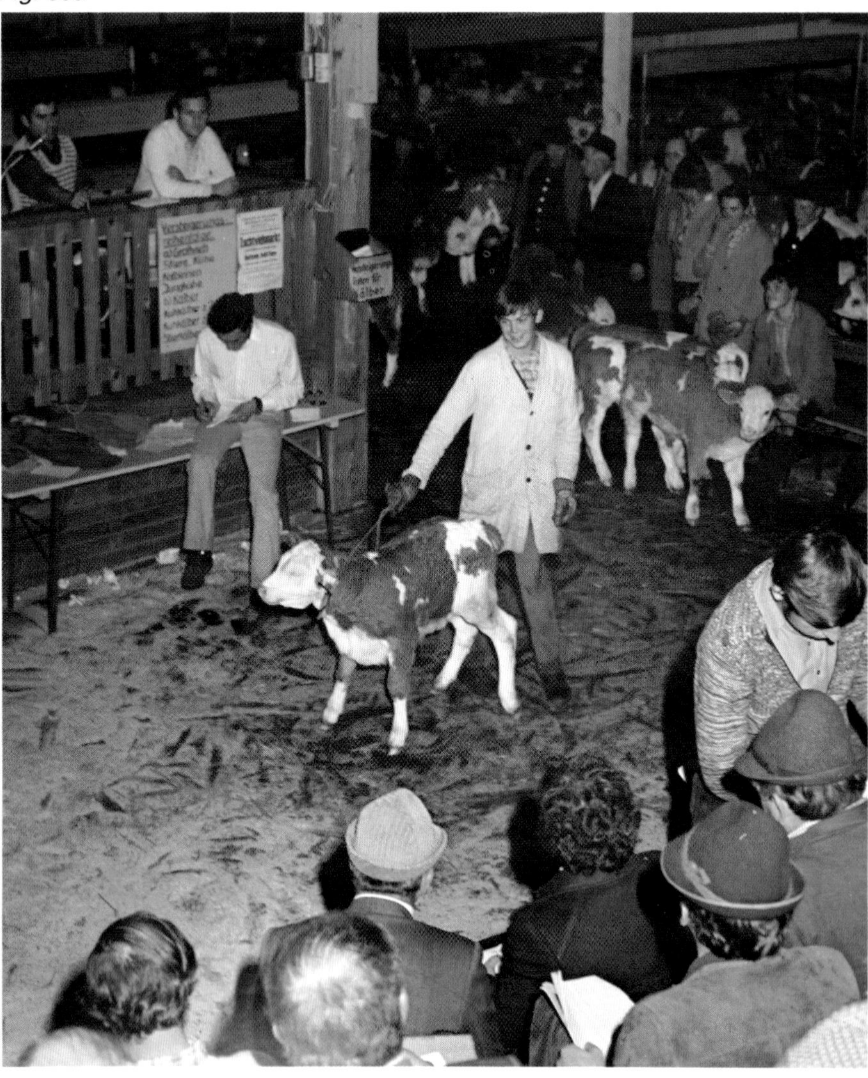

Purchase of calves

## Purchase of calves, examination on housing

■ It is during this period that calves are sold by dairy farms. The buyer should follow the routine examination procedure summarised in Fig. 510, in order to be able to make a quick and thorough assessment of the animals. See also sequence of photographs in the summaries on pages 12 to 24 and 68 to 80.

*Fig. 509: Auction of calves at the market: Rounding up, transport and rehousing in the new environment cause physical stress to the young animal.*

*Fig. 510: The most important characteristics of healthy and sick calves on rehousing.*

*Fig. 510*

| | Healthy calf | Sick calf |
|---|---|---|
| Total impression | Size and development corresponding to age; lively behaviour, upright posture, lively facial expression; alert eye and ear movements; short shining coat; calm, regular breathing. The animals are inquisitive and readily approach visitors. | Size and development not corresponding to age. Unduly large head, limp posture; abdomen drawn in; arched back, steep leg posture, lowered head, drooping ears, rough coat, beating of flanks or "pumping" respiration. Animal shows no interest in what is happening around it. |
| Head | Lively ear movement. Mucosae of eyes, nose and muzzle are pale pink and moist. | Drooping ears. Aqueous or mucopurulent discharge from the eyes and nose. Crusts around the eyes, nose and muzzle. |
| Examination of the palpebral conjunctivae (spreading with the fingers) | Palpebral conjunctiva pale pink. No protrusion of blood vessels. | Palpebral conjunctiva red, dark red or of porcelain colour. Protrusion of blood vessels of the sclera. |
| Checking the sucking reflex and opening the mouth | Strong sucking reflex. Buccal mucosa pale pink. | Weak or no sucking reflex. Buccal mucosa pale or reddened. |
| Skin. Checking the tension of the skin at the neck by raising a skin fold | Skin fold levels out immediately. Water balance normal. | Skin fold remains raised for some time. Sign of desiccation, e. g. with severe, prolonged diarrhoea. |
| Joints | Dry, stable. Corresponding joints on both sides of equal thickness. Correct leg posture. | Spongy, thickened joints. Painful changes. Shortening of tendons. |
| Navel | Umbilical cord well dried out. | Inflamed navel with swelling and reddening. Skin of the navel hairless; purulent secretion. Crusts. |
| Palpation of navel, abdominal wall and umbilical orifice | Umbilical cord approx. of pencil thickness. Abdominal wall closed. | Painful to the touch. Abdominal wall not closed (hernial orifice). |
| Anal region. Ascertaining the sex | Anus dry, closed. Area surrounding anus not soiled. | Anus inflamed, reddened. Straining in diarrhoea. Hairs on the inside of the thighs sticking together. Bald patches around the anus. |
| Body temperature | 38.5 to 39.5° C | Below 38.0° C; subnormal temperature. Above 39.5° C: fever (infection) |

Fig. 511

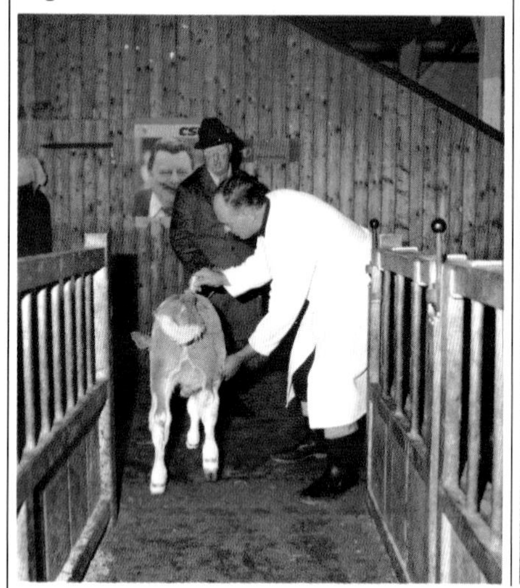

Fig. 512

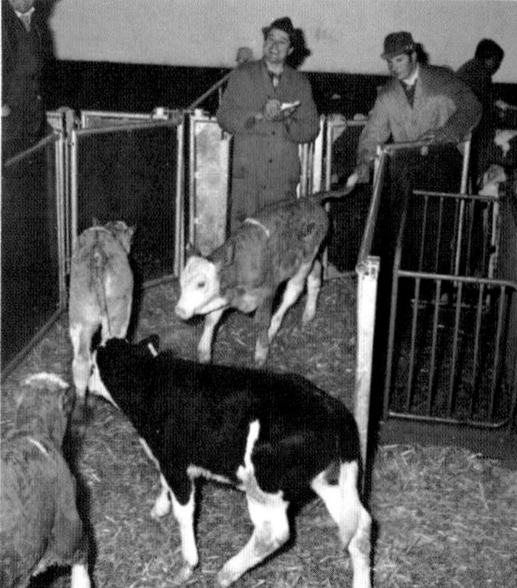

Fig. 513

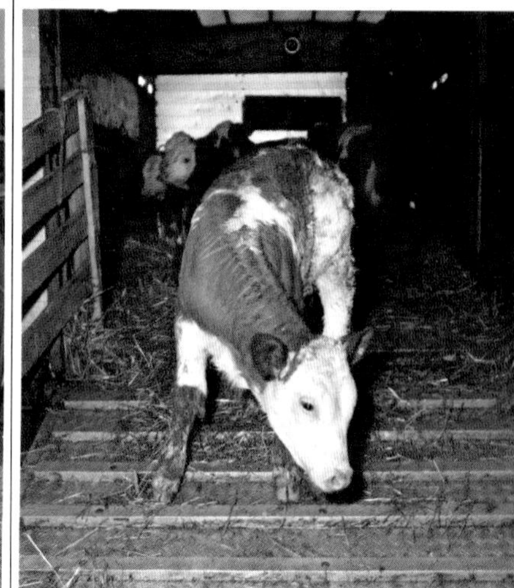



## Prophylaxis on housing

■ Calves after short transport (2 to 3 hours):

20 g CHEVICALF per animal/day for 14 days, to be stirred into the milk substitute. Careful observation of the calves. If general well-being is disturbed, take temperature.

■ Calves from market or dealer, arrival in the cattle house after approx. 12 hours:

1st day: Give tea with 25 g CHEVICALF and inject 10 ml VITIN per calf subcutaneously. Following 14 days: 20 g CHEVICALF per animal/day. Careful observation. Check body temperature for 5 days, if possible always at the same time, e. g. before drinking when the calves are restrained in the feeding rack.

■ Calves from market or dealer, long transport, arrival after 24 to 36 hours:

1st day: Electrolyte solution (ELRISAL) with 30 g BUSAL or 20 g MZI per calf/day and 5 ml TARDOMYOCEL, as well as subcutaneous injection of 10 ml VITIN per calf.
Following 5 days: 20 g BUSAL or 20 g MZI per animal/day. Then 20 g CHEVICALF per calf/day for 14 days. Careful observation of the animals. Check body temperature for 5 days.

*Fig. 511: An examination of the calves when they are brought to market, would be desirable, but is not always carried out. Visible faults are often announced before auction.*

*Figs. 512 and 513: Driving, weighing, loading and unloading are unavoidable, but constitute stress to the animals. Calm and thoughtful handling will reduce fear and agitation.*

*Fig. 514: Crowding causes agitation and sweating of the animals. They catch a chill in cold or draughty houses or during transport. Pathogens will then induce crowding disease.*

*Fig. 514*

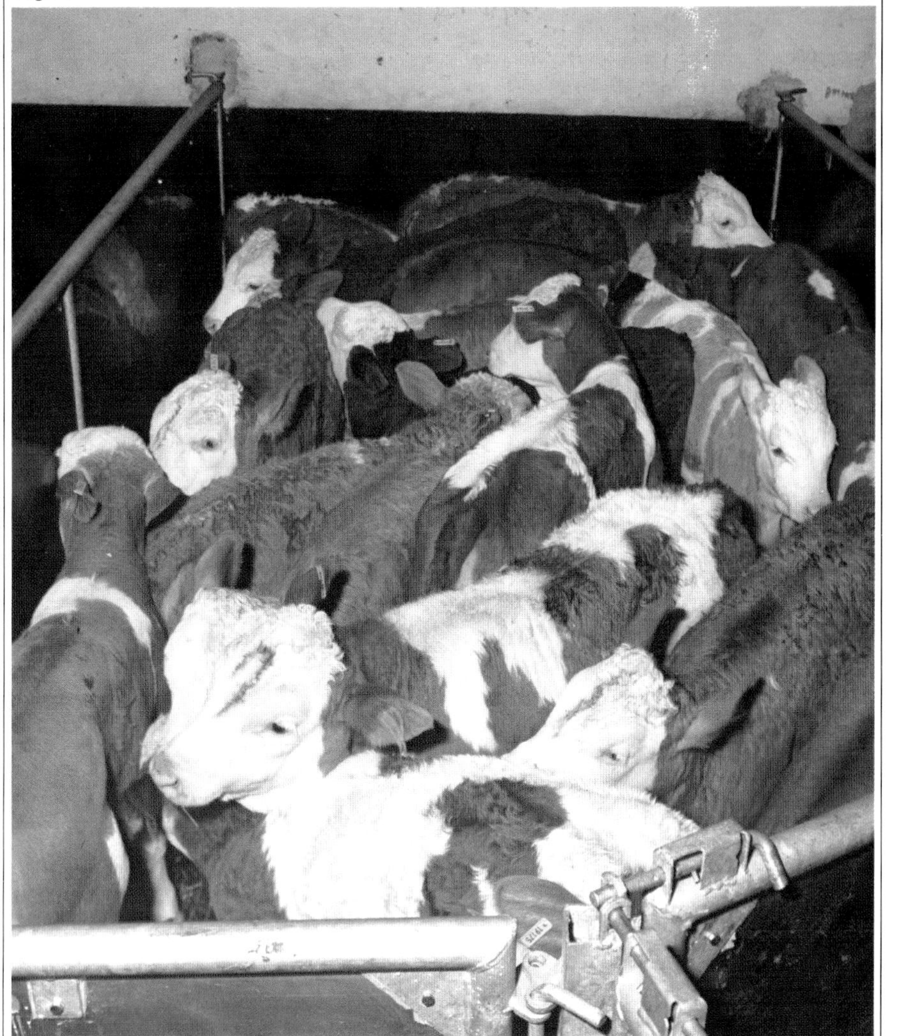

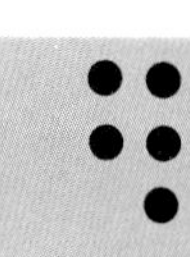

Fig. 515

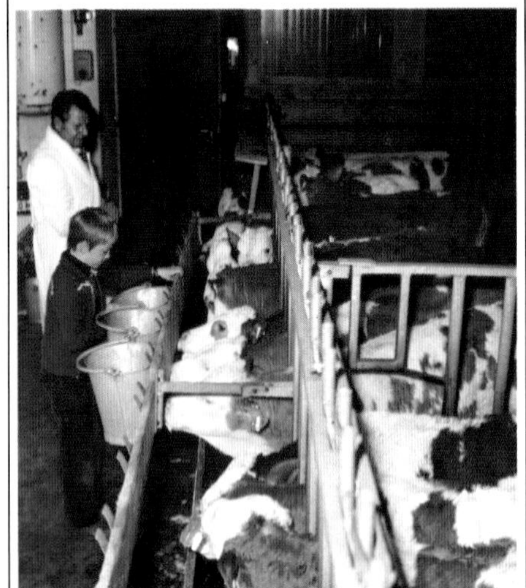

Fig. 516

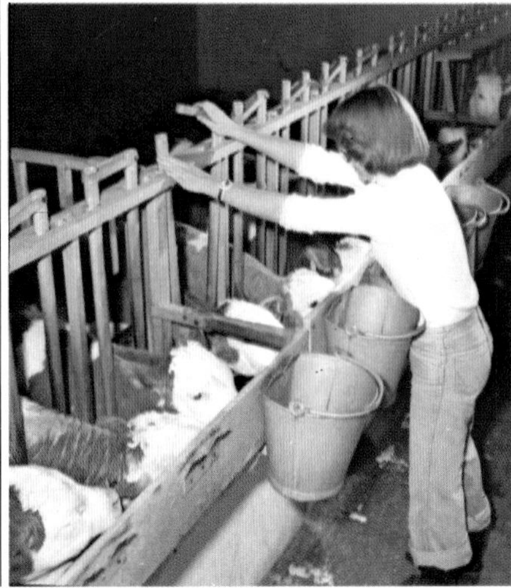

Fig. 517

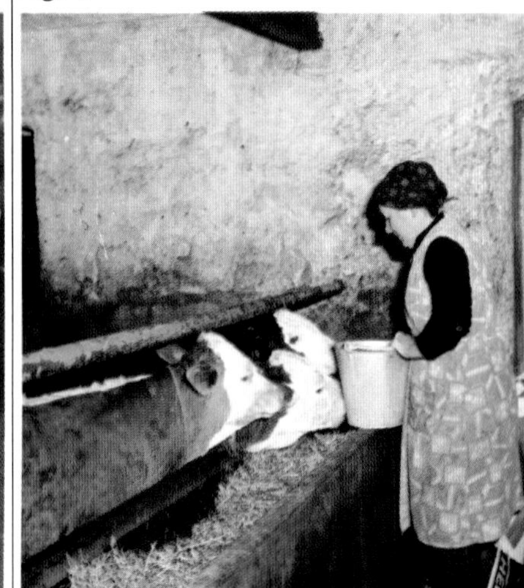

**Reception house**

## Requirements for a reception house

■ The reception house should be separate from the remaining cattle houses. After clearing and mucking out, it should be thoroughly cleaned and disinfected and the walls preferably whitewashed. Allow to stand empty for at least one week. "In-out" method. It must be possible to heat the house. Heat to 20–23° C before housing newly purchased animals.

■ Space requirements per calf: Minimum pen area 1 square metre, with a depth of 300 cm. Ceiling height 270 cm. Folding holders for buckets. Feeding racks to restrain calves during drinking are necessary. In this way the calves are confined for 15 to 20 minutes after drinking, and mutual licking and sucking are avoided, whilst early take-up of pelleted calf growing ration is promoted.

■ Housing in groups is better than individual penning. 5 to 10 animals per group.

■ Measurements of slatted floor: Width of planks: 10 cm, width of gaps: 2.5 to 3 cm. Planks must be laid level!

Fig. 518

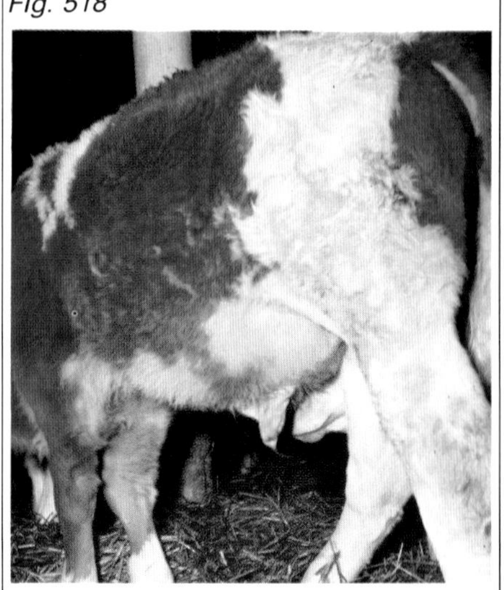

*Fig. 515: Calves in group pens. The bucket holders can be folded away. The feeding rack enables each animal to be restrained after drinking, which is a precondition for economic and easily monitored early weaning.*

*Fig. 516: Simple feeding rack. Each calf can be restrained separately.*

*Fig. 517: Labour-intensive, uneconomic drinking method. The calves are unable to drink without being disturbed by the other animals. In addition, milk is spilled and bad habits like mutual licking and sucking are promoted. The trough should be cleaned before drinking, so that the animals can be given growing ration in a clean trough after drinking.*

*Fig. 518: Sucking of the navel. This habit is often seen if the calves are able to move about freely immediately after drinking. With the reduced milk volume of 3 litres, the sucking reflex of the calves remains unsatisfied during early weaning and the calves therefore resort to mutual sucking as a substitute.*

*Fig. 519: Calf house with additional separation at the head of the animals. The calves are kept at the trough by means of a folding rack situated behind the animals.*

*Fig. 519*

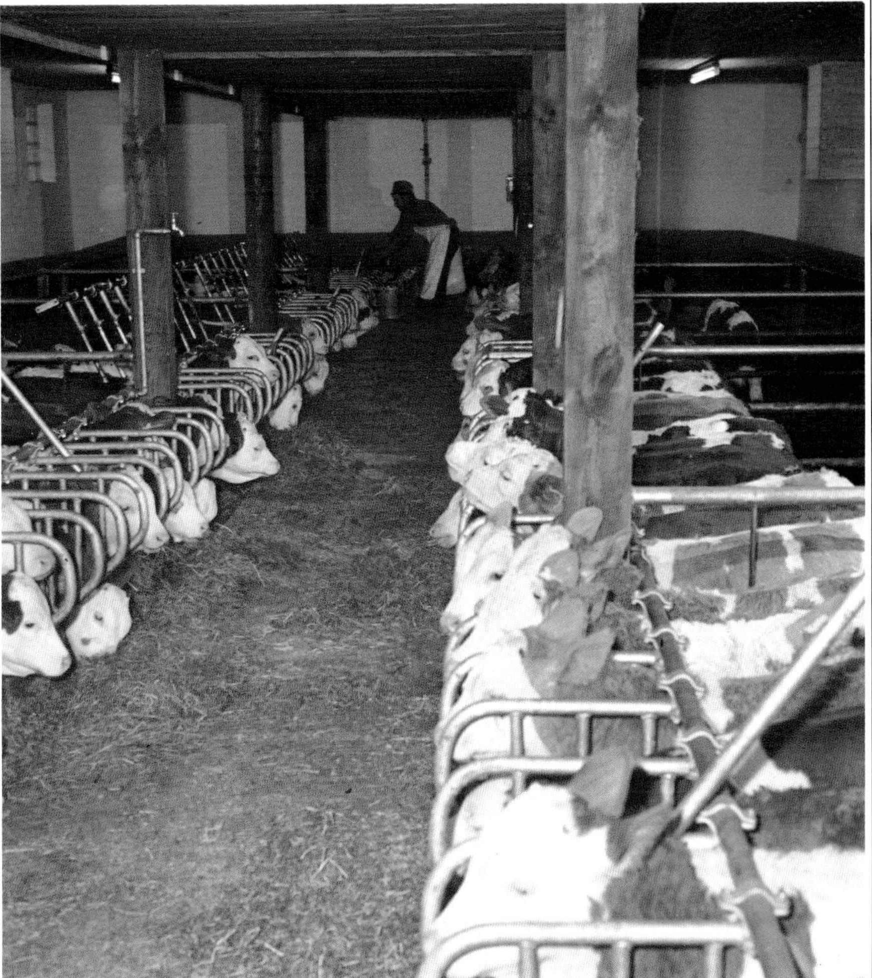

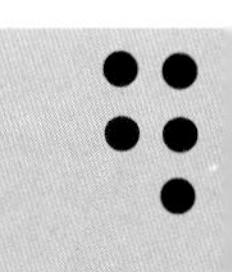



- Controlled environment: For straw litter, minimum temperature 16° C, optimum temperature 18 to 20° C. For slatted floor: 20 to 22° C. Air humidity: 60 to 80%. Maximum air movement: 0.2 m/sec. Concentration of noxious gases: Carbon dioxide 0.35% by volume, ammonia 0.003% by volume, hydrogen sulphide 0.001% by volume. Air space per calf: 6 to 7 $m^3$.

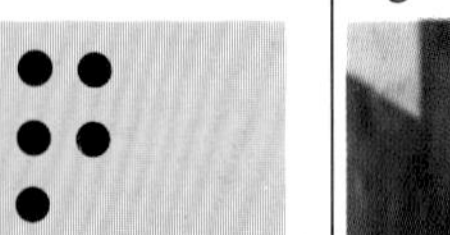

Fig. 520

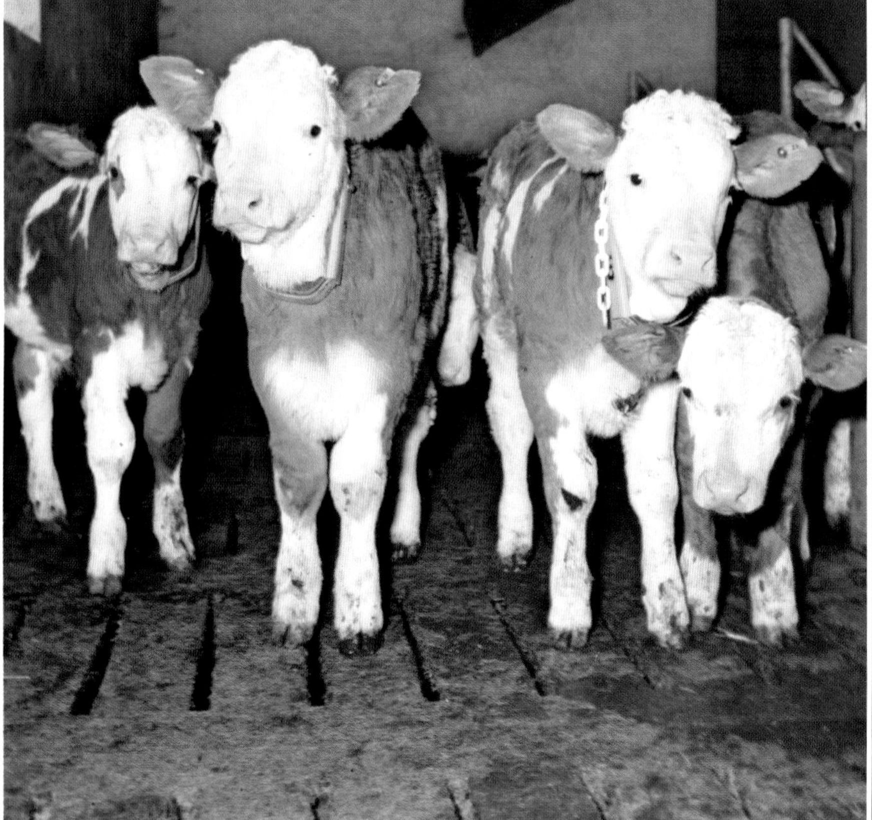

*Fig. 520: Early weaning on slatted floor. Fluctuations in temperature and air humidity should be balanced out quickly, so that the conditions mentioned (page 265) can be regularly maintained.*

*Figs. 521 to 523: Dehorning with cauterising iron. The iron must be sufficiently hot to ensure that the growth zone of the horn is rapidly obliterated. In that case, it is not necessary to remove the horn stump. After dehorning several calves, charred horn parts and hairs should be removed from the cauterising iron by means of a wire brush.*

**Change of feeding**

## Change-over to roughage

- To overcome difficulties in adjustment give 10 g CHEVIBULL per animal/day for at least 3 weeks.

**Docking of the tail**

## Docking of the tail

- In stocks where inflammation of the tail tip occurs frequently, dock tails by means of rubber rings by the 12th week of life at the latest.

Fig. 521

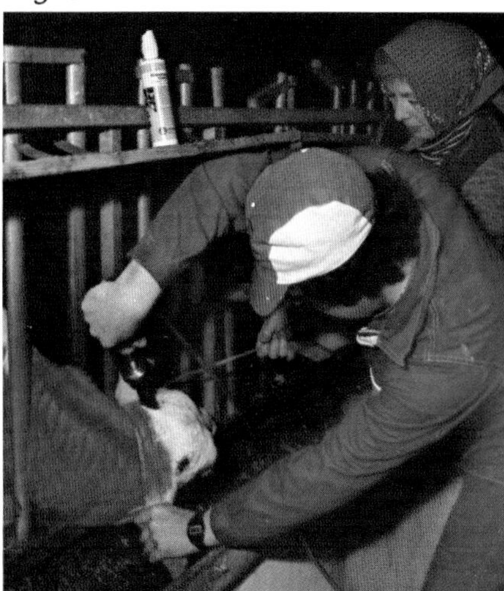

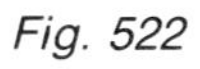

Fig. 522

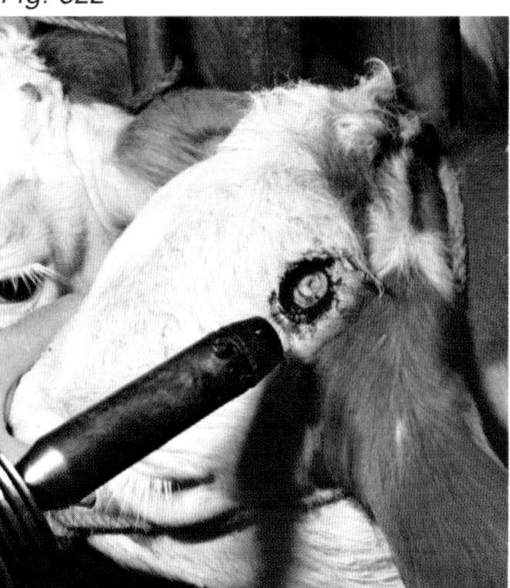

Fig. 523

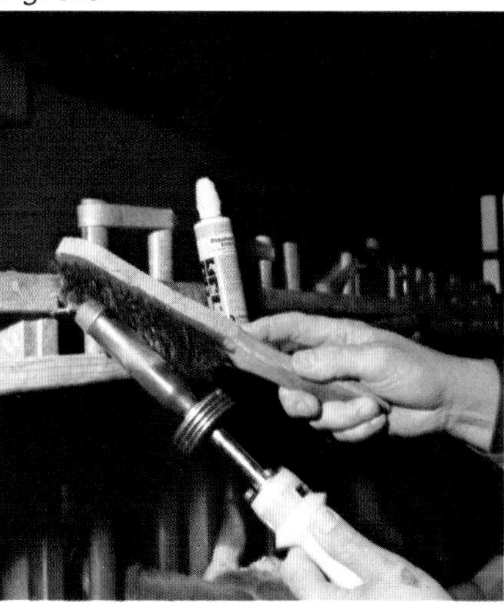

## Dehorning

- Dehorning with cauterising iron by the 12th or 13th week of life at the latest.

## Vaccinations

- Vaccination is possible against IBR, crowding disease, mucosal disease, parainfluenza III. Read up pages 91, 138, 152, 161 and 168.
- Time of vaccination: 2 to 3 weeks after housing. Parainfluenza III vaccination can be carried out immediately.
- Precondition of vaccination: Vaccinate only if all calves in the group are healthy.
- Necessary supportive measures: Calves fed on milk are given 20 g CHEVICALF per calf/day in the milk. Calves with developed compartmental stomach system (fattening calves) receive 10 g CHEVIBULL in the growing ration. Start 4 days before date of vaccination and continue up to 10th day after vaccination.

*Fig. 524*

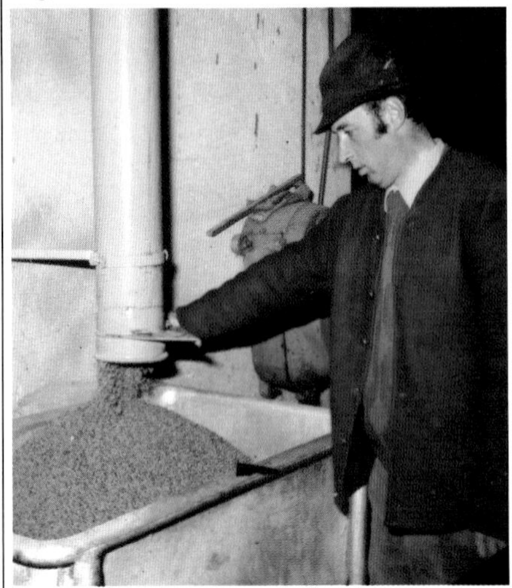

*Fig. 525*

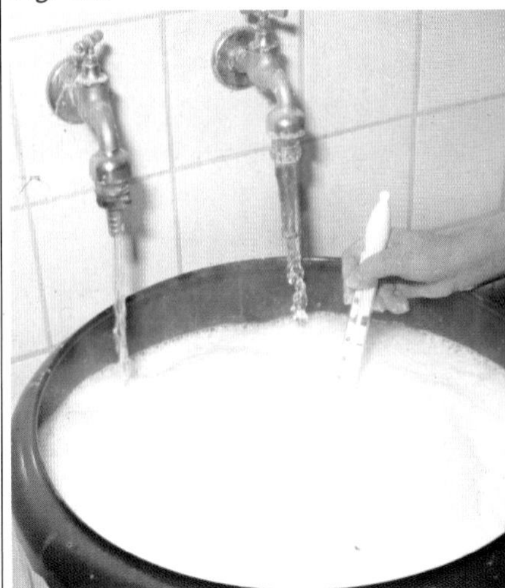

*Fig. 526*

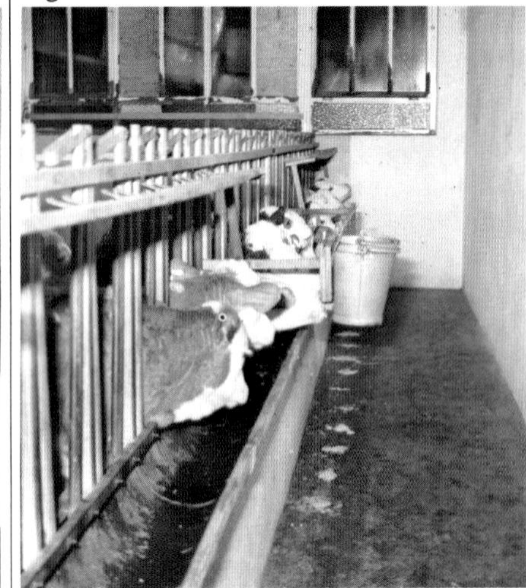



## Feeding requirements

- The early weaning method for rearing purchased bull calves enables the animals to become quickly accustomed to roughage as a result of the accelerated development of the stomach compartments.

- Total water requirement: 460 litres, of which approx. 200 litres are contained in the milk substitute and approx. 260 litres are given in addition.

- Total fodder consumption from the 5th to the 12th week of life, weight 70 to 120 kg: 25 to 30 kg milk substitute powder, 50 kg calf growing ration, compressed; 40 kg hay and 25 to 55 kg maize silage.

- Drinking temperature: 38 to 40° C. Stir milk substitute at 50° to 60° C, depending on make. Check drinking temperature regularly. Give sour milk at a temperature of 20 to 25° C.

- Note: After drinking, give fresh pelleted growing ration for every feed in cleaned trough. Store calf growing ration outside the cattle house. Restrain calves in the feeding rack for twenty minutes after drinking.

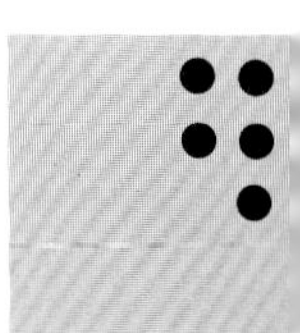



*Figs. 524 to 526: Important preconditions for successful early weaning:*

*Fig. 524: Dry storage of calf growing ration outside the cattle house. If the growing ration is stored in the house or at a moist place, the calves are reluctant to accept it. The photograph shows an outlet pipe for filling a feed trolley from a storage container.*

*Fig. 525: Stirring vat for milk substitute. Checking the stirring temperature and the drinking temperature is important to avoid indigestion.*

*Fig. 526: Feeding rack with holder for drinking bucket. The holder must be arranged in such a way that no milk drips into the feeding trough. Drips of milk form a growth medium for bacteria and cause indigestion if they become acidified and are then taken up by the animals.*

*Fig. 527: Early weaning of calves in single pens (Mastock Farm in Saudi Arabia). Each calf has a fodder bucket and a water bucket of its own. Fresh water is given at every feed. In our region, too, calves should always have water available during early weaning.*

*Fig. 527*

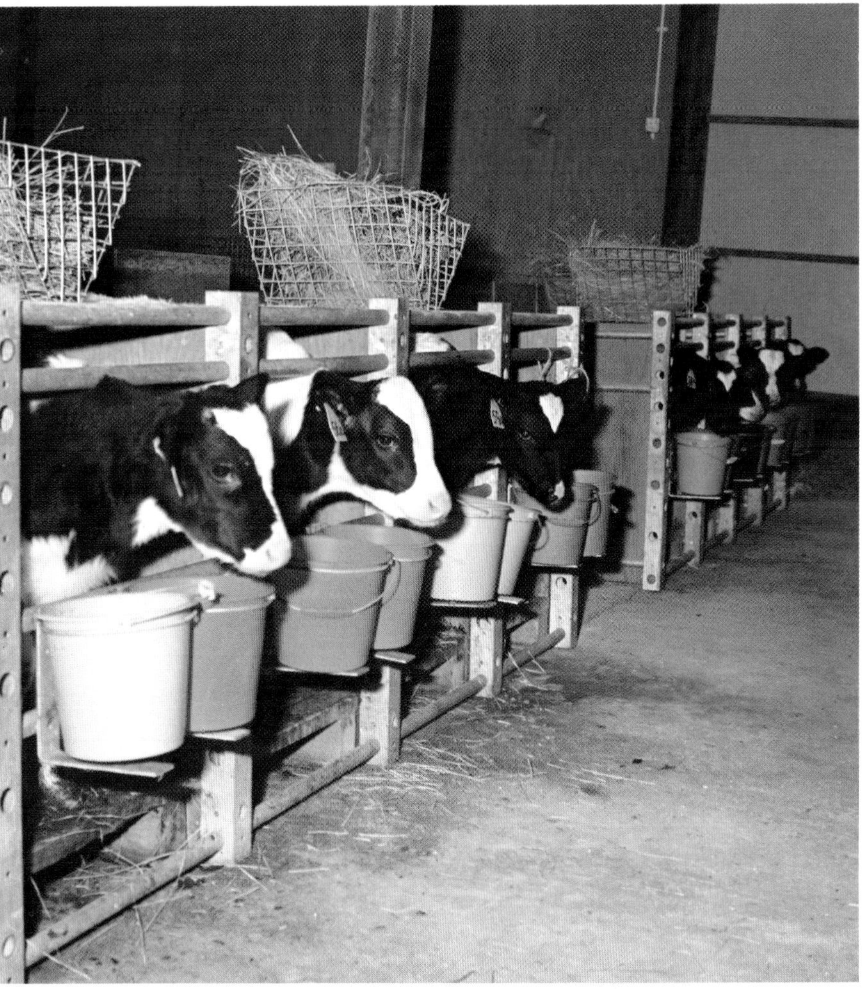

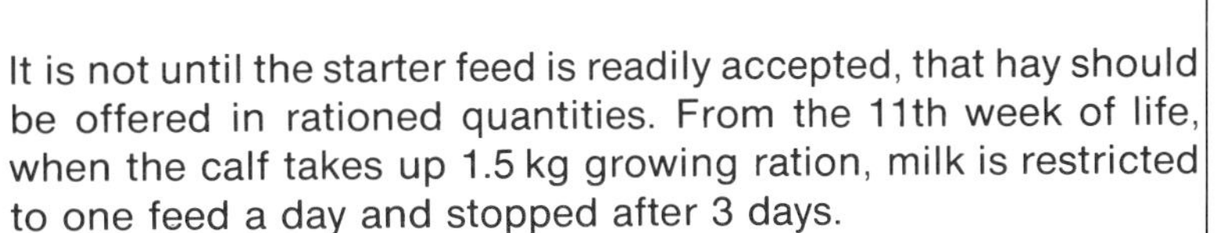

It is not until the starter feed is readily accepted, that hay should be offered in rationed quantities. From the 11th week of life, when the calf takes up 1.5 kg growing ration, milk is restricted to one feed a day and stopped after 3 days.

With proper weaning, the calf should have a fully functioning compartmental stomach system at the age of 12 weeks.

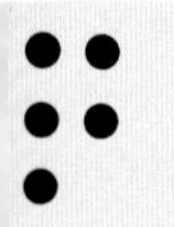

# Summary of preventive measures

## Calf fattening

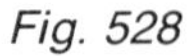

Fig. 528

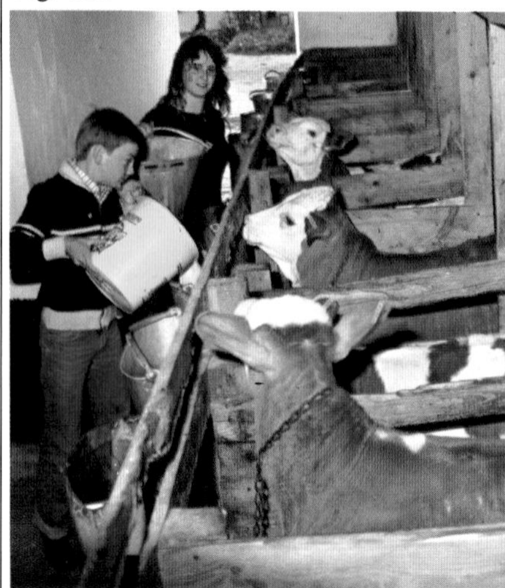

**Housing after purchase**

### Purchase of calves. Examination on housing

- Do not buy calves younger than 10 days old. Purchase in groups, so that the "in-out" method can be maintained in the cattle house compartments.
- The buyer should familiarise himself with the examination procedure outlined in Fig. 510, in order to obtain a rapid and thorough general assessment of the animals. See also the sequence of photographs in the summaries on pages 12 to 24 and 68 to 80. Mainly female animals are purchased. Hermaphrodites do not present any disadvantage.

**Prevention at time of purchase**

### Prophylaxis on housing

- After transport, the calves initially need fluids, not milk. On arrival give electrolyte solution (45 g ELRISAL per litre) with 10 g MZ I per 50 kg body-weight/day, then milk substitute with 10 g MZ I per 50 kg body-weight for 5 days, followed by milk substitute with MZ I in half this dosage for 10 days. For fattening stock fed with automatic feeding equipment, MZ I needs to be mixed with the milk substitute by the manufacturer.
- If prolonged treatment is necessary (influenza-type disease in calves; variations in controlled environment) during the remaining fattening period, the medicated feed MZ II or CHEVICALF is given in lieu of MZ I.

Fig. 529

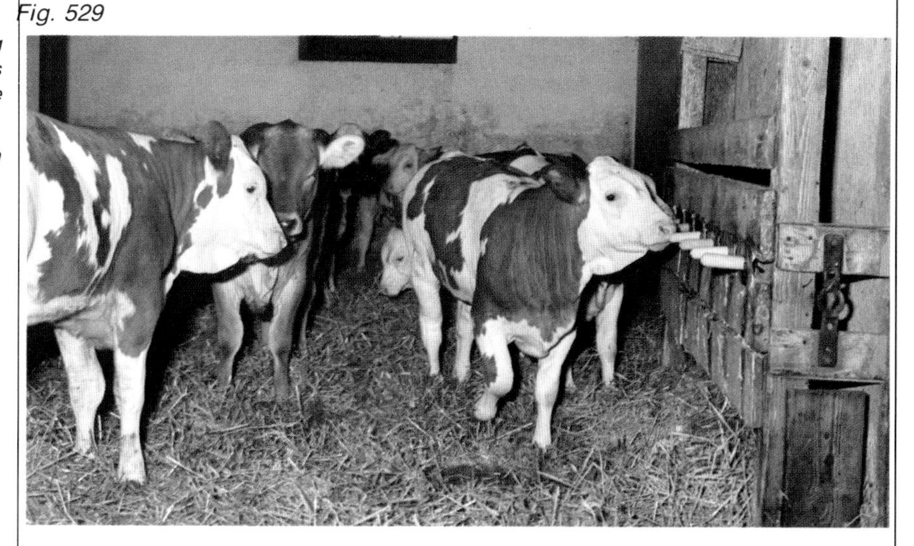

*Fig. 528: Calf fattening on floor grid, using drinking buckets. Here, too, small quantities of hay should be given, so as to improve health and general well-being.*

*Fig. 529: Calf fattening in covered yard with straw litter and automatic drinker.*

## Vaccination

**Vaccination**

- Additional preventive measure in stocks with a high incidence of influenza-type disease: Parainfluenza III vaccination on housing. Other vaccinations, particularly vaccination against crowding disease, are not indicated during calf fattening.

## Requirements for the calf fattening house

**Calf fattening house**

- Wherever possible, separate compartments should be used for fattening, to enable the "in-out" method to be carried out. After the calves have been sold, thorough cleaning and disinfection. Allow to stand empty for a few days. Heat to 20–23° C before housing new calves.
- Controlled environment: With straw litter: 18 to 20° C; without straw litter: 20 to 22° C. Air humidity: 60 to 80%. Maximum air movement: 0.2 m/sec. Suction of the ventilator per calf: 150 $m^3$ air per hour. Air space 7 to 8 $m^3$ per calf.

## Additional feeding of straw

**Additional feeding of straw**

- Small quantities of straw are not harmful to calves, but improve their health and general well-being. Iron deficiency (pale mucosae, scours) is reduced by the ingestion of straw, without affecting the (unfortunately) desired light colour of the meat.

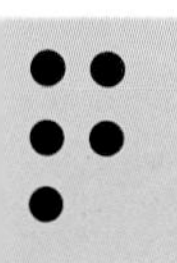

# Summary of preventive measures

from the 13th week of life
Rearing and fattening

Fig. 530

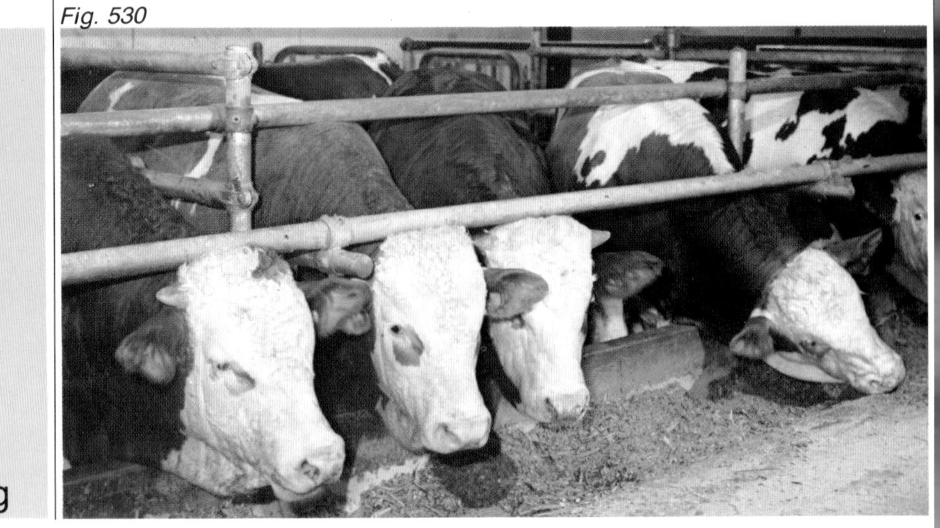

Rehousing

## Getting animals accustomed to slatted-floor house

- The resistance of the animals is reduced by the absence of the warm straw litter; the hard cold lying surface; the need to adapt the claws to the change from a soft elastic, non-slip floor surface to a hard unaccustomed slatted floor. To offset this stress, to improve vitality and to maintain the appetite, we give 10 g CHEVIBULL per animal/day for 3 weeks.

Purchase

## Purchase of weaned young cattle. Examination on housing

- On purchase (see Fig. 510 and summary on pages 68 to 80) check skin and coat, particularly for: trichophytosis, mange and lice.
- If purchased from warble fly-infested areas: Carry out anti-warble fly treatment before 1st December.
- Parasitological examination of faeces (random samples) for infestation with lungworms and gastrointestinal worms. Carry out anthelmintic treatment in accordance with findings.
- Careful observation of the animals during the first few weeks, looking particularly for any leg complaints.

Fig. 531

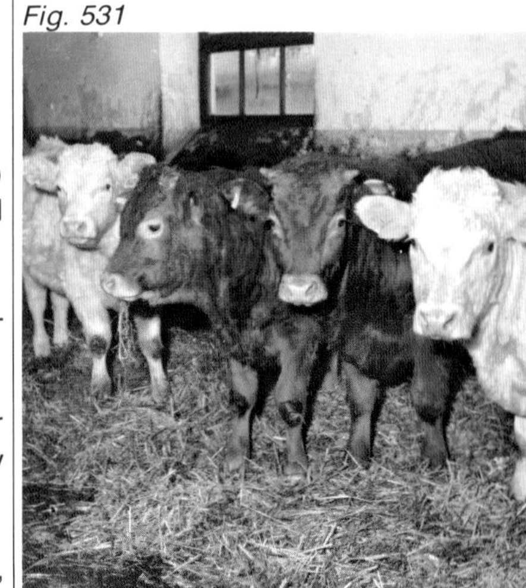

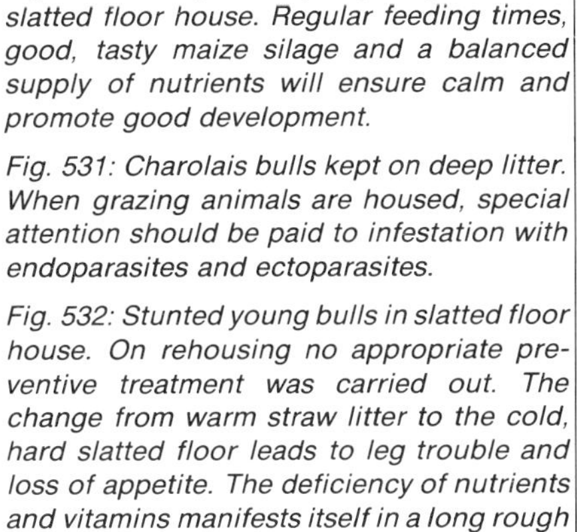
*Fig. 530: Evenly developed young bulls in a slatted floor house. Regular feeding times, good, tasty maize silage and a balanced supply of nutrients will ensure calm and promote good development.*

*Fig. 531: Charolais bulls kept on deep litter. When grazing animals are housed, special attention should be paid to infestation with endoparasites and ectoparasites.*

*Fig. 532: Stunted young bulls in slatted floor house. On rehousing no appropriate preventive treatment was carried out. The change from warm straw litter to the cold, hard slatted floor leads to leg trouble and loss of appetite. The deficiency of nutrients and vitamins manifests itself in a long rough coat, limp posture and a "run-down" appearance.*

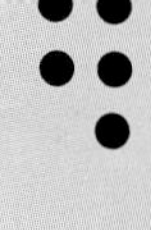

*Fig. 532*

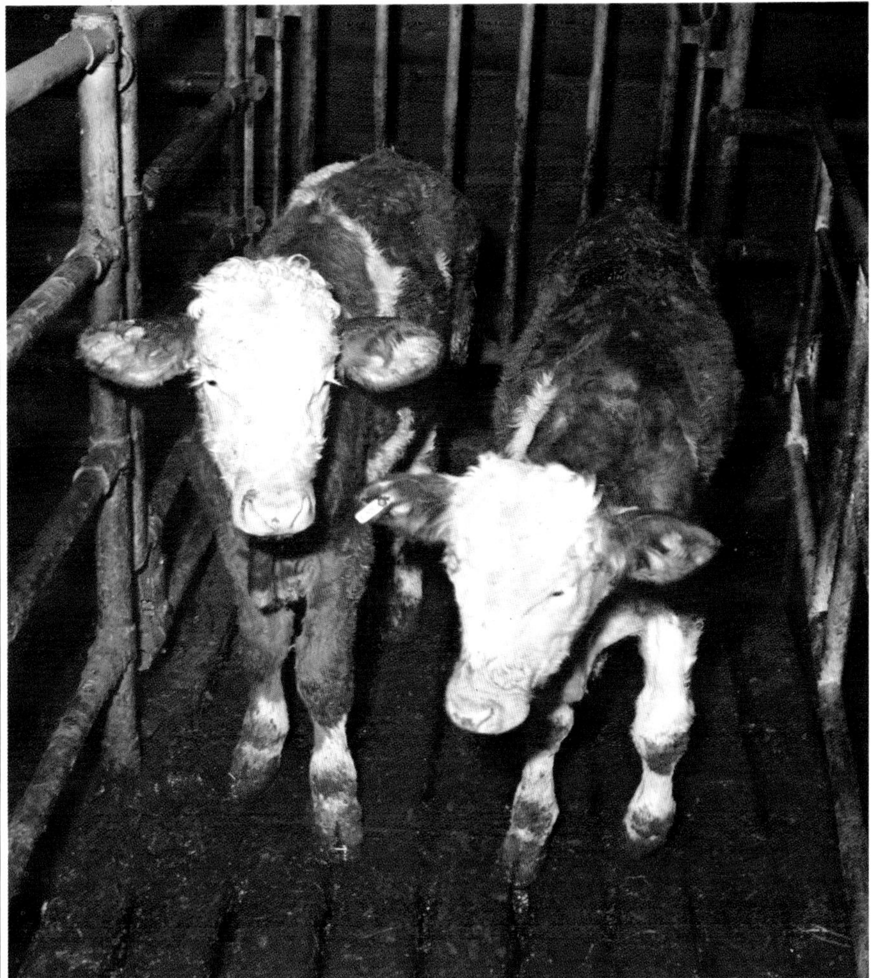

■ Prophylaxis on housing: Give 1 BOVIBOL per 150 kg bodyweight plus 10 g CHEVIBULL per animal/day mixed with the concentrates, for 3 weeks.

## "Influenza periods": Autumn and Spring

**Influenza periods**

■ To counteract the strain caused by prolonged temperature fluctuations which in turn produce variations in the controlled environment that are difficult to stabilise: Give 5 to 10 g CHEVIBULL per animal/day for 2 to 4 weeks, depending on the length of the period in which the animals are at risk.

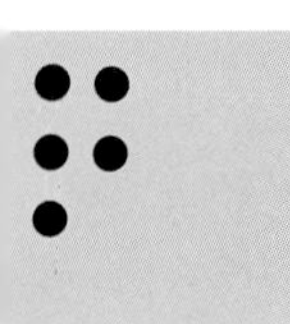

Vaccination

## Vaccinations

- Vaccination is possible against IBR, crowding disease, mucosal disease and foot-and-mouth disease; read up pages 91, 138, 152, 161, 168 and 170.
- Time of vaccination: Not earlier than 2 to 3 weeks after housing or rehousing.
- Condition: Vaccination should be carried out only if all cattle in the group are healthy.
- Necessary supportive measure: Give 10 g CHEVIBULL per animal/day, starting 4 days before vaccination and continuing up to the 10th day after vaccination.

Fig. 533

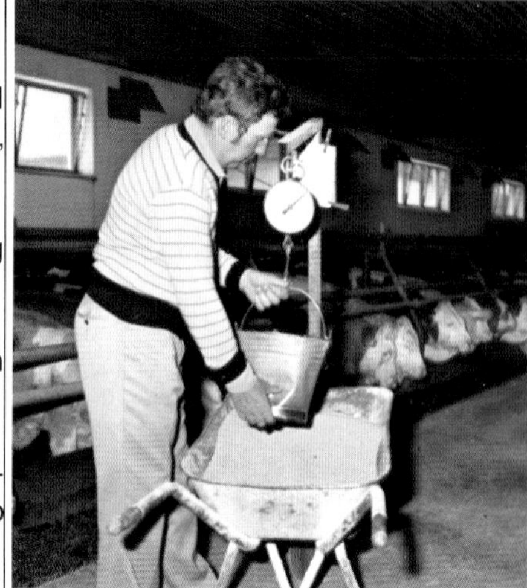

Cattle fattening house

## Requirements for cattle house, deep litter house and slatted floor house

- Space requirements (depending on body-weight): Length of trough: 50 to 65 cm per animal. Depth of pen: 350 to 400 cm. Lying area: 2 square metres per animal. Ceiling height: 300 cm.
- Measurements for slatted floor: Up to 200 kg body-weight: Width of plank 10 to 12 cm; width of gap 3 cm. From 200 kg body-weight: Width of plank 12 to 13 cm; width of gap 3.5 to 4 cm. Important: Planks must be laid completely level. No sharp or splintered edges. Surface providing a firm hold.
- Controlled environment: Optimum temperature of cattle house with straw litter 12 to 16° with slatted floor 16° C. Air humidity 60 to 80%; maximum air movement 0.2 m/sec. Concentration of noxious gases: carbon dioxide 0.35% by volume; ammonia 0.003% by volume; hydrogen sulphide 0.001% by volume. Air space per large-animal unit: 8 to 10 $m^3$.

*Fig. 533: Rationing the concentrates during the various fattening periods is the "secret" of intensive bull fattening.*

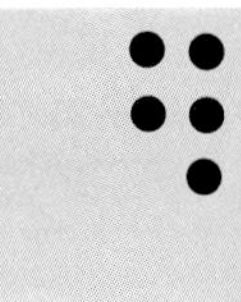

- Sick pen: In every covered yard, provision should be made for the accommodation of sick cattle in a sick pen where separate treatment can be carried out. In diseases of the claws, for instance, straw litter and the facility to tie up the animal are required.

## Feeding requirements in young bull fattening

Feeding

- Intensive feeding with a balanced supply of energy and nutrients will calm the animals. Keep to regular feeding times. Put together balanced groups. Avoid regrouping and rehousing. Ensure that drinking-water is always fresh. Check drinking trough at least once a day.

- Do not overfeed with concentrates during the middle fattening period, so as to ensure that sufficient maize is taken up. This promotes the development of the stomach compartments and delays the onset of sexual maturity.

- Good, tasty maize silage: Chaff length not less than 10 mm; optimum TS content 27 to 30%. Firm, dense storage of the silage. Inaccurate chaffing, loose storage, poor covering and excessive exposure to air on withdrawal will affect stability and taste. Pappy maize silage or silage with a dry substance content of more than 33% is not readily accepted.

## Weight checks

Weight checks

- These are necessary to assess the effect of balanced, purpose-related feeding. Should be carried out at least at the time of housing and rehousing and when the animals are sold; if possible every 100 days.

- Insufficient weight gain indicates the existence of latent disease or inappropriate management. Check animals for foul-in-the-foot and inflammation of the tail tip at the time of weighing.

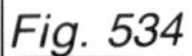

*Fig. 534*

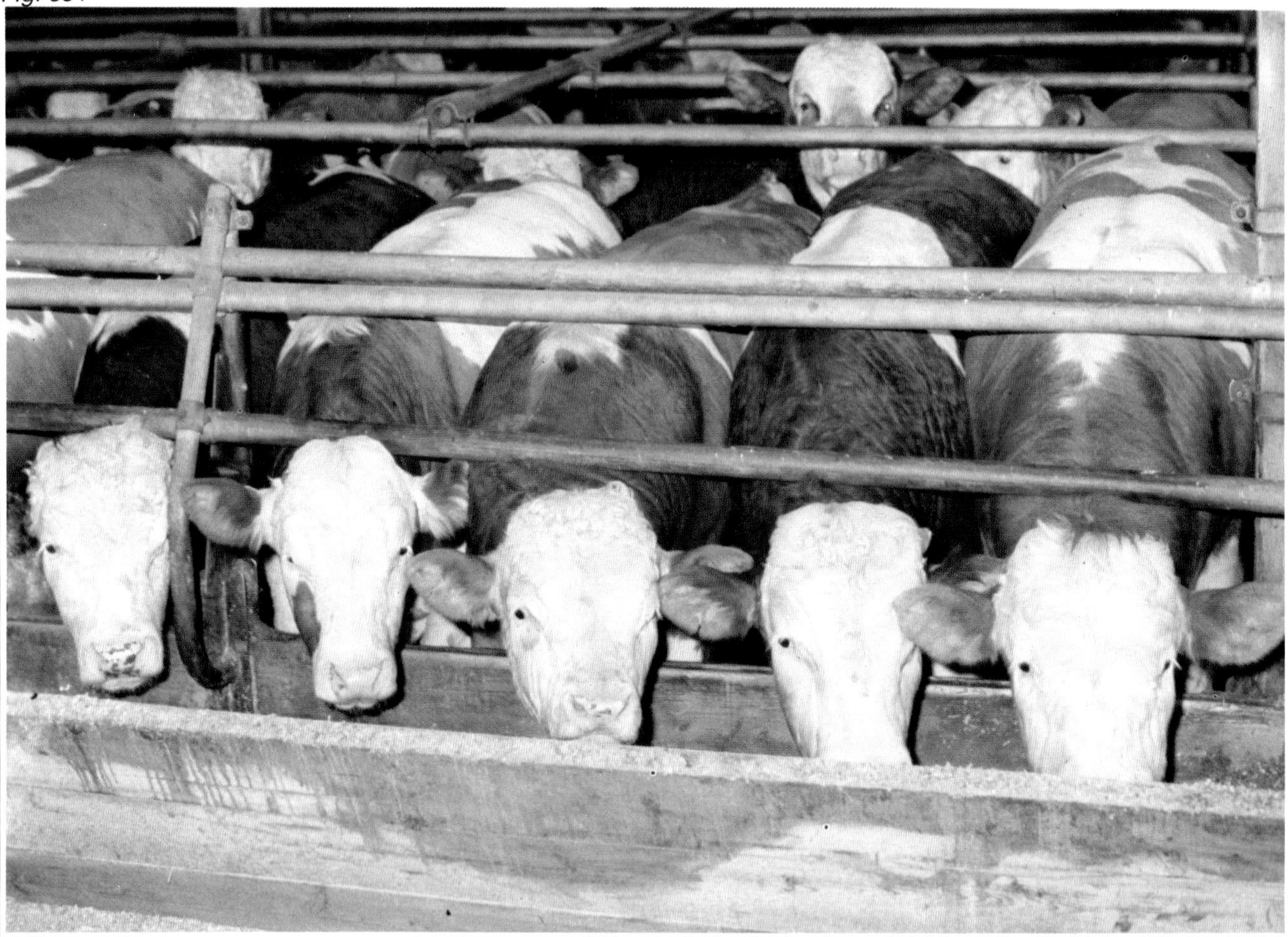

*Moderate feeding during the middle fattening period and rations adapted to the individual fattening periods on the basis of the animals' weight, will produce good weight gains during the entire fattening period.*